COCAINE ABUSE

New Directions
in
Treatment and Research

Edited by

Henry I. Spitz, M.D., F.A.P.A.

Associate Clinical Professor of Psychiatry,
Department of Psychiatry, Columbia University,
College of Physicians and Surgeons, New York, New York;
Director, Training Programs in Group Psychotherapy and
Marital Therapy, New York State Psychiatric Institute

and

Jeffrey S. Rosecan, M.D.

Assistant Clinical Professor of Psychiatry,
Department of Psychiatry, Columbia University,
College of Physicians and Surgeons, New York, New York;
Director, Cocaine Abuse Treatment and Research Program,
Columbia–Presbyterian Medical Center, New York, New York

BRUNNER/MAZEL, *Publishers* • New York

Cover photograph: Bill Ray

Library of Congress Cataloging-in-Publication Data

Cocaine abuse.

  Includes bibliographies and index.
  1. Cocaine habit—Treatment. I. Spitz, Henry I.,
1941–   . II. Rosecan, Jeffrey S., 1952–   .
[DNLM: 1. Cocaine. 2. Substance Abuse—therapy.
WM 280 C65932]
RC568.C6C627 1987   616.86´3   86-32676
ISBN 0-87630-461-7

Published by
BRUNNER/MAZEL, INC.
19 Union Square
New York, New York 10003

10 9 8 7 6 5 4 3 2

With love and appreciation
to Susan, Becky, and Jake
and
to Barbara

Foreword

The study of cocaine represents a field in which the integration of the neurosciences into clinical psychiatry is clearly visible. The interface between scientific research and its clinical application can be seen on several fronts. Investigators, starting with Freud and continuing through modern researchers, have been intrigued by the biochemical, physiological, and psychological aspects of cocaine.

Not until recently has basic laboratory research been conducted in a systematic effort to elucidate the effects of cocaine on brain and behavior. The data emerging from animal studies and the increased understanding of human neurochemistry and psychopharmacology have set the stage for a more scientific basis for clinical diagnosis and treatment planning in instances where cocaine is used to excess.

Data from varied sources converge and can be integrated to provide a comprehensive grasp of the biobehavioral phenomenology associated with cocaine. The clinician responsible for the treatment of cocaine-abusing individuals reaps rich rewards from the harvest of this information. Critical issues in the field of mental health crystallize around the themes of evaluation and treatment of the cocaine-abusing patient.

Current diagnostic thinking reflects advances in and updating of older notions of substance abuse and addiction. Accurate distinction between psychological and physiological manifestations of cocaine use is clouded during states of cocaine withdrawal and in toxic states associated with dependence on cocaine. The presence of affective disorders, commonly reported among users of psychoactive stimulants, further complicates the diagnostic picture. This, coupled with the possibility of concomitant use of marijuana, alcohol, and/or heroin, underscores the need for the clinician to be knowledgeable in many areas that bear on obtaining clarity in clinical diagnosis.

The avid interest in pharmacotherapy, psychotherapy, and combinations thereof highlights the importance of an open attitude on the clinician's part when considering the array of treatment options currently available. Individual, group, family, and marital psychotherapies are not only being utilized with increasing frequency, but are also moving into a firmer position in scientific inquiry. Psychotherapy research is progressing from the exclusively anecdotal model through the clinical-descriptive and currently into well-designed controlled studies that help elucidate the beneficial as well as potentially detrimental aspects of these forms of psychosocial intervention.

Finally, cocaine typifies a subject that invites cross-sectional research investigation. The interest in basic science, psychopharmacological, and psychotherapeutic research has increased almost exponentially in the past five years. The results emerging from these research efforts provide an exciting example of the confluence of expanded neuroscientific information, integrated and comprehensive clinical management, and thoughtfully constructed creative research designs which contribute to the growth of our knowledge.

In this book, the authors synthesize the bulk of the current theoretical and clinical information available about cocaine into a treatment-oriented framework. Drs. Spitz and Rosecan have made a valuable contribution to the advancement of our state of sophistication concerning major developments in the vanguard of modern psychiatry. Their work with cocaine abuse embodies the successful blending of neuroscience and psychologically based psychiatry into practical therapeutic models with broad clinical applicability.

At a time in our history when substance abuse in general, and cocaine use in particular, represent widespread, pressing social and health care problems, the need for this book is acute. The text is a welcome one for the insights it offers in helping to address the complex series of factors involved in the treatment of cocaine-related problems.

Herbert M. Pardes, M.D.,
Lawrence C. Kolb Professor and Chairman,
Department of Psychiatry, Columbia University,
College of Physicians and Surgeons,
New York, New York

Contents

I. BACKGROUND ISSUES

II. NEUROSCIENCE ISSUES

III. TREATMENT ISSUES

IV. FUTURE DIRECTIONS

Contributors

Nori Geary, Ph.D.
Assistant Professor, Department of Psychology, Columbia University, New York, NY

Barbara Gross, M.A.
Research Associate, Cocaine Abuse Treatment Program, Columbia–Presbyterian Medical Center, New York, NY

Robert M. Kertzner, M.D.
Assistant Clinical Professor of Psychiatry, Columbia University, College of Physicians and Surgeons; and Director of Services, Columbia–Presbyterian Psychiatric Associates, New York, NY

Donald F. Klein, M.D.
Professor of Psychiatry, Columbia University, College of Physicians and Surgeons; and Director of Psychiatric Research, New York State Psychiatric Institute

Edward V. Nunes, M.D.
Instructor of Clinical Psychiatry, Columbia University, College of Physicians and Surgeons; Research Fellow, Depression Evaluation Service, New York State Psychiatric Institute; and Director of Research, Cocaine Abuse Treatment Program, Columbia–Presbyterian Medical Center, New York, NY

Jeffrey S. Rosecan, M.D.
Assistant Clinical Professor of Psychiatry, Columbia University, College of Physicians and Surgeons; and Director, Cocaine Abuse Treatment Program, Columbia–Presbyterian Medical Center, New York, NY

Michael Sheehy, M.D.
Associate Clinical Professor of Psychiatry, Columbia University, College of Physicians and Surgeons, New York, NY; and Medical and Executive Director, Silver Hill Foundation, New Canaan, CT

Andrew E. Skodol, M.D.
Associate Clinical Professor of Psychiatry, Columbia University, College of Physicians and Surgeons, New York, NY

Henry I. Spitz, M.D., F.A.P.A.
Associate Clinical Professor of Psychiatry, Columbia University, College of Physicians and Surgeons, New York, NY; and Director, Training Programs in Group Psychotherapy and Marital Therapy, New York State Psychiatric Institute

Susan T. Spitz, M.S.W.
Coordinator, Couples Therapy Program, Columbia–Presbyterian Psychiatric Associates, New York, NY

Preface

Cocaine abuse has reached epidemic proportions in this country. Current estimates suggest that 20–24 million Americans have experimented with cocaine. Four to five million people are considered to be regular users, and the amount of cocaine used in this country increases by 10–20% each year.

Cocaine cuts across class lines and is no longer exclusively a drug for the affluent. Cocaine-related emergency room deaths have increased 200% since 1976, and cocaine-related admissions to government treatment programs have increased 500% over the same period. Emergency rooms, general hospitals, and psychiatric facilities are increasingly confronted with a patient population which many professionals feel ill-equipped or lacking in current knowledge to treat definitively.

In addition to the health care problems, virtually no segment of our society is unaware of or unaffected by the spread of cocaine abuse. Families face growing concern about children's involvement with drugs, as do the educational, legal, and criminal justice sectors. Cocaine-related tragedies involving both the famous and the "person next door" have become a regular part of contemporary news media coverage.

The need for dissemination of new information about cocaine is acute and prompted the creation of this book. Our purpose is to present the major issues related to the current state of scientific knowledge about cocaine, starting in basic science and progressing through diagnosis, clinical management, treatment, and research. An effort has been made to present theoretical, laboratory, and research data in a fashion that will be understandable and of practical value to front-line practitioners, administration, family members, and others seeking information to incorporate into their work or personal lives.

The format of the text has been divided into four major sections: Background Issues, Neuroscience Issues, Treatment Issues, and Future Directions. Chapter 1 sets the questions related to cocaine use in a historical perspective and reviews fundamental issues concerning cocaine abuse which will be amplified in many sections of the text that follows.

The neuroscience section begins with basic animal research studies on cocaine and, along with its companion chapter on human neurochemistry, delineates the physiological, biochemical, and behavioral findings that form the basis for cocaine's propensity for misuse by selected individuals.

The bulk of the book concentrates on themes related to the treatment of cocaine abuse. Chapter 4 provides a broad overview of the current psychological and biological treatment formats available to the practitioner. The chapters included in the treatment section take each specific element of treatment and put them under higher magnification. Chapter 5 is an in-depth presentation of the importance of clarity in clinical diagnosis of cocaine abusers. Differential diagnosis becomes a critical area since cocaine abuse has been known to cause clinical confusion, owing to cocaine's ability to "mimic" other psychological and medical conditions.

Chapters 6, 7, and 8 are devoted to theoretical and clinical principles of the major forms of psychotherapeutic intervention used with cocaine abusers. The rationale for and the common therapeutic considerations encountered in the application of individual, group, and family therapy to the problem of cocaine abuse are discussed in these chapters.

The problems unique to the treatment of the cocaine abuser in the hospital setting are presented in Chapter 9. The criteria for in-patient treatment of cocaine abuse and the medical and psychological symptoms that require close monitoring are discussed in a clinical context.

The section on treatment concludes with an overview of the major pharmacological approaches to the management of cocaine abuse. Chapter 10 summarizes what is known about the use of psychotropic medication as a component of a cocaine abuse treatment program. This chapter builds on basic science information from Chapters 2 and 3, diagnostic issues discussed in Chapter 5, and serves as a model for integrating neuroscientific understanding into comprehensive patient care.

The final section of the book contains a chapter on research related to cocaine. The growing edge of the cocaine abuse field is reflected in the research questions and answers offered in Chapter 11. The book concludes with a chapter that addresses a representative cross-section of contemporary issues touched by cocaine. The topics discussed in the last chapter are: "crack"; women and cocaine; cocaine, pregnancy, and the fetus; cocaine and sports; cocaine in the workplace; and the cocaine-abusing health care professional.

The "living laboratory" from which many of the authors' ideas and experience originated is located at the Cocaine Abuse Treatment Program of the Department of Psychiatry, Columbia University, College of Physicians and Surgeons. While we have evolved a preference for an eclectic treatment model combining cognitive, educational, supportive, behavioral, medication, and psychotherapeutic elements in a family and group setting, our purpose in the writing of this text was not to present our program, but rather to provide a fair rendering of representative work in the clinical and research arenas. In so doing, it is our hope to create a "state-of-the-art" cocaine book that will contribute to increased understanding and improved treatment options for those whose lives are adversely affected by cocaine use.

Acknowledgments

The process of writing a contemporary cocaine text owes its success to many influences. The authors would like to express their appreciation to several people whose contributions were critical to the success of the project.

Drs. Richard Sauber and Jerry Maxmen helped demystify the complex tangle of factors involved in the mechanics of publishing a book and encouraged our initial hopes for this venture.

Drs. Irving Bieber and Robert Toborowsky "looked over our shoulders," offered sage advice, and made important suggestions regarding the form and content of the book.

Albert Gross was of invaluable assistance in the areas of nutrition and brain chemistry.

David Lane, of the New York State Psychiatric Institute Library, was instrumental in simplifying the enormous task of reviewing the scientific literature on a host of subjects contained in the book.

Camille Atkins and Lisa Mahoney bore with us through numerous deadlines and provided consistently cheerful and capable secretarial support.

Finally, to all those members of our personal and professional networks who gave of their time, talents, and perspective, we are sincerely grateful.

COCAINE ABUSE

New Directions
in
Treatment and Research

I
Background Issues

Chapter 1

Cocaine Reconceptualized: Historical Overview

Jeffrey S. Rosecan, M.D.,
and Henry I. Spitz, M.D.

S.F. is a brilliant young physician attending a case conference at a metropolitan medical center where he is a resident. He has been on-call for 36 hours and cannot concentrate on the presentation. S.F. is lonely, depressed, and overworked. All he can think about is his fiancée, who is several hundred miles away. He knows that her father will not permit her to marry until he is able to support her, and with his loans and meager salary that could take years. He excuses himself from the conference, takes a needle and syringe from the nurses' station, and locks himself in a bathroom stall. He fills the syringe with cocaine and plunges the needle into his arm. Within seconds, the young doctor feels a rush of euphoria. His tears dry up; he regains his composure and quickly rejoins the conference.

The date is 1884, the place is Vienna, and the doctor is Sigmund Freud in this fictionalized clinical vignette. As Byck notes in Freud's *Cocaine Papers* (1974), Freud himself used cocaine beginning in 1884 as a curiosity, as a research interest in experimental pharmacology, and probably as self-medication for his own depression. On June 2, 1884, he wrote to his fiancée Martha Bernays:

> Woe to you, my Princess, when I come I will kiss you quite red and
> feed you till you are plump. And if you are forward you shall see

who is stronger, a gentle little girl who doesn't eat enough or a big wild man who has cocaine in his body. In my last severe depression I took coca again and a small dose lifted me to the heights in a wonderful fashion. I am just now busy collecting the literature for a song of praise to this magical substance. (pp. 10–11)

This "song of praise" was *Über Coca,* Freud's 1884 monograph on cocaine which advocated its use in the treatment of alcoholism, morphine addiction, asthma, and gastrointestinal disturbances, in addition to depression. Freud used cocaine to treat the morphine addiction of his friend Von Fleishl after reading reports of clinical successes in American medical journals. The results were disastrous; Von Fleishl ended up not only addicted to cocaine, but also experiencing the first documented case of cocaine psychosis ("delirium tremens with white snakes creeping over his skin").

Freud also ran a series of experiments on himself in 1884 (Freud, 1885). While going about his duties at the hospital in Vienna, he administered cocaine to himself and documented the effects on reaction time and muscle strength (see Table 1.1).

These experiments are landmarks in the history of psychopharmacology and represent, to the authors' knowledge, the only human experiments of their kind. Freud found that cocaine increased muscle strength (as measured by a dynamometer) for four hours and decreased reaction time. Freud hypothesized that these were central, not peripheral, actions of cocaine. Many contemporary cocaine users feel that cocaine initially enhances performance and reduces fatigue. Users also report euphoria and an increased sense of well-being, which was best described by Freud in *Über Coca* in 1884:

The psychic effect of cocaine . . . consists of exhilaration and lasting euphoria, which does not differ in any way from the normal euphoria of a healthy person. . . . One senses an increase of self control and feels more vigorous and more capable of work. . . . One is simply normal, and soon finds it difficult to believe that one is under the influence of any drug at all. (p. 60)

Clearly, the pioneering work done by Freud in eludicating the physiological and psychological effects of cocaine in human subjects needs to be continued.

Freud's glowing reports of cocaine and his assertion that it was nonaddicting became quite controversial by the end of the nineteenth century. Although cocaine was used in patent medicines, liqueurs, and soft drinks such as Coca-Cola, there were many reports of cocaine toxicity

Table 1.1
Freud's Experiments with Cocaine[†]

Experiment of November 9, 1884. Dynamometer for two hands;

Time	Pressures	Max.	Average	Remarks
8:00	66–65–60	66	63.6	fasting
10:00	67–55–50	67	57.3	after morning rounds
10:22	67–63–56	67	62	after breakfast
10:30	65–58–67	67	63.6	—
10:33	0.10 *cocaïnum muriaticum**			
10:45	82–75–69	82	75.3	first ruptus
10:55	76–69–64	76	69.6	tired
11:20	78–71–77	78	75.3	euphoria
12:30	72–66–74	74	70.6	before lunch
12:55	77–73–67	77	72.6	—
1:35	75–66–74	75	71.6	after lunch
1:50	76–71–61	76	69.3	—
3:35	65–58–62	65	61.6	euphoria over

†From S. Freud, Über Coca, in Cocaine Papers, R. Byck, editor, 1974. Reprinted with permission.
*Freud did not state the measurement here but it was almost certainly grams, as later specified in his experiment of November 26, 1884. *Ed*.

(*continued*)

Table 1.1 (*continued*)
Experiment of November 10, 1884. [Same apparatus.]

Time	Pressures	Max.	Average	Remarks
8:00	60	60	60	tired
10:00	73–63–67	73	67.6	after rounds
—	thereupon, a small indeterminate quantity of cocaine			
10:20	76–70–76	76	74	cheerful
10:30	73–70–68	73	70.3	—
11:35	72–72–74	74	72.6	—
12:50	74–73–63	74	70	—
2:20	70–68–69	70	69	—
4:00	76–74–75	76	75	normal condition
6:00	67–64–58	67	63	after strenuous work
8:30	74–64–67	74	68.3	somewhat tired
—	thereupon, 0.10 *cocaïnum muriaticum**			
8:43	80–73–74	80	75.6	ruptus
8;58	79–76–71	79	75.3	—
9:18	77–72–67	77	72	buoyant feeling

* Once again, Freud did not state the measurement here but it was almost certainly grams. *Ed.*

Table 1.1 *(continued)*

Experiment of November 26, 1884.

Time	Reaction times	Max.	Min.	Av.	Remarks
7:10	15½–21½–19–21–18½–24–24	24	15½	20.5	motor energy, 36—, tired
about 7:30, 0.10g *cocaïn. mur.*					
7:38	17–21½–16–21–17–16	21½	16	18	motor energy, 39+
8:05	17–17–18–17	18	17	17.2	a little more cocaine
8:15	13½–11–16–15–16–12	16	11	13.9	euphoria
10:30	15½–14½–15–13½–17½	17½	14½	15.2	remaining good feeling motor energy, 37.5

Experiment of December 4, 1884. Well-being. No cocaine.

Time	Reaction times	Max.	Min.	Av.	Remarks
8:15	13½–13–14½–13½	14½	13	13.6	motor energy, 38–39k
8:30	15–14–14–19–15½–15½	19	14	15.5	during 4th reaction a disturbing sound
8:45	11½–13½–14½–12½–16½	16½	12½	13.7	—
9:00	12½–13–13–15½–14–18½	18½	12½	14.2	motor energy, 38

and addiction. This eventually led to its being made illegal in 1914 with the Harrison Narcotic Act. As Musto (1986) has stated,

> This first epidemic lasted from 1885 until the 1920's, about 35 years. There were three stages: an initial euphoria about an apparently harmless, indeed a valuable and helpful stimulant; a middle period of dispersion and multiplying instances of prolonged use; and finally, a powerful rejection of cocaine as its popular image became as negative as it had once been positive. This last stage was so effective in discouraging the use of cocaine that the drug had faded into obscurity until recently. (p. 1)

Between 1920 and the 1970s, cocaine use was not widespread and for the most part was restricted to artists, jazz musicians, and the avant garde. The stimulants of choice for most of the population were amphetamines, which were synthesized in the 1930s and were legally prescribed by physicians as diet pills and "pep pills." With the resurgence of wisespread illicit drug use in the 1960s, cocaine gained a new respectability as the "champagne" of drugs. Although still illegal, cocaine was felt to be relatively safe and nonaddicting, especially when snorted. This was the prevailing view of the medical and psychiatric establishment through the early 1980s. In the March 1982 issue of *Scientific American*, Van Dyck and Byck assert,

> Dependence on intranasal cocaine manifests itself in a pattern of continued use while supplies are available and in simple abstention when supplies are lacking. The pattern of behavior is comparable to that experienced by many people with peanuts or potato chips. It may interfere with other activities of the individual, but it may be a source of enjoyment as well. (p. 138)

The definitive *Comprehensive Textbook of Psychiatry* (Kaplan, Freedman, & Sadock, 1980) stated, "If it is used no more than two or three times a week, cocaine creates no serious problems" (p. 1621).

The American Psychiatric Association's *Diagnostic and Statistical Manual of Mental Disorders*, Third Edition (DSM-III, APA, 1980) has a diagnostic category for cocaine abuse, not cocaine dependence, implying a less serious addiction. Heroin, amphetamines, and even cigarettes warrant dependence diagnoses. The proposed revision of DSM-III (DSM-III-R), reviewed in Chapter 5 by Skodol, eliminates the distinction between abuse and dependence. However, until very recently the general public and the medical community felt that cocaine was generally safe and nonaddicting, especially when snorted. Why has cocaine reemerged as a major drug of abuse after a relatively quiescent period of 60 years? Is it addictive, and if so, how? How and why do people become addicted to cocaine? We shall attempt to answer these questions in this and other chapters of this volume.

Cocaine is a stimulant derived from the leaves of the coca plant. Coca leaves have been ritually chewed by South American peoples for thousands of years; however, it was not until 1860 that cocaine was first extracted from the coca leaf. Coca was believed to be a mystical drug and was used in religious rituals by the Incas in ancient Peru (see Grinspoon & Bakalar, 1985, and Petersen, 1977, for reviews). The plant was believed to be of divine origin, and there are several myths to account for its appearance on earth. During the period of Incan rule, coca was felt to be a magical offering from the gods to ensure a safe passage through the Andes.

After the decline of the Incan empire in the fifteenth century, the Spanish conquistadors took over the cultivation and distribution of coca and used it to force the Andean Indians to work under adverse conditions of brutal labor and little food. The Spaniards learned to enjoy coca themselves, and eventually introduced it to Europe. Pizarro brought it from Peru to the Spanish court, yet it was not until the extraction of cocaine from the coca leaf by the Austrian chemist Niemann in 1860 that Europeans discovered cocaine. The Italian neurologist Mantegazza described the effect of cocaine as follows: "I felt deeply joyful and intensely alive. . . . I would rather have a life span of ten years with coca than one of 1,000,000 centuries without coca." Similar glowing reports from Europe and the United States set the stage for Freud's experiments with cocaine.

Coca was also chewed by Andean natives to suppress their appetite and increase their endurance for work under adverse conditions in the high altitudes. In Chapter 12, we present a contemporary perspective on these issues: some women begin their dependence on cocaine by using it as an appetite suppressant, and many female cocaine abusers appear to have eating disorders, such as bulimia. Cocaine may also improve performance initially, and many users gradually learn to rely on it to perform, whether athletically, sexually, at a party, or at work. The problem is that when cocaine is abused or used chronically, performance invariably suffers.

IS COCAINE ADDICTING?

This question was also asked in the 1880s, was also very controversial, and was never answered definitively. Alcohol and opiates (i.e., morphine, heroin) are and were generally considered to be addicting for two reasons: they could control and debilitate the drug addict or alcoholic completely, and their withdrawal syndromes (i.e., delirium tremens in the alcoholic) were dramatic and required medical intervention. Although there have consistently been case reports of uncontrollable cocaine abuse in the medical literature over the past century, the lack of a dramatic withdrawal syndrome and the relative infrequency of these reports have kept the general public and the scientific community from accepting cocaine as addicting. From the 1860s until the advent of amphetamines in the 1930s, cocaine was the main central nervous system (CNS) stimulant available. During this period, the major drugs of abuse were the CNS depressants alcohol and morphine. Cocaine does not conform to the same criteria for dependence as the CNS depressants (i.e., tolerance, withdrawal); hence its addictive potential was controversial. Cocaine does, however, have its own unique CNS actions, both acute and chronic (see Table 1.2). These actions, over time, appear to produce neurochemical changes that can create a need for more cocaine. This need can become an all-consuming cocaine craving in some individuals, causing problems at work and in interpersonal relationships. In laboratory animals, cocaine is the most reinforcing of drugs and is consistently self-administered until death. This is not true with heroin or alcohol. These studies are reviewed by Geary in Chapter 2. The cocaine withdrawal syndrome, consisting of lethargy, depression, oversleeping, and overeating, and eventually the craving for more cocaine, can also be explained by these neurochemical changes produced by chronic cocaine use. The CNS depressant withdrawal syndromes, with autonomic arousal as their hallmark, bear little resemblance to this cocaine withdrawal syndrome. Nunes and Rosecan review the neurochemistry of cocaine, the craving, and the withdrawal syndrome in Chapter 3.

Based on the proposed DSM-III-R criteria, cocaine is addicting, and

Table 1.2
Acute and Chronic Actions of Cocaine in Neurotransmitters

Acute	Chronic
1. Reuptake blockade (presynaptic)	1. Depletion of neurostransmitters
2. Release of preformed neuro-transmitters into the synapse	2. Supersensitivity of postsynaptic receptors for neuro-transmitters
3. Increased synthesis of neurotrans-mitters (probable)	

cocaine dependence should finally enter this official nosology of mental disorders. This reclassification is based on a reconceptualization of cocaine as a drug that can produce subtle imbalances in brain chemistry which create a need for more cocaine. Viewed this way, cocaine is deceptively, though powerfully, addicting over time in a manner that is unique among subtances of abuse.

HOW AND WHY DO PEOPLE BECOME ADDICTED TO COCAINE?

Addiction to any substance is a complicated process which can be conceptualized as an interaction between the individual, the environment, and the substance. (See Table 1.3.)

The Individual

Certain individuals are at risk to develop problems of addiction because of their psychological predisposition. Many cocaine abusers use cocaine as self-medication for painful emotional states. Often cocaine is used to cope with the loss of a love relationship (as was the case with SF at the beginning of this chapter), loss of a job, or a financial loss. Cocaine abusers are often masking underlying insecurities and self-esteem defects when they use cocaine for performance, whether athletic, sexual, at a party, or at work. As noted previously, cocaine can improve performance acutely while impairing it chronically. In this way, users can become psychologically dependent on cocaine before the physical dependence sets in.

Table 1.3
Factors Involved in the Development of an Addiction

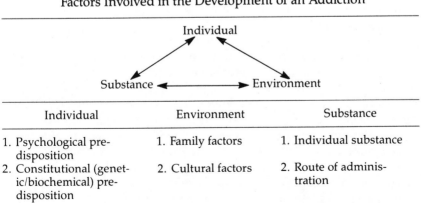

Individual	Environment	Substance
1. Psychological predisposition	1. Family factors	1. Individual substance
2. Constitutional (genetic/biochemical) predisposition	2. Cultural factors	2. Route of administration

Other individuals are at risk for the development of cocaine dependence because of their constitutional or biochemical predisposition. The complicated relationship between psychiatric disorders and cocaine dependence can be summarized as follows. Cocaine abusers self-medicate not just painful emotional states, but also affective disorders (depression, cyclothymia, etc.) and behavioral disorders (such as residual attention deficit disorder) (Khantzian, 1985). Several studies (Gawin & Kleber, 1986; Mirin et al., 1984; Nunes et al., 1986) have shown a greater incidence of these disorders in cocaine abusers than that reported in other substance abusers. In these studies, preexisting or coexisting affective disorders were found in more than 50% of the samples. Another important factor in this interrelationship between cocaine dependence and psychiatric disorders is that for many individuals, chronic cocaine use is depressogenic. This may be related to the neurochemical changes produced by chronic cocaine use, which in preliminary studies resemble those seen in depression. Although there are no published family history or twin studies of cocaine abusers, it is likely that future studies will show genetic loading for affective illness.

In summary, certain individuals, because of psychological or constitutional factors, appear to be predisposed to cocaine dependence. Systematic research is clearly needed in this area to more clearly define the specific individual elements that result in excessive use of cocaine.

The Environment

The family is the mediator between an individual and his or her culture. We believe that family factors are involved in the development and treatment of cocaine dependence. Cocaine abuse can be one of the indicators of family dysfunction; hence treatment of the cocaine addict should involve active treatment of the family. This is reviewed by Spitz and Spitz in Chapter 8.

Other cultural factors are important in cocaine's widespread use today. Over the past century, cocaine has been portrayed as a glamorous, high-status drug. Angelo Mariani, an Italian chemist, developed a coca wine in 1863, which he named Vin Mariani. He promoted it widely over the next 40 years and used testimonials from physicians and celebrities, ranging from Thomas Edison and Jules Verne to the Pope, in advertisements. Recently, cocaine use has been publicized among performing artists, professional athletes, and the rich and famous. Cocaine has had a mystique of its own for most of its history, and this status is an important factor in its current popularity, since users often feel they have entered a privileged group. Adolescents are particularly vulnerable to this pressure and will often experiment with cocaine and other drugs in order to be accepted by their peers. It is the authors' opinion that the cocaine mystique must be challenged and confronted before the current epidemic of cocaine abuse will subside. Well-formulated anticocaine campaigns similar to the antismoking messages currently in the media are necessary as a component of an effort to deromanticize the "glamorous" aspects of cocaine use. A prevailing cultural climate that fails to address these issues automatically puts its population at higher risk of exposure to the negative consequences of experimentation with cocaine.

The Substance

Cocaine, regardless of route of administration, carries a high potential for abuse. Cocaine can gradually create a need for itself, which in susceptible individuals can supplant other interests and become an addiction. Although many appear to use it safely, or "recreationally," the cumulative neurochemical changes produced, combined with a progressive psychological reliance on the drug, can lead even the most casual user to compulsive use. Cocaine is potently reinforcing in animals and will produce more debilitation and a greater mortality than heroin in self-administration studies (Bozarth & Wise, 1985).

In this chapter, we reconceptualize cocaine as a uniquely addicting drug, based on its neurochemical actions. Although the cocaine addict resembles the alcoholic, heroin, or amphetamine addict, there are important differences. Treatment of the cocaine-dependent patient should follow the general guidelines of substance abuse treatment outlined in Chapter 4, but should at the same time respect the uniqueness of cocaine the substance.

Comprehensive and definitive treatment of cocaine abuse requires the successful integration of individual and environmental factors combined with up-to-date knowledge of the emerging neurobiological fund of information related to properties of cocaine itself.

REFERENCES

American Psychiatric Association: Diagnostic and Statistical Manual of Mental Disorders, 3rd ed, Washington, DC, American Psychiatric Association, 1980.

Bozarth MA, Wise RA: Toxicity associated with long-term intravenous heroin and cocaine administration in the rat. JAMA 254(1):81–83, 1985.

Freud S: Über Coca, in Cocaine Papers, edited by Byck R, New York, Stonehill Publishing Co., 1974, pp 49–73.

Freud S: Contribution to the knowledge of the effect of cocaine. Wien Medi Wochenschr 35(5):129–133, 1885.

Gawin FH, Kleber HD: Abstinence symptomatology and psychiatric diagnosis in cocaine abusers. Clinical observations. Arch Gen Psychiatry 43(2):107–113, 1986.

Grinspoon L, Bakalar JB: Cocaine: A Drug and Its Social Evolution, New York, Basic Books, 1985.

Kaplan HI, Freedman AM, Sadock BJ: Comprehensive Textbook of Psychiatry/III, Baltimore/London, Williams & Wilkins, 1980, p 1621.

Khantzian EJ: The self-medication hypothesis of addictive disorders: focus on heroin and cocaine dependence. Am J Psychiatry 142(11):1259–1264, 1985.

Mirin SM, Weiss RD, Sollogub A, Michael J: Affective illness in substance abusers, in Mirin SM, ed: Substance Abuse and Psychopathology, Washington DC, American Psychiatric Press, 1984, pp 57–78.

Musto DF: Lessons of the first cocaine epidemic. Wall Street Journal, June 11, 1986.

Nunes E, Quitkin F, Rosecan J: Psychiatric diagnosis in cocaine abuse: evidence for biological heterogeneity. Presented at the British Association for Psychopharmacology, Cambridge, England, July 14, 1986.

Petersen RC: History of cocaine, in Petersen RC, Stillman RC, eds: Cocaine, Washington DC, US Govt Printing Office, 1977, pp 17–34.

Van Dyck C, Byck R: Cocaine. Sci Am, pp 128–141, March 1982.

II
Neuroscience Issues

Chapter 2

Cocaine: Animal Research Studies

Nori Geary, Ph.D.

Cocaine administration in rodents, carnivores, and nonhuman primates has a variety of dramatic behavioral effects. Depending on dosage and injection regimen, cocaine elicits motor responses including increased locomotion, stereotypic behavior, dyskinesia, and convulsions. Cocaine also affects learned behavior. For example, animals readily learn to use cocaine's interoceptive effects as discriminative stimuli to guide behavior, and this opens the drug's stimulus properties to analysis. Cocaine's most dramatic behavioral effect, however, is its unparalleled rewarding potency. Animals become more readily addicted to cocaine than to any other drug, and cocaine-addicted animals suffer more dysfunctional and lethal consequences than animals dependent on other drugs.

This chapter reviews these effects of cocaine on animal behavior. An attempt is made to focus on animal research relevant to the analysis of cocaine's most prominent and problematic subjective and behavioral effects in humans, including euphoria, craving, dependence, and disruption of adaptive behavior. Three strong currents that relate to these issues emerge: the extremely potent rewarding effects of cocaine, the different behavioral effects of low and high cocaine dosages or cocaine availability, and cocaine's ultimate debilitating consequences. It is concluded that cocaine potently influences numerous fundamental brain mechanisms regulating affect and behavior in animals as well as in humans, and that both the behavioral effects and their neuroendocrine mechanisms are accessible to convergent routes of experimental analysis.

MOTOR EFFECTS OF COCAINE

Cocaine administration in humans produces, in addition to its effects on mood, the classic signs of psychomotor stimulation, including perception of increased energy and alertness, inhibition of REM and non-REM sleep, and motor, verbal, and ideational hyperactivity (Byck & Van Dyck, 1977; Freud, 1884, 1970; Post & Contel, 1983). Cocaine elicits similar behavioral effects in animals, as do most drugs with dopamine agonist activity, for example, amphetamine. Both locomotor activity and the incidence of repeated stereotypic behavior increase in rats and monkeys after only one or two injections of as little as 10 mg/kg cocaine (Kilbey & Ellinwood, 1977; Post & Contel, 1983; Post & Rose, 1976; Roy et al., 1978) and as little as 1 mg/kg in cats (Collins et al., 1979) (1 mg = 3 μmol). Stereotypic behavior patterns in animals include repetitive, relatively invariant, and intense responses, such as exploratory or orienting responses (vertical rearing, sniffing, etc), grooming, gnawing, nose poking, head bobbing or waving, locomotion, or, in animals trained to perform conditioned responses, fragments of learned response sequences. Interestingly, if cocaine is administered during the performance of learned behaviors, then the learned responses or fragments of them are much more likely to become stereotyped than are the unconditioned behaviors described above (Ellinwood & Kilbey, 1975; Collins et al., 1979). This suggests that the motor activity elicited by cocaine stimulation is at least in part organized by the behavioral context in which cocaine is administered.

Higher cocaine dosages increase the intensity of stereotypic behaviors and also elicit prolonged staring, visual tracking movements in the absence of moving stimuli, dyskinesias, grand mal convulsions, ataxia, and catalepsy (Downs & Eddy, 1932; Tatum & Seevers, 1929). Acute cocaine seizures are often fatal. Surprisingly, such motor effects are also produced if moderate cocaine dosages are administered only once a day for several days (Post & Contel, 1983; Post & Rose, 1976; Roy et al., 1978; Stripling & Ellinwood, 1977a,b). This is known as cocaine-induced behavioral sensitization. Its development is illustrated in Figures 2.1 and 2.2, which depict the results of experiments by Post and Rose (1976). Rats that were injected with 10 mg/kg cocaine daily displayed progressive increases in activity and stereotypy scores over the course of 10–20 tests.

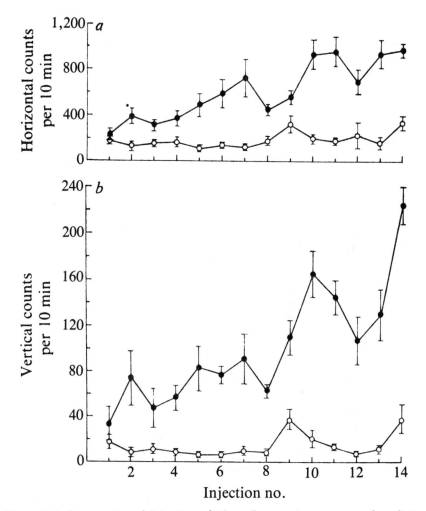

Figure 2.1. Intraperitoneal injection of 10 mg/kg cocaine once per day elicits progressive increases in horizontal activity (a) and vertical activity (b). Data shown are mean ± SEM of eight rats treated with cocaine (filled circles) and eight rats treated with saline (open circles). Behavior was monitored for 90 minutes after injections. Horizontal activity was measured with a grid of infrared photoelectric cells on the cage floor that registered slight movements as well as gross locomotor activity. Vertical activity was measured by photoelectric cells placed 13 cm above the floor. (From Post & Rose, 1976. Reproduced with permission.)

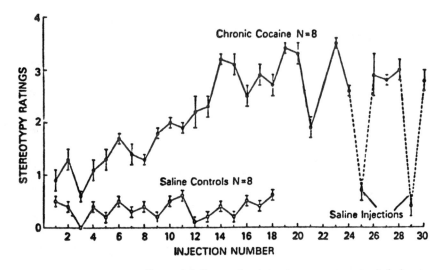

Figure 2.2. Progressive effects of daily cocaine injections on stereotypic behavior in rats. Stereotypy was rated each 10 minutes for 90 minutes after intraperitoneal injections of 10 mg/kg cocaine. No stereotypy was scored 0; intense, continuous stereotypic patterns were scored 4. Initially, rats displayed mild repetitive sequences, such as moving from corner to corner and quick circular movements of the head. After chronic cocaine treatment, these patterns became more intense, invariant, and prolonged. Rats would, for example, frantically rotate or bob their heads while lying prone for periods of up to 15 minutes. When cocaine-treated rats were administered saline instead of cocaine on days 25 and 29, behavior was normal. (From Post & Contel, 1983; Post & Rose, 1976. Reproduced with permission.)

Both the intensity and the duration of motor responses increased severalfold in sensitized rats. Cocaine's street name "Bolivian marching powder" (McInerney, 1984) does not appear unjustified! In rhesus monkeys, daily injection of 10–17 mg/kg cocaine produced similar initial sensitization effects (Post et al., 1976). After reaching maximal levels in the fourth week, stereotypy and hyperactivity were replaced by the emergence of motor responses that were not initially present, including lingual and buccal dyskinesias, staring, visual tracking, ataxia, catalepsy, and convulsions.

Similar motor sensitization effects have been reported for psychomotor stimulants and dopamine agonists other than cocaine (see Post & Contel, 1983, for a review). These studies indicate that hyperactivity and stereotypy are specifically sensitized, whereas most of the physiological effects of psychomotor stimulants that are shared by cocaine, such as hypertension and tachycardia, as well as other behavioral effects, such as anorexia and drug stimulus properties (see below), do not become sensitized or show tolerance. Thus, the motor and nonmotor effects of cocaine appear to be mediated by at least partly independent neuroendocrine mechanisms.

In contrast to the motor sensitizatiion effects that are produced by repeated, intermittent cocaine treatment, continuous infusions or more frequent daily injections have often failed to produce sensitization (Leith & Barrett, 1976; Nelson & Ellison, 1978). This surprising result suggests that sensitization is not simply due to an accumulation of drug in the blood or brain, but results from some sort of dynamic neuroendocrine response to repeated cocaine challenges. Cocaine's short biological half-life (Javaid et al., 1983; Mulé & Misra, 1977) also argues against the drug accumulation hypothesis. This conclusion is further supported by the observations that different motor effects emerge at different times during sensitization, that some effects show tolerance rather than sensitization, and that sensitized responses persist even when weeks or months intervene between drug treatments (Post & Contel, 1983; Segal & Mandell, 1974; Stripling & Ellinwood, 1977a). Motor sensitization also seems not to be a primarily learned effect, since when a placebo is substituted for cocaine in sensitized animals, hyperactivity and stereotypy scores return immediately to control levels (see, for example, Figure 2.2, days 25 and 29). Learning may, however, play an at least permissive role. Rats sensitized to cocaine in their home cages failed to show sensitization during the first test outside the home cage (Post et al., 1981a). Thus, development of some form of habituation to the environmental context in which cocaine is administered may be necessary for the expression of motor sensitization.

In addition to displaying properties similar to psychomotor stimulants, cocaine shares the local anesthetic actions of drugs like lidocaine. Post and his colleagues originally hypothesized that some action, possibly central, that is shared by cocaine and local anesthetics may mediate motor sensitization because lidocaine injected once daily also elicits motor sensitization (Post et al., 1975). Further, rats sensitized to lidocaine show cross-sensitization to cocaine (Squillace et al., 1982). In contrast, such cross-sensitization does not occur from amphetamine to cocaine (Short & Shuster, 1976) or from cocaine to amphetamine (Shuster et al., 1977). Cocaine, like lidocaine, can also facilitate electrophysiologically kindled convulsions or limbic system EEG spindles (Kilbey et al., 1979; Post et al., 1981b; Stripling & Russell, 1985; Stripling et al., 1983). Electrophysiological kindling and motor sensitization are procedurally similar in that both involve repeated stimulation. Nevertheless, Post and

Contel (1983) finally concluded that kindling and sensitization are unlikely to share a common neuroendocrine substrate because kindling
phenomena occur only with much higher dosages than required for
sensitization.

The motor effects of cocaine and other psychomotor stimulants have
been linked most frequently to dopaminergic brain mechanisms, although cocaine also affects other neurotransmitter systems (Dackis &
Gold, 1985; Mandell & Knapp, 1979; Post & Contel, 1983; Wise, 1984a;
also see Nunes & Rosecan, Chapter 3). Little is known, however, about
which brain dopamine systems or what changes in dopamine neurons
mediate the various behavioral effects. One interesting possibility is that
cocaine-induced sensitization of stereotypy may be related to desensiti-
zation of presynaptic dopamine autoreceptors rather than stimulation of
post-synaptic receptors (Post et al., 1974; Schwartz et al., 1978). Sensitization may also be influenced by the depletion of presynaptic stores of
dopamine, epinephrine, or serotonin (Mandell & Knapp, 1979; Scheel-
Kruger et al., 1977; Whitby et al., 1960). Another possible mechanism of
stereotypy involves the neurotransmitter γ-aminobutyric acid (GABA).
Cocaine appears to antagonize GABA neurotransmission (Cohen, 1984),
and administration of the GABA agonist muscimol eliminated the stereotypic responses elicited by high doses of cocaine while facilitating
locomotor activity (Bachus & Gale, 1984, 1985). The locomotor effects of
low doses of cocaine are also potentiated by caffeine (Misra et al., 1986).

Finally, Glick and his colleagues (Glick & Hinds, 1984; Glick et al.,
1983) have investigated another dimension of cocaine's locomotor effects. They showed that intraperitoneal injections of 10–40 mg/kg cocaine elicit circling in rats tethered in cylindrical cages and that this
stimulatory effect exhibits a sex-dependent interaction with the rats' preferred rotation direction. Females biased toward rotating to the right
rotated more and showed a stronger bias after cocaine than left-biased
females, whereas the opposite was true of males. Furthermore, in females but not in males, a single cocaine injection sensitized the effect of
subsequent injections administered up to a week later. Because direc-
tional circling preferences have been associated with asymmetries in
nigrostriatal dopamine function, Glick et al. suggest that brain asymmetry may be an important determinant of cocaine's psychomotor effects.
The hippocampus is another possible site for such an effect. In the
hippocampus there are left-right asymmetries in the concentrations of
the neurotransmitter 5-hydroxytryptamine (serotonin), its precursor
tryptophan, and its breakdown product 5-hydroxyindoleacetic acid, and
cocaine injection increased each of these asymmetries (Mandell &

Knapp, 1979). Whether such effects may underlie individual differences in human susceptibility to cocaine or whether individual differences might be related to sex or cerebral lateralization would be fascinating to study.

In conclusion, cocaine elicits a constellation of motor effects in animals that parallel its psychomotor stimulant effects in humans. Repeated administration of moderate cocaine dosages sensitize these effects and, like single injections of large doses, can result in extreme behavioral toxicity and death. Little is known about the neuroendocrine mechanisms of these effects. Because the dosages of cocaine used by humans for recreational purposes and the pattern of such use are clearly sufficient to elicit similarly severe consequences (Brinkley, 1986; Mittleman & Wetli, 1984; Myers & Earnest, 1984), this is a problem of great clinical importance.

Cocaine's motor effects in animals may also be of more general theoretical significance because these effects are temporally dynamic and because they interact with behavioral and contextual factors. In humans, cocaine can elicit bipolar subjective effects, with initial euphoria replaced by subsequent anxiety and dysphoria after either acute or chronic administration (Dackis & Gold, 1985; Post & Contel, 1983; Resnick et al., 1977). Psychomotor stimulant abuse can also lead to delusions, including the classic cocaine-induced formication delusion (which is associated with behaviors similar to those observed in cocaine-sensitized monkeys), and to psychosis (Bell, 1973; Lewin, 1931; Post, 1975). The motor effects described here may provide a useful animal model of possible neuroendocrine bases of such dynamic subjective effects of cocaine in humans.

STIMULUS PROPERTIES OF COCAINE

Although animals' subjective experiences of drug states are not directly accessible, they can be indirectly assessed using the drug discrimination procedure. This technique employs the interoceptive stimuli produced by drug administration as discriminative stimuli for operant conditioning. During conditioning, two or more drug states are used to signal the availability of some reward, usually food or water, if the response appropriate to the state occurs. For example, hungry animals might receive food only if they press one bar after cocaine injection and a different bar after saline injection.

Two tests of drug discrimination are possible. First, the aquisition of differential responding to the training states indicates that the states are discriminably different, although appropriate controls are necessary to ensure that differential responding is not due to changes in response capacity or other direct drug effects. Second, after acquisition of a discrimination, the animals' ability to detect substitution of test drugs for the training drugs can be probed. If animals respond differently during a test drug state than during the training drug state, then it is concluded that the interoceptive stimulus properties of the two states are discriminably different; if the animals respond similarly, then it is concluded that the two states are, at least to a degree, similar (for detailed discussions of method and theory, see Colpaert, 1977; Ho & Silverman, 1978; Stolerman & D'Mello, 1981). Thus, classes of drugs with shared stimulus properties can be defined. To the extent that the subjective experience of the drug contributes to its stimulus properties, the drug discrimination procedure can also be used to model animals' drug experiences.

Drug discrimination studies have demonstrated that cocaine administration in rats produces a discriminable drug stimulus similar to that produced by other psychomotor stimulants. Rats learn to discriminate cocaine from saline and, once trained to do so, then generalize the trained cocaine stimulus to different doses of cocaine, as well as to amphetamine, methylphenidate, phencyclidine, and cathinone, but not to nonstimulants (Colpaert et al., 1976, 1978b; Cunningham & Appel, 1982; D'Mello & Stolerman, 1977, 1978; Ellinwood & Kilbey, 1977; Ho & Silverman, 1978; Schechter & Glennon, 1985). That humans also often fail to discriminate cocaine from amphetamine (Fischman & Schuster, 1982; Martin et al., 1971) supports the contention that animals discriminate drugs on the basis of the perceptual effects similar to those occurring in humans. The generalization between cocaine and amphetamine is not, however, complete. D'Mello and Stolerman (1977) trained one group of rats to discriminate cocaine from saline and another to discriminate amphetamine from saline before determining dose-response curves for both drugs. Decreasing the dose of the drug used as the training stimulus produced much smaller response decrements then decreasing the dose of the crossover drug. This indicates that the cocaine and amphetamine stimuli are similar, but not identical, in the rat.

The drug discrimination paradigm has also been used to investigate the neuroendocrine substrate of cocaine's stimulus properties. Two sets of findings suggest the importance of dopamine neurotransmission. First, cocaine-trained rats generalize responding to dopaminergic agonists such as apomorphine and methylphenidate (Colpaert et al., 1976, 1978a,b). Second, pretreatment with dopaminergic receptor blockers antagonizes the stimulus control exerted by stimulants, whereas antagonism of other neurotransmitter systems is less effective (Colpaert et al., 1978b; Ho & Silverman, 1978; Jarbe, 1978). Some evidence for a noradrenergic contribution to cocaine's stimulus properties has also been reported (Colpaert et al., 1978b; Wood et al., 1985).

Another possibility is that cocaine's stimulus properties derive from its similarity to neurally active endogenous biogenic amines other than the classic neurotransmitters. Colpaert et al. (1980) provided evidence for this by demonstrating that the potency of various substances to induce stimulus generalization with cocaine correlated with the substances' potency to inhibit type B monoamine oxidase (MAO), but did not correlate with inhibition of type A MAO. This is evidence against a dopaminergic mediation of cocaine's stimulus properties because dopamine is a common substrate for both MAO types. Similarly, norepinephrine and 5-hydroxytryptamine are preferred substrates for type A, not type B, MAO. In contrast, the endogenous amine β-phenylethylamine (PEA) is a highly preferred substrate for type B MAO. PEA also shares pharmacological similarities with psychomotor stimulants (Moja et al., 1978). Therefore, these data are indirect support for the hypothesis that the stimulus properties and possibly the mood effects of cocaine result from its similarity to PEA.

An interesting possible insight into cocaine's dysphoric effects is provided by a drug discrimination test done by Shearman and Lal (1981). They demonstrated that pentylenetetrazol, an anxiogenic drug, generalizes to cocaine and that the stimulus properties of both cocaine and pentylenetetrazol are antagonized by diazepam. These results may reflect a link to PEA, insofar as PEA has also been hypothesized to be involved in the mediation of affect (Sabelli et al., 1986).

The stimulus properties of cocaine also generalize to morphine (Ando & Yanagita, 1978; Colpaert et al., 1978b), although it will require much more work to determine the extent to which the subjective and rewarding effects of cocaine (or other psychomotor stimulants) and opiates share common mechanisms. For example, generalization to morphine has only been tested after training animals to discriminate cocaine from saline. Thus, the drug states of the respective drugs could be very different, yet still be more similar to each other than either is to saline. Indeed, although the similarity of the rewarding actions of cocaine and the opiates has often been emphasized in the animal literature (Stein, 1978; Wise, 1984a), their subjective and addictive effects in humans are different.

In contrast to the opiates, the pharmacological properties that cocaine shares with local anesthetics are apparently not important components of cocaine's stimulus properties. Neither procaine nor lidocaine generalizes to cocaine (Colpaert et al., 1978b). This parallels their very weak potencies to elicit euphoric experiences in humans (Fischman et al., 1983a,b) or to maintain self-administration in monkeys (De La Garza & Johanson, 1982; Johanson & Aigner, 1981).

These studies exemplify several advantages of the drug discrimination procedure for the study of cocaine's effects in animals. Drug discrimination tests permit descriptions of stimulus properties that are likely to be largely due to cocaine's perceptual effects and permit comparisons between cocaine and other drugs. Finally, combination of cocaine with other pharmacological agents permits analyses of the neuroendocrine substrate of cocaine's stimulus properties. Unfortunately, there is one inherent complication in the use of the drug discrimination procedure as a model of subjective experiences elicited by cocaine: it is very difficult to determine or influence which of the many interoceptive effects of a drug acquire discriminative control of behavior. Efforts in this direction are especially important in the case of a drug with as many effects as cocaine, but little progress has been made. For example, not a single experiment has yet assessed the possible contribution of cocaine's cardiovascular effects to its stimulus properties.

REWARDING EFFECTS OF COCAINE

Self-Administration of Cocaine

Cocaine is rewarding in humans in two senses. Cocaine produces subjective feelings of euphoria, friendliness, and vitality (Ellinwood & Kilbey, 1977; Freud, 1884, 1970; Post & Contel, 1983). Cocaine also controls voluntary behavior. Cocaine users devote time, energy, and money toward an active, indeed all too often frenetic and obsessive pursuit of the drug. Although the subjective aspects of cocaine reward cannot be studied directly in animals, the rewarding effect that energizes and directs behavior is accessible to animal research, and its study has been instructive.

A canon law of the experimental psychology of learning is that voluntary behavior is shaped by its consequences. If rewarding consequences are made contingent on particular behaviors, those behaviors tend to increase in frequency. Conversely, if animals learn to perform an arbitrary behavioral response to produce some outcome, then the behavior is said to be motivated and the outcome is said to be rewarding (Teitelbaum, 1966). This is the rationale of the most persuasive animal model of drug reward and dependence, the voluntary self-administration paradigm.

A self-administration test is arranged simply by programming drug delivery to be contingent on some response by the animal. Biologically irrelevant responses that have low spontaneous rates, such as pressing a lever mounted in the cage wall, are usually used, and drugs are usually infused automatically via chronic intravenous catheters. Refinements of the basic paradigm include delivering the drug according to some intermittent schedule, for example rewarding only every tenth response, programming stimuli to signal periods when responses will or will not be rewarded, and inserting second manipulanda upon which responses are rewarded differently or not at all. Every species of animal tested, including rats, dogs, and several species of monkey, readily learns to self-administer cocaine (see Johanson, 1984, for a review). The pattern of responding and the behavioral and physiological effects of cocaine self-administration, however, depend critically on test conditions.

Several early investigations of cocaine self-administration were done under conditions of limited drug access. This work suggested that animals autoregulate cocaine delivery. For example, eight rhesus monkeys that self-administered cocaine during four-hour daily tests in which each lever press resulted in the delivery of 0.1–1.2 mg/kg cocaine achieved relatively constant mean cocaine intakes per session (17–26 mg/kg) by adjusting response rate inversely with the concentration of cocaine infused per reward (Wilson et al., 1971). Neither tolerance nor sensitivity developed over a period of months.

Regulation of cocaine intake is also suggested by experiments in which cocaine dose was varied and bar presses were rewarded only once each nine minutes (FI 9) (Balster & Schuster, 1973) or on the average of once each two and a half minutes (VI 2.5) (Woods & Schuster, 1968). Monkeys self-administered about 15–25 mg/kg/day cocaine in these studies. Similarly, rats barpressing 14 hours/day self-administered nearly constant amounts of cocaine when the dose was varied from 0.25 to 1.5 mg/kg or when the response requirement was varied from 1 to 20 presses per reward (FR 1–20) (Pickens & Thompson, 1968). Figure 2.3 shows some representative data from this experiment. Although rats' total drug intake, about 70–100 mg/kg/day, was higher than monkeys', rats, like monkeys, appear to modulate responding in order to maintain drug intake at a constant level.

Investigation of several further conditions established the specificity of cocaine's effects (Pickens & Thompson, 1968). When cocaine infusions were discontinued, rats greatly increased their response rates for a short

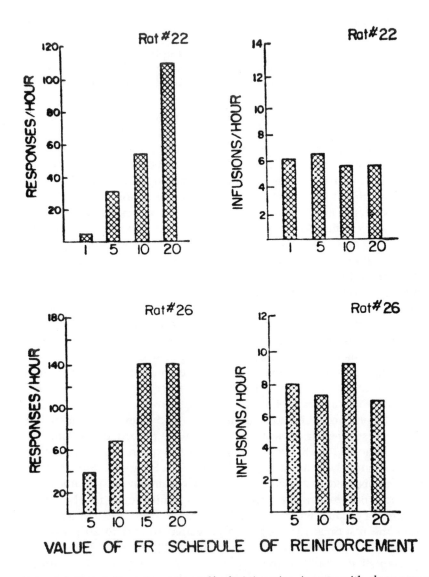

Figure 2.3. Regulation of cocaine self-administration in rats with drug access limited to 14 hours/day. One to 20 responses were required for intravenous infusions of 1 mg/kg cocaine delivered in 0.5 ml over 50 seconds. Response rate varied with the response requirement so as to achieve a nearly constant cocaine intake. (From Pickens & Thompson, 1968. Reproduced with permission.)

time, then slowed, and finally stopped responding. This extinction frustration effect is typical of natural rewards. Rats also ceased responding when cocaine infusions were delivered without a lever-pressing requirement. Finally, in a choice test in which a second, unrewarded response bar was made available, rats pressed only the bar that produced cocaine infusions and switched bars quickly if the bars were reversed. In similar choice tests in which the two bars were associated with different cocaine doses, rhesus monkeys allocated their responses on the two bars in proportion to the amount of cocaine each produced (Iglauer & Woods, 1974; Johanson & Schuster, 1975; Llewellyn et al., 1976). These results indicate that animals respond for cocaine in an organized, purposeful fashion under these conditions.

A classic test of the potency of a reward is to increase the effort necessary to obtain it. Yanagita (1973) found that the number of bar presses required for infusion of 0.5 mg/kg cocaine could be increased to 6,400–12,800 responses/infusion before monkeys would not maintain self-administration. No other drug, including opiates and amphetamine, has been reported to be more potent than cocaine in such tests (Johanson, 1984). Cocaine reward also withstands explicit punishment. Monkeys continued to self-administer cocaine when each infusion of cocaine was accompanied by an electric shock (Bergman & Johanson, 1981; Grove & Schuster, 1974). In a discrete trials choice test, monkeys also chose higher cocaine doses that were accompanied by shock over doses half as large that were not punished (Johanson, 1977). For monkeys, the psychological costs of effort and punishment seem low in comparison to the value of cocaine.

Goeders and Smith (1983) have used self-administration tests to investigate the brain mechanisms mediating cocaine reward. Rats implanted with microinjection cannulas learned to bar-press for injections of 25–100 pmol cocaine into the medial prefrontal cortex. As in experiments involving peripheral self-administration, when an inactive bar was present, rats pressed only the bar producing cocaine, and when the response requirement was increased from one to 10 responses per reward, they increased their response rate proportionally.

Because the medial prefrontal cortex is one of the major terminal fields of the mesocortical dopaminergic system, Goeders and Smith next investigated the involvement of dopaminergic neurons in intracranial cocaine self-administration. Self-administration was greatly attenuated when the dopamine receptor blocker sulpiride was injected together with cocaine, suggesting that dopaminergic blockade prevented cocaine's rewarding effect. (In contrast, rats pretreated with similar dopamine antagonists increased rates of self-administration, suggesting an effort to overcome the preexisting blockade [Roberts & Vickers, 1984; Woolverton, 1986].)

Goeders and Smith (1984) next lesioned presynaptic dopaminergic neurons at the self-administration site with 6-hydroxydopamine. This eliminated cocaine self-administration, although the animals would still self-administer dopamine. This suggests that the dopaminergic projection to the medial prefrontal cortex is necessary for intracranial cocaine self-administration (for a conflicting result, however, see Szostak et al., 1984).

Whether other dopaminergic systems are involved in cocaine self-administration is unclear. Lesions of the nucleus accumbens, which is part of the mesolimbic dopamine system, temporarily reduced the potency of intravenous cocaine to maintain self-administration (Roberts et al., 1977, 1980), although, paradoxically, cocaine injection into either the nucleus accumbens or ventral tegmental area, which are also parts of the mesolimbic dopamine system, did not support self-administration (Goeders & Smith, 1983). This and other mysteries concerning the neural basis of cocaine reward have been reviewed recently by Wise (1984a).

Cocaine's local anesthetic properties have been hypothesized to contribute to its rewarding effect because rhesus monkeys will self-administer procaine and other local anesthetics (Ford & Balster, 1977; Hammerbeck & Mitchell, 1978; Johanson, 1980). The rewarding effect of local anesthetics other than cocaine, however, is weak in that higher doses are required to support self-administration. A simultaneous choice test demonstrated this point in another way. Rhesus monkeys chose cocaine injection almost exclusively over procaine injection, even when the procaine dose was 16 times higher than the cocaine dose (Johanson & Aigner, 1981). This suggests that the relatively high response rates emitted in one-bar tests in which procaine is the only reward may be deceptive. The mechanisms of cocaine and procaine self-administration also have been dissociated. Blockade of dopaminergic receptors with low doses of haloperidol decreased the rate of procaine self-administration but increased cocaine self-administration, as if more cocaine was needed for the reward effect (De La Garza & Johanson, 1982).

Finally, cocaine may be rewarding because it mimics novel endogenous neurotransmitter or neuromodulatory substances. Intravenous infusion of three such substances, PEA, phenylethanolamine, or *N*-methyl phenylethylamine, supports vigorous self-administration in dogs (Risner & Jones, 1977; Shannon & DeGregorio, 1982). As described above, cocaine's stimulus properties may also be related to PEA agonism

(Colpaert et al., 1980). The possibility that cocaine reward is mediated by PEA is especially intriguing in light of hypotheses that variations in levels of PEA or a similar endogenous substance modulate affect in humans (Sabelli et al., 1986).

The self-administration studies reviewed to this point clearly demonstrate that intravenous cocaine infusion is powerfully rewarding. Although cocaine's stimulatory effects may account for some aspects of the pattern of responding under certain infusion contingencies (Balster & Schuster, 1973; Goldberg & Kelleher, 1976; Johanson & Schuster, 1981), psychomotor stimulation cannot explain the apparent regulation of the amount of cocaine self-administered or the necessity of a contingent relation between response and drug delivery for response maintenance. Similarly, there is no evidence that self-administration was maintained by negative reinforcement. That is, animals do not appear to respond for cocaine administration in order to avoid some aversive consequence of cocaine abstinence (although a report that squirrel monkeys will simultaneously respond on one bar for cocaine self-administration and on another bar for brief timeouts from the opportunity to respond on the first bar suggests that monkeys prefer intermittent cocaine administration to continuous administration [Spealman, 1979]).

Cocaine did not produce signs of physical dependence, and even if such consequences existed, drug-naive animals learned to self-administer at high rates before any dependence would have had time to develop (Deneau et al., 1969; Woods & Schuster, 1968). (Self-administration of drugs that do produce physical dependence also develops and can be maintained in the absence of signs of dependence.) Rather, cocaine self-administration under these conditions has all the signs of organized, voluntary, and goal-directed behavior that is similar to behaviors organized by natural rewards such as food. Although it cannot be concluded with certainty, an attractive hypothesis is that cocaine reward is mediated in animals and humans alike through an intense euphoric, mood-elevating effect.

Note, however, that in all the self-administration studies discussed to this point, the animals' access to cocaine has been limited. Removing this restraint reveals an effect even more compelling than cocaine's rewarding effect. Unlimited access to cocaine is lethal.

Deneau, Yanagita, and Seevers (1969; Yanagita et al., 1965) tested self-administration of 0.25–1.0 mg/kg cocaine/reward in rhesus monkeys that were given 24 hour/day drug access. The monkeys quickly learned the response and then proceeded to self-administer cocaine around the clock at high, erratic rates (up to 180 mg/kg/day) until, after two to five days, exhaustion overtook them. After periods of 12 hours to five days of abstinence, the cycle was reinitiated. Under these conditions, self-administration behavior failed to display the appearance of organization and regulation typical of the limited-access experiments discussed previously. Animals rarely ate or slept while responding for cocaine. Response rate, and consequently the rate of drug delivery, was highly erratic, with days of uninterrupted self-administration alternating with periods of abstinence. It is interesting to note that human intravenous stimulant abuse apparently follows a similar course (Kramer et al., 1967).

In addition, the full range of psychomotor effects, including stereotypy, hyperactivity, dyskinesia, ataxia, staring, scratching and biting of the skin, and convulsions, interfered with self-administration. Periods of abstinence, for example, usually began when the monkeys suffered states of exhaustion or seizures. Despite this degree of toxicity, monkeys did not become physically dependent on cocaine. If cocaine availability was withdrawn, they quickly returned to a normal, healthy state. The effects of unlimited cocaine access have been replicated in rats as well as monkeys (Bozarth & Wise, 1985; Johanson et al., 1976). Although limited- and unlimited-access conditions have not been compared directly, animals appear to self-administer about two to five times as much cocaine when access is unrestrained than when it is restrained (Aigner & Balster, 1978; Bozarth & Wise, 1985; Deneau et al., 1969; Johanson et al., 1976; Johanson & Schuster, 1975; Pickens & Thompson, 1968; Wilson et al., 1971; Woods & Schuster, 1968).

Experiments with two response bars further demonstrate the dissolution produced by cocaine. When access was completely unlimited, but only one bar produced cocaine, monkeys pressed the inactive bar as often or nearly as often as the active bar during periods of intense self-administration (Deneau et al., 1969; Johanson et al., 1976). When a choice between a bar producing food and a bar producing cocaine was made available once each 15 minutes, monkeys chose cocaine almost exclusively and completely ignored their only source of food for over a week (Aigner & Balster, 1978).

The behavioral and physiological dysfunctional effects of unlimited cocaine self-administration are more severe than those of stimulants such as caffeine or nicotine, of pentobarbitol, or of opiates (Deneau et al., 1969). For example, although monkeys self-administering morphine became physically dependent on the drug, they regulated self-administration accurately, ate and slept regularly, and maintained themselves in good health for periods of over a year. Figures 2.4 and 2.5 demonstrate the contrasting results in monkeys self-administering morphine and co-

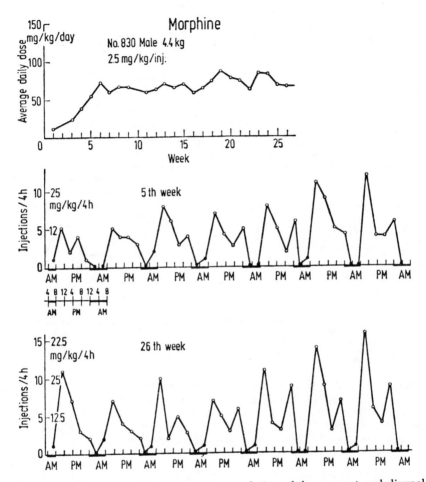

Figure 2.4. Typical example of long-term regulation of the amount and diurnal pattern of morphine self-administration in a rhesus monkey with unlimited drug access; compare to the effects of cocaine demonstrated in Figure 2.5. Each response was rewarded with 2.5 mg/kg morphine infused in 0.25 ml over about six seconds. This consistent pattern of self-administration was maintained throughout experiments of up to 16 months' duration. When morphine access was interrupted, the monkeys displayed severe withdrawal signs. (From Deneau et al., 1969. Reproduced with permission.)

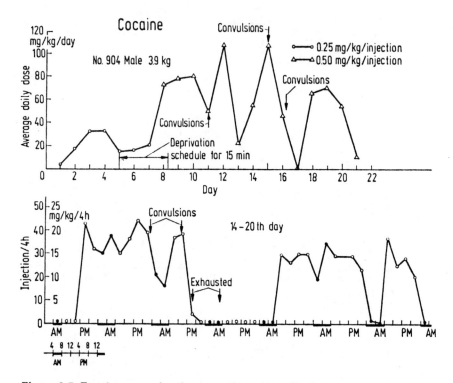

Figure 2.5. Erratic, unregulated course of cocaine self-administration in a rhesus monkey with unlimited drug access. Responses were rewarded with 0.25–0.5 mg/kg cocaine infused as described in Figure 2.4. Cocaine self-administration was accompanied by behavioral and physiological deterioration and death. (From Deneau et al., 1969. Reproduced with permission.)

caine. Unlimited access to other psychomotor stimulants, such as amphetamine, appears to have effects that are similar to that of cocaine, although toxicity may be somewhat milder (Deneau et al., 1969; Johanson et al., 1976; Pickens & Harris, 1968).

The ultimate consequence of unlimited cocaine access is death. In Deneau et al.'s study (1969), in which the operation of the infusion apparatus may have limited cocaine availability to one infusion per 50 seconds, all monkeys died within 30 days. They survived if drug access was restricted to one infusion per hour. Two rhesus monkeys allowed to self-administer 0.2 mg/kg cocaine every 10 seconds died in less than five days (Johanson et al., 1976). Cocaine is equally lethal in rats. As shown in Figure 2.6, mortality was almost three times higher in rats self-administering cocaine than in rats self-administering heroin (Bozarth & Wise, 1985).

To summarize, self-administration reveals three aspects of voluntary cocaine use. First, when cocaine availability is limited, animals organize their behavior to maintain high, regular rates of cocaine intake. As in humans, not only is the cocaine experience highly rewarding, but it is also capable of maintaining energetic drug-seeking behavior. Self-administration effects can be analyzed at the neuroendocrine as well as the

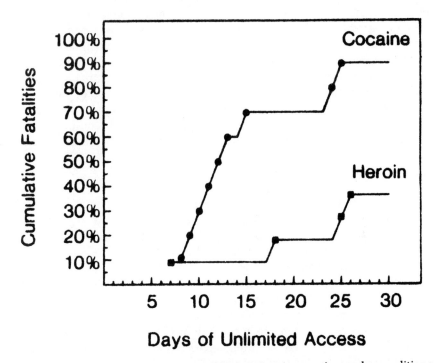

Days of Unlimited Access

Figure 2.6. Extreme mortality in rats self-administering cocaine under conditions of unlimited access. Circles show the survival times for 10 rats that learned to self-administer cocaine, 1 mg/kg/response, and squares for 11 rats that self-administered heroine, 0.1 mg/kg/response. Drugs were delivered in 0.25 ml over 10 seconds. Cocaine was erratically self-administered in amounts of up to 250 mg/kg/day, whereas heroin was self-administered in a regular pattern in amounts of about 10 mg/kg/day. (From Bozarth & Wise, 1985. Reproduced with permission.)

behavioral level (Johanson, 1984; Wise, 1984a; Woods, 1978). Several lines of pharmacological research suggest that dopaminergic brain mechanisms may contribute importantly to cocaine reward (Dackis & Gold, 1985; Stein, 1978; Wise, 1984a,b), although this is not yet proven nor the participation of other neuroendocrine mechanisms eliminated.

Second, even under conditions of limited access, cocaine self-administration is often sufficient to elicit motor and toxic effects. These may be severe enough to disrupt self-administration, but are not usually debilitating. Furthermore, they are not sufficiently aversive to disorganize or inhibit self-administration.

Third, in sharp contrast to limited-access conditions, free access to cocaine is as debilitating as it is rewarding. Behavior is dominated by obsessive and disorganized cocaine self-administration. In this sense, cocaine appears more addicting than opiates and other drugs that produce physical dependence. In fact, despite the lack of signs of physical dependence, animals continue to self-administer cocaine until death. Cocaine is not only severely toxic, but is so in quantities that are voluntarily administered. It gives pause, and underlines the potential importance of this area of research, to consider that the amounts of cocaine self-administered by animals are similar to the amounts found effective by human abusers (Fischman et al., 1977; Fischman & Schuster, 1982).

Conditioned Place Preferences

The self-administration paradigm graphically demonstrates cocaine's powerful effects on ongoing behavior, but cannot be used to analyze its effects on behavior in the nondrugged state. Place conditioning is an alternative procedure that has attracted recent interest because preference for the drug experience can be measured in nondrugged animals. The conditioning procedure consists of pairing drug administration with one set of distinctive environmental stimuli and control injections with another set. One or several pairs of drug and control conditioning trials are done before a preference test, in which nondrugged animals are allowed to choose to expose themselves either to the drug-associated environment or to the control environment. Preference for the drug-associated environment indicates that the drug experience was rewarding.

Spyraki et al. (1982) tested rats' preference for two sides of a shuttle box that differed in wall brightness and floor texture after they had received four cocaine injections in one environment and four saline injections in the other. Rats that received 2.5–20 mg/kg cocaine during the conditioning trials spent significantly more time in the cocaine-associated environment than in the saline-associated environment.

There have been only a few investigations of the neuroendocrine mechanisms of cocaine place conditioning, and these have produced conflicting results. Intraperitoneal cocaine injections still elicited conditioned place preferences in rats that were pretreated with the dopamine receptor blockers haloperidol, pimozide, or flupenthixol and in rats with dopamine-depleting 6-hydroxydopamine lesions of the nucleus accumbens, although in the lesion studies the degree of dopamine depletion (less than 75%) may not have been sufficient to elicit a functional deficit (Mackey & Van Der Kooy, 1985; Spyraki et al., 1982). Dopamine receptor blockade with flupenthixol or haloperidol, however, also appeared to dissociate cocaine-induced place preferences, which were not prevented, from amphetamine-induced place preferences, which were (Mackey & Van Der Kooy, 1985). These results suggest dopaminergic neurons, in particular dopaminergic neurons on the nucleus accumbens, are not necessary for the conditioned place preferences produced by peripheral cocaine injections.

Some investigations of place preferences produced by central cocaine administration, however, suggest just the opposite conclusion. In one study a conditioned place preference was produced by cocaine microinjections into the nucleus accumbens, and the preference was attenuated when flupenthixol was added to the cocaine (Aulisi & Hoebel, 1983), and in another, microinjection of cocaine into the lateral cerebral ventricle produced a place preference that was attenuated by pimozide pretreatment (Morency & Beninger, 1985). Thus, central cocaine administration may elicit place preferences through a dopaminergic mechanism, although dopamine has not yet been implicated in peripheral cocaine place preferences.

Cocaine's local anesthetic properties have also been implicated in the place preferences elicited by peripheral cocaine injection. In Spyraki et al.'s (1982) experiment, intraperitoneal injections of procaine elicited place preferences that were as large as those elicited by cocaine. Because local anesthetics also have central actions (see Post & Contel, 1983; Ritchie et al., 1970, and the "Motor Effects" section above), however, this is not compelling evidence that cocaine acts peripherally to condition place preferences. Furthermore, even if a peripheral action of cocaine were sufficient to produce a place preference, it would not explain why central, but not peripheral, cocaine place preferences are sensitive to disruption by dopamine antagonists, because peripheral cocaine should also produce central effects.

Finally, cocaine microinjection into the medial prefrontal cortex, which receives projections from the mesocortical dopamine system, supports not only self-administration responding (Goeders & Smith, 1983), but also a conditioned place preference (Isaac et al., 1984).

To summarize, the conditioned place preference technique provides a simple behavioral model of cocaine reward. Its advantages include simplicity, relative sensitivity, and, perhaps most useful, a means to test cocaine's rewarding effect in drug-free animals. This precludes drug effects not related to reward processes, such as, perhaps, psychomotor stimulation, from influencing the behavioral index of reward. The possibility of measuring cocaine reward in the drug-free state appears to be of potential theoretical significance as a model of the intense craving for cocaine that many humans report to occur between bouts of cocaine use. A cautionary note is also in order, however, because cocaine-induced place preferences appear surprisingly fragile. In the typical shuttlebox apparatus, rats' initial preference, usually for the darker side, seems nearly as strong as the cocaine-conditioned preferences, and seemingly trivial procedural changes can block the formation of place preferences (Mucha et al., 1982; Pap et al., 1986; Spyraki et al., 1982; Schenk et al., 1984).

SUMMARY AND CONCLUSIONS

This chapter has reviewed cocaine's several effects on animal behavior. Like other psychomotor stimulants, cocaine elicits a variety of motor effects, ranging from hyperactivity and stereotypy to highly toxic effects. These are not merely simple motor responses, but include an important psychological dimension. Their nature and intensity, for example, depend on drug history and behavioral context. The most dramatic such effect is the sensitization of motor effects elicited by repeated, intermittent treatment with moderate dosages of cocaine.

Cocaine is also highly rewarding to animals. This is demonstrated powerfully in the self-administration paradigm, in which animals work for cocaine injections. When drug access is limited, cocaine reward maintains energetic and organized goal-directed behavior. Cocaine is perhaps the most rewarding of all drugs in such tests. When drug access is unlimited, larger amounts of cocaine are self-administered and self-regulation deteriorates. Animals enter a frenetic cycle of self-administration to the point of exhaustion, which is repeated until they die. Cocaine is "psychologically addicting" only in that detoxification is not associated with physiological withdrawal signs; in fact, animals find it the most lethal of drugs.

The memory of the cocaine experience can also shape behavior. Animals readily learn to use the interoceptive stimuli produced by cocaine injection to guide responses maintained by other rewards, as shown by drug discrimination studies. Animals also prefer environments in which they previously experienced cocaine.

These data suggest several generalizations. First, there are interesting and accessible animal models for cocaine's effects in humans. Models, or potential models, of cocaine euphoria, reward, craving, addiction, dysphoria, and toxicity have been discussed and are developed further in Chapter 11.

Second, the behavior mechanisms influenced by cocaine are powerful. Several lines of evidence demonstrate the extreme reward, and abuse, potential of cocaine in animals. Furthermore, both these rewarding effects as well as cocaine's motor effects can dominate and distort normal function. These behavioral mechanisms are undoubtedly related to the drug's analogous and equally prominent effects in humans. Therefore, the analysis of animal behavior is likely to further understanding of human cocaine use and abuse.

Third, the doses and conditions in which cocaine elicits its various effects, in particular its rewarding and toxic effects, overlap. Cocaine is still rewarding even though simultaneously toxic. Unless external constraints are imposed on cocaine access, animals indulge in cocaine beyond the point of no return. This suggests that humans' attempts to titrate their cocaine use so as to integrate it into their lives is inherently risky, and that the more material resources that people have, the riskier it is.

Fourth, several of cocaine's effects are dynamic. They depend on both the history and environmental context of cocaine administration. This is especially evident in the case of cocaine's motor effects, which can become sensitized under appropriate regimens. This suggests that certain patterns of use of even moderate amounts of cocaine can produce high risks of toxicity.

Fifth, animal studies can be used to determine the brain mechanisms of cocaine's behavioral effects. Several research strategies to relate brain and behavior have been discussed. Dopaminergic mechanisms have been implicated in many of cocaine's behavioral actions, but these lines of research need much more work.

Such animal research is likely to facilitate the development of effective pharmacological interventions of cocaine-related clinical problems, an effort now in only the earliest stages (see Chapter 10).

REFERENCES

Aigner TG, Balster RL: Choice behavior in rhesus monkeys: cocaine versus food. Science, 201:534–535, 1978.

Ando K, Yanagita T: The discriminative stimulus properties of intravenously administered cocaine in rhesus monkeys, in Colpaert FC, Rosecrans JA, eds: Stimulus Properties of Drugs: Ten Years of Progress, Amsterdam-New York, North-Holland Publish. Co., 1978, pp 125–136.

Aulisi EF, Hoebel BG: Rewarding effects of amphetamine and cocaine in the nucleus accumbens and block by flupenthixol. Soc Neurosci Abstr 9:121, 1983.

Bachus SE, Gale K: Muscimol in the nigrotegmental target area blocks selected components of stereotypy elicited by amphetamine or cocaine. Soc Neurosci Abstr 10:414, 1984.

Bachus SE, Gale K: Behavioral sensitization to dopamine stimulants induced by chronic neuroleptic and chronic cocaine treatment: role of nigral GABA receptors. Soc Neurosci Abstr 11:1249, 1985.

Balster RL, Schuster CR: Fixed-interval schedule of cocaine reinforcement: effect of dose and infusion duration. J Exp Anal Behav 20:119–129, 1973.

Bell DS: The experimental reproduction of amphetamine psychosis. Arch Gen Psychiatry 29:35–40, 1973.

Bergman J, Johanson CE: The effects of electric shock on responding maintained by cocaine in rhesus monkeys. Pharmacol Biochem Behav 14:423–426, 1981.

Bozarth MA, Wise RA: Toxicity associated with long-term intravenous heroin and cocaine self-administration in the rat. JAMA, 254:81–83, 1985.

Brinkley J: U.S. says cocaine-related deaths are rising. New York Times, July 11, 1986, p A1.

Byck R, Van Dyck C: What are the effects of cocaine in man? in Petersen RC, Stillman RC, eds: Cocaine, NIDA Research Monograph, Washington, DC, U.S. Government Printing Office, 1977.

Cohen SA: Cocaine antagonism of gamma-aminobutryic acid action on cultured hippocampal neurons. Soc Neurosci Abstr 10:1208, 1984.

Collins JP, Lesse H, Dagan LA: Behavioral antecedents of cocaine-induced stereotypy. Pharmacol Biochem Behav 11:683–687, 1979.

Colpaert FC: Drug-produced cues and states: some theoretical and methodological inferences, in Lal H, ed: Discriminative Stimulus Properties of Drugs, New York and London, Plenum Press, 1977, pp 5–21.

Colpaert FC, Niemegeers CJE, Janssen PAJ: Cocaine cue in rats as it relates to subjective drug effects: a preliminary report. Eur J Pharmacol 40:195–199, 1976.

Colpaert FC, Niemegeers CJE, Janssen PAJ: Discriminative stimulus properties of cocaine and D-amphetamine, and antagonism by haloperidol: a comparative study. Neuropharmacology 17:937–942, 1978a.

Colpeart FC, Niemegeers CJE, Janssen PAJ: Discriminative stimulus properties of cocaine: neuropharmacological characteristics as derived from stimulus generalization experiments. Pharmacol Biochem Behav 10:535–546, 1978b.

Colpaert FC, Niemegeers CJE, Janssen PAJ: Evidence that a preferred substrate for type B monoamine oxidase mediates stimulus properties of MAO inhibitors: a possible role for beta-phenylethylamine in the cocaine cue. Pharmacol Biochem Behav 13:513–517, 1980.

Cunningham KA, Appel JB: Discriminative stimulus properties of cocaine and phencyclidine: similarity in the mechanism of action, in Colpaert FC, Slangen JL, eds: Drug Discrimination: Applications in CNS Pharmacology, Amsterdam Elsevier Biomedical Press, 1982, pp 181–192.

Dackis CA, Gold MS: New concepts in cocaine addiction: the dopamine depletion hypothesis. Neurosci Behav Rev 9:496–477, 1985.

De La Garza R, Johanson CE: Effects of haloperidol and physostigmine on self-administration of local anesthetics. Pharmacol Biochem Behav 17:1295–1299, 1982.

Deneau G, Yanagita T, Seevers MH: Self-administration of psychoactive substances by the monkey. Psychopharmacology 16:30–48, 1969.

D'Mello GD, Stolerman IP: Comparison of the discriminative stimulus properties of cocaine and amphetamine in rats. Br J Pharmacol 61:415–422, 1977.

Downs AW, Eddy NB: The effect of repeated doses of cocaine on the rat. J Pharmacol Exp Ther 46:199, 1932.

Ellinwood EH, Kilbey MM: Amphetamine stereotypy: the influence of environmental factors and prepotent behavioral patterns on its topography and development. Biol. Psychiatry 10:3–16, 1975.

Ellinwood EH, Kilbey MM: Chronic stimulant intoxication models of psychosis, in Hanin I, Usdin E, eds: Animal Models in Psychiatry and Neurology, New York, Pergamon Press, 1977, pp 61–74.

Fischman MW, Schuster CR: Cocaine self-administration in humans. Fed Proc 41:241–246, 1982.

Fischman MW, Schuster CR, Krasnegor NA: Physiological and behavioral effects of intravenous cocaine in man. Adv Behav Biol 21:647–664, 1977.

Fischman MW, Schuster CR, Hatano Y: A comparison of the subjective and cardiovascular effects of cocaine and lidocaine in humans. Pharmacol Biochem Behav 18:123–127, 1983a.

Fischman MW, Schuster CR, Rajfer S: A comparison of the subjective and cardiovascular effects of cocaine and procaine in humans. Pharmacol Biochem Behav 18:711–716, 1983b.

Ford RD, Balster RL: Reinforcing properties of intravenous procaine in rhesus monkeys. Pharmocol Biochem Bhev 6:289–296, 1977.

Freud S: Über Coca. Zentrbl Ther 2:289–314, 1884. Translation: Freud S. On the general effects of cocaine. Drug Depend 5:15–28, 1970.

Goeders NE, Smith JE: Cortical dopaminergic involvement in cocaine reinforcement. Science 221:773–775, 1983.

Goeders NE, Smith JE: Effects of 6-hydroxydopamine lesions of the medial prefrontal cortex on intracranial cocaine self-administration. Soc Neurosci Abstr 10:1206, 1984.

Glick SD, Hinds PA: Sex differences in sensitization to cocaine-induced rotation. Eur J Pharmacol 99:119–121, 1984.

Glick SD, Hinds PA, Shapiro RM: Cocaine-induced rotation: sex-dependent differences between left- and right-sided rats. Science 221:775–777, 1983.

Goldberg SR, Kelleher RT: Behavior controlled by scheduled injections of cocaine in squirrel and rhesus monkeys. J Exp Anal Behav 25:93–104, 1976.

Grove RN, Schuster CR: Suppression of cocaine self-administratiion by extinction and punishment. Pharmacol Biochem Behav 2:199–208, 1974.

Hammerbeck DM, Mitchell CL: The reinforcing properties of procaine and D-amphetamine compared in rhesus monkeys. J Pharmacol Exp Ther 204:558–569, 1978.

Ho BT, Silverman PB: Stimulants as discriminative stimuli, in: Colpaert FC, Rosecrans JA, eds: Stimulus Properties of Drugs: Ten Years of Progress, Amsterdam, Elsevier/North-Holland Biomedical Press, 1978, pp 53–68.

Iglauer C, Woods JH: Concurrent performances: reinforcement by different doses of cocaine in rhesus monkeys. J Exp Anal Behav 22:179–196, 1974.

Isaac W, Neiswander J, Landers T, Alcala R, Bardo M, Nonneman A: Mesocortical dopamine system lesions disrupt cocaine reinforced conditioned place preference. Soc Neurosci Abstr 10:1206, 1984.

Jarbe TUC: Cocaine as a discriminative cue in rats: interactions with neuroleptics and other drugs. Psychopharmacology 59:183–187, 1978.

Javaid JI, Musca MN, Fischman, M, Schuster CR, Davis JM: Kinetics of cocaine in humans after intravenous and intranasal administration. Biochem Drug Dispos 4:9–18, 1983.

Johanson CE: The effects of electric shock on responding maintained by cocaine injections in a choice procedure on the rhesus monkey. Psychopharmacology 53:277–282, 1977.

Johanson CE: The reinforcing properties of procaine and proparacaine in rhesus monkeys.

Psychopharmacology 67:189–194, 1980.

Johanson CE: Assessment of the dependence potential of cocaine in animals. Natl Inst Drug Abuse Res Monogr Ser 50:54–71, 1984.

Johanson CE, Aigner T: Comparison of the reinforcing properties of cocaine and procaine in rhesus monkeys. Pharmacol Biochem Behav 15:49–53, 1981.

Johanson CE, Schuster CR: A choice procedure for drug reinforcers: cocaine and methylphenidate in the rhesus monkey. J Pharmacol Exp Ther 193:676–688, 1975.

Johanson CE, Schuster CR: Animal models of drug administration, in Mello K, ed: Advances in Substance Abuse: Behavioral and Biological Research, Vol II, Greenwich, CT, JAI Press, 1981, pp 219–297.

Johanson CE, Balster RL, Bonese K: Self-administration of psychomotor stimulant drugs: the effects of unlimited access. Pharmacol Biochem Behav 4:45–51, 1976.

Kilbey MM, Ellinwood EH: Chronic administration of stimulant drugs: response modification, in Ellinwood EH, Kilbey MM, eds: Advances in Behavioral Biology, Vol. 21. Cocaine and Other Stimulants, New York, Plenum Press, 1977, pp 409–430.

Kilbey MM, Ellinwood EH, Easler ME: Effect of chronic cocaine pretreatment in kindled seizures and behavioral stereotypies. Exp Neurol 64:306–314, 1979.

Kramer JC, Fischman VS, Littlefield DC: Amphetamine abuse. JAMA 201:89–93, 1967.

Leith NJ, Barrett RJ: Amphetamine and the reward system: evidence for tolerance and post-drug depression. Psychopharmacology (Berlin) 46:19–25, 1976.

Lewin L: Euphoria: mental sedatives, codeine and its derivatives, dionine, heroin, eucodal, chlorodyne, in Phantastica, Narcotic and Stimulating Drugs: Their Use and Abuse, translated by Wirth PHA, New York, Dutton, 1931, pp 75–88.

Llewellyn ME, Iglauer C, Woods JH: Relative reinforcer magnitude under a nonindependent concurrent schedule of cocaine reinforcement in rhesus monkeys. J Exp Anal Behav 25:81–91, 1976.

Mackey WB, Van Der Kooy D: Neuroleptics block the positive reinforcing effects of amphetamine but not of morphine as measured by place conditioning. Pharmacol Biochem Behav 22:101–105, 1985.

Mandell AJ, Knapp S: Asymmetry and mood, emergent properties of serotonic regulation. Arch Gen Psychiatry 36:909–916, 1979.

Martin WR, Sloan JW, Sapira JD, Jasinski DR: Physiological, subjective, and behavioral effects of amphetamine, methamphetamine, ephdrine, phenmetrazine, and methylphenidate in man. Clin Pharmacol Ther 12:245–258, 1971.

McInerney J: Bright Lights, Big City, New York, Vintage, 1984.

Misra AL, Vadlamani NL, Pontani RB: Effect of caffeine on cocaine locomotor stimulant activity in rats. Pharmacol Biochem Behav 24:761–764, 1986.

Mittleman RE, Wetli CW: Death caused by recreational cocaine use. JAMA 252:1889–1893, 1984.

Moja EA, Stoff DM, Gillin JM, Wyatt RI: Beta-phenylethylamine and animal behavior, in Mosnaim AD, Wolf ME, eds: Noncatecholic Phenylethylamines, Part 1, New York, Marcel Dekker, 1978, pp 315–343.

Morency MA, Beninger RJ: Conditioned place preference induced by intracerebroventricular microinjections of cocaine: possible involvement of contral dopamine. Soc Neurosci Abstr 11:718, 1985.

Mucha RF, Van Der Kooy D, O'Shaughnessy M, Bucenieks P: Drug reinforcement studied by the use of place conditioning in rat. Brain Res 243:91–105, 1982.

Mulé SJ, Misra AL: Cocaine: distribution and metabolism in animals. Adv Behav Biol 21:215–228, 1977.

Myers JA, Earnest MP: Generalized seizures and cocaine abuse. Neurology 34:675–676, 1984.

Nelson LR, Ellison G: Enhanced stereotypies after repeated injections but not continuous amphetamines. Neuropharmacology 17:1081–1084, 1978.

Pap Z, Hinton V, Benarroch R, Rosecan J, Geary N: Acute imipramine treatment enhances a conditioned place preference for cocaine in a novel test. Soc Neurosci Abstr 12:1986.

Pickens R, Harris WC: Self-administration of D-amphetamine by rats. Psychopharmacology 12:158–163, 1968.
Pickens R, Thompson T: Cocaine-reinforced behavior in rats: effects of reinforcement magnitude and fixed-ratio size. J Pharmacol Exp Ther 161:122–129, 1968.
Post RM: Cocaine psychosis: a continuum model. Am J Psychiatry 132:225–231, 1975.
Post RM, Contel NR: Human and animal studies of cocaine: implications for development of behavioral pathology, in Creese I, ed: Stimulants: Neurochemical, Behavioral, and Clinical Perspectives, New York, Raven Press, 1983, pp 169–202.
Post RN, Rose H: Increasing effects of repetitive cocaine administration in the rat. Nature 260:731–732, 1976.
Post RM, Kotin J, Goodman FK: The effects of cocaine on depressed patients. Am J Psychiatry 131:511–517, 1974.
Post RM, Kopanda RT, Lee A: Progressive behavioral changes during chronic lidocaine administration: relationship to kindling. Life Sci 17:943, 1975.
Post RM, Kopanda RT, Black KE: Progressive effects of cocaine on behavior and central amine metabolism in rhesus monkeys: relationship to kindling and psychoses. Biol Psychiatry 11:403–419, 1976.
Post RM, Lockfeld A, Squillace KM, Contel NR: Drug-environment interaction: context dependency of cocaine-induced behavioral sensitization. Life Sci 28:755–760, 1981a.
Post RM, Squillace KM, Pert, A, Sass W: Effect of amygdala kindling on spontaneous and cocaine-induced motor activity and lidocaine seizures. Psychopharmacology (Berlin) 72:189–196, 1981b.
Resnick RB, Kestenbaum RS, Schwartz LK: Acute systemic effects of cocaine in man: a controlled study of intranasal and intravenous routes. Science 195:696–698, 1977.
Risner ME, Jones BE: Characteristics of beta-phenethylene self-administration by dogs. Pharmacol Biochem Behav 6:689–696, 1977.
Ritchie JM, Cohen PJ, Dripps RD: Cocaine, procaine and other synthetic local anesthetics, in Goodman LS, Gilman A, eds: The Pharmacological Basis of Therapeutics, Toronto, Macmillan, 1970, pp 371–402.
Roberts DCS, Vickers G: Atypical neuroleptics increase self-administration of cocaine: an evaluation of a behavioural screen for antipsychotic activity. Psychopharmacology 82:135–139, 1984.
Roberts DCS, Corcoran ME, Fibiger HC: On the role of ascending catecholaminergic systems on intravenous self-administration of cocaine. Pharmacol Biochem Behav 6:615–620, 1977.
Roberts DCS, Koob GF, Klonoff, P, Fibiger HC: Extinction and recovery of cocaine self-administration following 6-hydroxydopamine lesions of the nucleus accumbens. Pharmacol Biochem Behav 12:781–787, 1980.
Roy SN, Bhattacharyya AK, Pradhan S, Pradhan SN: Behavioral and neurochemical effects of repeated administration of cocaine in rats. Neuropharmacology 17:559–564, 1978.
Sabelli HC, Fawcett J, Gusovsky F, et al.: Clinical studies on the phenylethylamine hypothesis of affective disorder: urine and blood phenylacetic acid and phenylalanine dietary supplements. J Clin Psychiatry 47:66–70, 1986.
Schecter MD, Glennon RA: Cathinone, cocaine, and methamphetamine: similarity of behavioral effects. Pharmacol Biochem Behav 22:913–916, 1985.
Scheel-Kruger J, Baestrup C, Nielson M, Golembrowska K, Mogilnicka E: Cocaine: discussion on the role of dopamine in the biochemical mechanism of action. Adv Behav Biol 21:373–408, 1977.
Schenk S, Hunt T, Malvechko R, Robertson A, Amit Z: Cocaine conditioning on the place preference paradigm. Soc Neurosci Abstr 10:1207, 1984.
Schwartz PJC, Constentin J, Martres MP, Pritais P, Baudry M: Modulation of receptor mechanisms in the CNS: hyper- and hyposensitivity to catecholamines. Neuropharmacology 17:665–685, 1978.
Segal DS, Mandell AJ: Long-term administration of D-amphetamine: progressive augmen-

tation of motor activity and stereotypy. Pharmacol Biochem Behav 2:249–255, 1974.

Shannon HE, DeGregorio CM: Self-administration of the endogenous trace amines beta-phenylethylamine, N-methyl phenylethylamine and phenylethanolamine in dogs. J Pharmacol Exp Ther 222:52–60, 1982.

Shearman GT, Lal H: Discriminative stimulus properties of cocaine related to an anxiogenic action. Prog Neuropsychopharmacol 5:57–63, 1981.

Short PH, Shuster L: Changes in brain norepinephrine associated with sensitization to D-amphetamine. Psychopharmacology 48:59–67, 1976.

Shuster L, Yu G, Bates A: Sensitization to cocaine stimulation in mice. Psychopharmacology 52:185–190, 1977.

Spealman RD: Behavior maintained by termination of a schedule of self-administered cocaine. Science 204:1231–1233, 1979.

Spyraki C, Fibiger HC, Phillips AG: Cocaine-induced place preference conditioning: lack of effects of neuroleptics and 6-hydroxydopamine lesions. Brain Res 253:195–203, 1982.

Squillace KM, Post RM, Pert A: Effect of lidocaine pretreatment on cocaine-induced behavior in normal and amygdala-lesioned rats. Neuropsychology 8:113–122, 1982.

Stein L: Reward transmitters: catecholamines and opioid peptides, in Lipton MA, DiMascio A, Killam KF, eds: Psychopharmacology: A Generation of Progress, New York, Raven Press, 1978, pp 569–587.

Stolerman IP, D'Mello GD: Role of training conditions in discrimination of central nervous stimulants by rats. Psychopharmacology (Berlin) 73:295–303, 1981.

Stripling JS, Ellinwood EH Jr: Potentiation of the behavioral and convulsant effects of cocaine by chronic administration in the rat. Pharmacol Biochem Behav 6:571–579, 1977a.

Stripling JS, Ellinwood EH Jr: Sensitization to cocaine following chronic administration in the rat. Adv Behav Biol 21:327–351, 1977b.

Stripling JS, Russell RD: Effect of cocaine and pentylenetetrazol on cortical kindling. Pharmacol Biochem Behav 23:573–581, 1985.

Stripling JS, Gramlich CA, Cunningham MG: Effect of cocaine and lidocaine on the development of kindled seizures. Soc Neurosci Abstr 9:486, 1983.

Szostak C, Matin-Iverson MT, Fibiger HC: Effects of 6-hydroxydopamine lesions of the medial prefrontal cortex on cocaine self-administration. Soc Neurosci Abstr 10:1167, 1984.

Tatum AL, Seevers MH: Experimental cocaine addiction. J Pharmacol Exp Ther 36:401–410, 1929.

Teitelbaum P: The use of operant methods in the assessment and control of motivational states, in Honig WK, ed: Operant Behavior: Areas of Research and Application, New York, Appleton-Century-Crofts, 1966, pp 565–608.

Whitby LG, Hetzling G, Axelrod J: Effect of cocaine on the disposition of noradrenaline labeled with tritium. Nature 187:604–605, 1960.

Wilson MC, Hitomi M, Schuster CR: Self-administration of psychomotor stimulants as a function of unit dosage. Psychopharmacology (Berlin) 22:271–281, 1971.

Wise RA: Neural mechanisms of the reinforcing action of cocaine. Natl Inst Drug Abuse Res Monogr Ser 50:15–33, 1984a.

Wise RA: Neuroleptics and operant behavior: the anhedonia hypothesis. Behav Brain Sci 5:39–53, 1984b.

Wood DM, Lal H, Yaden S, Emmet-Oglesby MW: One-way generalization of clonidine to the discriminative stimulus produced by cocaine. Pharmacol Biochem Behav 23:529–533, 1985.

Woods JH: Behavioral pharmacology of drug self-administration, in Lipton MA, Killam KF, eds: Psychopharmacology: A Generation of Progress, New York, Raven Press, 1978, pp 595–612.

Woods JH, Schuster CR: Reinforcement properties of morphine, cocaine, and SPA as a function of unit dose. Int J Addictions 3:231–237, 1968.

Woolverton WL: Effects of a D1 and a D2 dopamine agonist on the self-administration of cocaine and piribedil by rhesus monkeys. Pharmacol Biochem Behav 24:531–535, 1986.

Yanagita T: An experimental framework for evaluation of dependence liability in various types of drugs in monkeys. Bull Narc 25:57–64, 1973.

Yanagita T, Deneau GA, Seevers MH: Evaluation of pharmacologic agents in the monkey by long term intravenous self or programmed administration, Excerpta Med Int Cong Ser, 87:453–457, 1965.

Chapter 3

Human Neurobiology
of Cocaine

Edward V. Nunes, M.D., and Jeffrey S. Rosecan, M.D.

Cocaine has wide-ranging and powerful effects on behavior and emotion and is highly addictive. Chapter 2 has shown how laboratory animal models can be used to understand these effects and to begin to delineate the neuronal substrate. In this chapter we shall extend this line of inquiry to humans and attempt an understanding of cocaine neurobiology based on animal and human evidence. This exercise is especially important, because it forms a basis for proposing and evaluating psychopharmacological interventions for cocaine abuse. In Chapter 2, Geary emphasizes the capacity of cocaine to usurp other "natural" rewards and become an organism's most powerful and sought-after reinforcer in self-administration paradigms. He also describes the resistance of cocaine self-administration to behavioral interventions and the implication that somatic, i.e., pharmacological interventions may be critically important in the control of cocaine abuse.

We shall begin by reviewing the phenomenology of human cocaine use from euphoria to dysphoria to craving to addiction. The remainder of the chapter will be devoted to exploring how these phenomena can be understood in neurobiological terms. The basic pharmacology of cocaine will be described at the synaptic level and at the level of neuron and nerve circuitry. This will be integrated with the animal behavior data presented in Geary's chapter. Finally, human neurobiological data will be presented. This information comes in three forms: neuroendocrine studies, psychiatric diagnostic studies, and studies of psychopharmacological interventions in cocaine abuse. The theoretical underpinnings of the various psychopharmacological interventions will be discussed. This will lay the foundation for Chapter 10, which discusses the psychopharmacological treatment of cocaine abuse.

Several main themes will emerge. Cocaine induces the entire range of pathological emotions in humans, from extreme euphoria and grandiosity to depression and anxiety to severe paranoia. Cocaine also significantly alters functioning in central transmitter systems, such as the dopaminergic, noradrenergic, and serotonergic systems, which are thought to be critically involved in mood regulation and in affective disorders in humans according to current theories in biological psychiatry. Cocaine abuse may then be looked on as a natural experiment in affective illness, and cocaine may emerge as an important tool for the study of affective illness. Another important point is that despite recent technological advances and accelerating progress, neurobiology remains a nascent field. Our understanding of brain function is still rudimentary. In all likelihood, we are aware of only a few of hundreds of important neurotransmitter and neuroregulatory systems, let alone their interconnections. Furthermore, much remains to be learned even about known neuronal systems. Thus, our understanding of cocaine neurobiology must be at best partial and incomplete.

PHENOMENOLOGY OF HUMAN COCAINE USE

Cocaine use originated several thousand years ago in the Andean Indian civilizations. They had no written language with which to record their experience of cocaine's effects. However, archaeological records and observations of the conquistadors provide some detail. The Indians chewed coca leaves together with an alkaline substance such as ash, which helps extract the alkaloid and increase dosage. One Incan myth holds that the coca plant sprang up from the blood of a beautiful woman who was executed for adultery. It was to be chewed by men to remind them of her. Another myth holds that coca was handed to men by the gods to help them endure earthly existence (Petersen, 1977). The myths suggest that chewing coca was sensuous, seductive (like the woman), dangerous (adultery), and highly rewarding.

Coca was apparently controlled by the ruling classes and distributed as a reward to soldiers and workers, suggesting that it was highly valued. There is also evidence that it was used as a local anesthetic in surgical procedures and folk remedies. After the Spanish conquest, coca was used to recruit and motivate the natives for arduous work in mines and fields. Coca chewing was observed to create a euphoria and permit the Indians to labor all day with little food or water (Petersen, 1977).

The early medical literature dating from the turn of the century to the 1950s contains a wealth of clinical and experimental observations of cocaine's effects on humans. Much of this literature has been gathered in an annotated bibliography published by NIDA in 1976 (NIDA, 1976). In addition to euphoria, cocaine's addictive, depressive, and toxic effects are described in detail. Selected studies have been summarized and compiled in Table 3.1. Routes of administration were either sniffing, chewing, ingestion, or injection. Doses, when reported, are on the order of hundreds of milligrams, roughly corresponding to doses consumed by today's users.

Acute psychic effects described (see Table 3.1) include euphoria, giddiness, talkativeness, increased self-confidence, restlessness, anorexia, and insomnia reminiscent of hypomania. A wealth of unpleasant effects, generally associated with higher doses, are also described. These include agitation, crying, anger, visual, auditory, and tactile hallucinations, paranoid delusions, amnesia, and delirium and stupor. Physiological effects include tachycardia, perspiration, and increased muscular strength at lower doses suggestive of sympathetic nervous system arousal, and convulsions and death at higher doses. These findings are strikingly similar to modern clinical reports of cocaine toxicity and death (Coleman, et al., 1982; Nanji & Filipenko, 1984; Rappolt, et al., 1977; Schachne, et al., 1983).

A consistent picture of chronic cocaine use also emerges from these reports (see Table 3.1). Many of the unpleasant effects listed above persist, such as insomnia, hallucinations, and paranoia. In addition, depression, exhaustion, lethargy, irritability, impotence, muscular twitches and tremors, and muscular weakness often occur. Craving and tenacious addiction are frequently described. Freud initially suggested that addiction was only a risk in prior morphine addicts. However, subsequent case series report that many cocaine addicts had no prior history of drug abuse. Thievery and moral deterioration are noted. Malnutrition and weight loss and nasal ulcers and bleeding are also described. Interestingly, several studies report evidence of persistent intellectual deterioration, including mental dullness (Bose, 1902), acalculia (Gordon, 1908), and dementia (Gordon, 1908). A more recent study comparing coca-chewing and nonchewing Andean Indians also found evidence of intellectual deterioration (Negrete & Murphy, 1967). It is not clear whether this is the result of ongoing drug use or permanent brain damage.

Table 3.1

Early Studies of Cocaine Use in Humans

Reference	N	Subjects, Methods	Cocaine Dose and Route	Findings
Freud, 1885	?	Administration to self and healthy subjects	50–100 mg acute	Wide range of effects from none to *euphoria* with talkativeness, giddiness, insomnia, anorexia, increased muscular strength, vigor, lasting 4–5 hours
	1	Morphine addict	400 mg/day	Morphine addiction resolved, no cocaine addiction
Freud, 1887	?	Clinical observations in morphine addicts; literature review	Up to 1,000 mg/day	Describes *"toxicity"*: stupor, tachycardia, anorexia, insomnia, hallucinations, "persecution mania," delirium, describes *addiction*, asserts this only possible in those previously addicted to another drug
Hammond, 1887	1	Self-administration and observation	From 65 to 1,170 mg/day, subcutaneous	*Lower doses*: euphoria, more able to write, tachycardia, tremor, insomnia, lasting 12 hours; headache next day *Higher doses*: rapid thoughts, talkativeness, insomnia, fear, fearlessness, agitation, loss of control, irregular heart rate; exhaustion, poor concentration, headache next day
Bose, 1902	10	Cocaine addicts, 4 from "medicinal" cocaine use; clinical observations	Chronic 0.5–7 g/day, chewing	*Acute effects*: stimulation followed by *rebound depression and craving* *Chronic effects*: *addiction*, anorexia, weakness, insomnia, mental dullness, impotence, weight loss, amnesia, sweating, tachycardia, acute mania, paranoid psychosis, hallucinations, incoherence, convulsions, death

(*continued*)

Table 3.1 (continued)

Reference	N	Subjects, Methods	Cocaine Dose and Route	Findings
Bose, 1902 (cont'd)				"The only solution lies in locking inebriates up in asylums and stopping their cocaine completely"
Bose, 1913	4	Cocaine addicts; clinical observations	? dose, oral or chewing	Collapse and *death*
Gordon, 1908	15	Acute cocaine intoxication; clinical observations	?	Tachycardia, cold sweats, agitation, talkativeness, crying, anger, depression, delirium, stupor, hallucinations, *suicide attempts*, persistent aculculia, *convulsions*, *death*
	10	Chronic intoxication	? dose, nasal	Tachycardia, impotence, insomnia, restlessness, paranoid delusions, hallucinations, *dementia*; *abstinence syndrome* of malaise, anxiety, depression
Owens, 1912	23	Clinical observations	? dose, nasal, s.c., i.v.	*Acute effects*: excitement, tachycardia, insomnia, anorexia, twitching, hallucinations, paranoid delusions, *convulsions*, withdrawal *Chronic effects*: anorexia, poor concentration, weight loss, *nasal ulcers*, nosebleeds
Chopra & Chopra, 1930/1931	22	Clinical observations	? dose, oral chewing	*Addiction, abstinence syndrome* of craving, restlessness, irritability, poor concentration, lethargy *Chronic effects*: physical wasting, impotence, paranoid delusions, hallucinations, "*moral deterioration*"

Study	N	Population/Setting	Dose	Effects
Ortiz, 1944	26	Normal subjects and cocaine addicts, laboratory setting	0.5–6 mg/kg oral	*Normals*: increased speed of performance in attention test with increased errors. *Addicts*: increased speed of performance in attention test with less errors, increased heart rate, blood pressure
Lindemann & Malamud, 1933/1934	6	4 schizophrenics, 2 neurotics, acute administration	30–50 mg. subcutaneous	More talkative, increased self-confidence, demanding, critical, aggressive, increased psychotic material in schizophrenics
Chopra & Chopra, 1958	200	Clinical observations	? dose, chewing	*Acute effects*: pleasure, excitement, confidence, grandiosity, lasting 45 minutes to 2 hours. *Addiction*. *Abstinence*: depression, fatigue, headaches, drug seeking. *Toxicity*: hallucinations, paranoid delusions, paresthesias, nausea, vomiting, muscle cramps
Negrete & Murphy, 1967	92	Chronic coca chewers vs. nonchewers in northern Argentina		Chronic chewers did less well on some psychological tests of intellectual functioning, suggesting *brain damage* or *depressant* effect of chronic cocaine
Buck et al., 1968	102	Chronic coca chewers vs. nonchewers		Chronic chewers: less well nourished, poorer hygiene, more absences from work, more illness and malnutrition.

s.c. = subcutaneous; i.v. = intravenous.

A withdrawal or abstinence syndrome is also frequently noted. Hammond, in his dramatic self-administration experiment, described rebound depression and craving following single doses of cocaine and described headache and a state of exhaustion and difficulty concentrating lasting for several days after his highest dose (more than 1 gram) (Hammond, 1887). Several subsequent authors described a similar abstinence syndrome consisting of fatigue, depression, lethargy, headache, poor concentration, irritability, craving, and improvement in delusions (Bose, 1902; Gordon, 1908 ; Chopra 1930, 1931, 1958).

Most contemporary literature on the effects of cocaine in humans is based on clinical observations from the epidemic of cocaine abuse that has swept the United States over the past five to 10 years (Kleber & Gawin, 1984b; Smith, 1984). These observations are quite consistent with the older literature. The acute euphoriant and stimulant effects are contrasted with chronic effects of depression, irritability, personality change, sociopathic behavior, craving, and paranoid psychosis. Severe addiction can occur across a wide range of dosages. An abstinence syndrome of depression, lethargy, and craving is variably described. Severe toxicity, including convulsions, myocardial infarction, and death are increasingly reported (Coleman et al., 1982; Nanji & Filipenko, 1984; Schachne et al., 1983; Jonsson et al., 1983; Myers & Earnest, 1984). The modern technique of free-base smoking permits the rapid achievement of very high blood levels and probably contributes to an increasing incidence of toxic behavioral and physical effects (Perez-Reyes et al., 1982).

What is missing from the clinical observations is more precise delineation of dose-response relationships and of the timing of acute and chronic cocaine effects. In the past decade a group of experiments has been carried out in which cocaine was administered to human volunteers while psychic and somatic responses were carefully measured. These studies have been summarized and compiled in Table 3.2. Nasal (i.n.) doses of 50–100 mg and intravenous (i.v.) doses of 15–30mg produce predictable increases in pulse and blood pressure and in various mood scales reflecting euphoria, energy, and self-confidence. Freebase (f.b.) cocaine has also been administered in the laboratory and found to be similar to i.v., if not slightly more powerful (Perez-Reyes et al.,1982). These effects peak within 15 minutes for i.v. and 30 minutes for i.n. doses and vanish within one to two hours. Blood levels of cocaine persist well after arousal has disappeared. The half-life of cocaine in the serum is brief, on the order of one hour (Van Dyck et al., 1982; Javaid et al., 1978; Rowbotham et al., 1984). The phenomenon of acute tolerance has been demonstrated after a single 96-mg i.n. dose of cocaine (Fischman et al., 1985). The phenomenon of rebound depression was observed in only a minority of studies and subjects (Fischman & Schuster, 1980; Resnick et al., 1977a). This effect may require higher doses or may reflect individual differences in response to cocaine. For example, many of Post's depressed patients exhibited a dramatic, paradoxical dysphoric response to i.v. cocaine (Post et al., 1974). Thus susceptibility to depression might be linked to dysphoric reactions to cocaine.

The subjective experience of cocaine was found to resemble that of amphetamine and morphine based on the Addiction Research Center Inventory (ARCI) (see Table 3.2). Interestingly, procaine and lidocaine are reported in several experiments to produce mild euphoria and to be confused with cocaine by some subjects (Van Dyke et al., 1982; Fischman & Schuster, 1983a).

Chronic and higher-dose cocaine use have not been studied in the laboratory. As noted above, modern clinical observations are consistent with the older literature, portraying a variety of toxic effects, tolerance, and craving and addiction. Gawin and Kleber have improved our understanding of chronic cocaine effects by systematically documenting abstinence symptomatology in a series of 30 cocaine abusers seeking treatment (Gawin & Kleber, 1986). Their observations span months following an index binge and provide the most complete description yet available in the literature. Their model is displayed in Figure 3.1. Several features are especially notable. The aftereffects of cocaine can last for several months, and subtle effects, such as spontaneous or triggered craving, may persist indefinitely. Also, the symptoms shift and oscillate. In phase 1, agitation gives way to fatigue. Insomnia and anorexia give way to hypersomnia and hypherphagia. Depression is high in phase 1 and disappears early in phase 2, although a state of anhedonia and anergia returns later in phase 2. Cocaine craving is high early in phase 1, disappears through late phase 1 and early phase 2, but returns later in phase 2 and recurs indefinitely on an episodic basis. Anxiety is low early in phase 2 but emerges later together with craving.

A summary model of the phenomenology of human cocaine use is presented in Figure 3.2. Lower doses taken over a short period of time lead to a brief euphoria, which is highly rewarding. This in itself may create a strong drive to take cocaine, promoting addiction. Higher, repeated doses result in acute tolerance to the euphoria and the development of unpleasant effects such as rebound depression, paranoia, and toxicity. Addiction also develops, either as an attempt to reverse the unpleasant effects, or because of the intense craving for the cocaine euphoria that users typically describe. Upon abstinence there is a shifting series of symptoms of depression, anxiety, and craving, which can persist and oscillate over weeks to months.

Table 3.2

Laboratory Studies of Acute Cocaine Administration in Humans

Reference	N	Route	Dose (mg)	Pulse (/min)	SBP (mm Hg)	Subjective and Other Effects
Fischman & Schuster, 1980	8	i.n.	96	+20		Stimulant effects (ARCI*) high over 1st 2 hours, then lower over next 6 hours, suggesting rebound effect Cocaine reverses some sleep deprivation effects, such as confusion, low arousal, slow reaction time
Van Dyck et al., 1982		i.n.	100			Peak high at 15–30 minutes; $t_{1/2}$ of high = 48 minutes; cocaine blood levels peak at 60 minutes; $t_{1/2}$ = 78 minutes; high (AR-CI) resembles morphine and amphetamine with euphoria and increased self-confidence Lidocaine produced a high resembling 14-mg cocaine dose
Rowbotham et al., 1984	8	p.o.	140	+27	+27	Peak high at 50 minutes Peak cocaine blood level at 50 minutes; $t_{1/2}$ = 77 minutes Plasma epinephrine and norepinephrine increased
Post et al., 1974	10	p.o.	30–200/day			No consistent effects on mood or vital signs Dose-dependent reduction in REM sleep Subjects were depressed inpatients
	12	i.v.	2.5–25	+	+	Peak arousal at 10–20 minutes; moderate doses produced feeling of well-being; higher doses produced mixed states including dysphoria, tearfulness, an anesthetic sense of relief from problems; subjects were depressed inpatients
Resnick et al., 1977a	19	i.n.	100	+20	+20	Vital sign effects peaked within 20 minutes Pleasant high peaked at 15 minutes Rebound dysphoria in 2 subjects at 45–60 minutes

Reference	N	Route				
Resnick et al., 1977a (cont'd)		i.v.	25	+30	+25	Vital sign effects peaked within 10 minutes Pleasant high peaked within 5 minutes Rebound dysphoria in 4 subjects at 20–30 minutes
Javaid et al., 1978	10	i.n.	96	+25%		Peak heart rate at 10–20 minutes; peak plasma level at 30 minutes Peak high at 20 minutes, vanished at 90 minutes
		i.v.	32	+50%		Peak heart rate at 15 minutes; plasma $t_{1/2}$=16–87 minutes Peak high at 3–5 minutes, vanished at 40 minutes Large intersubject variation in cocaine plasma levels
Fischman et al., 1976	9	i.v.	24	+30%	+10	Vital signs peak at 5–20 minutes; high resembles morphine and amphetamine (ARCI) with increased friendliness and vigor
Fischman & Schuster, 1983a	4	i.v.	32	30–60		Peak high within 15 minutes; resembles (ARCI) morphine and amphetamine Lidocaine produced no high or vital sign effects
Fischman & Schuster, 1983b	4	i.v.	32	++		High resembles morphine and amphetamine by ARCI; procaine produced mild high, confused with cocaine by 3/4 subjects
Perez-Reyes et al., 1982	6	f.b.	50			Effects resemble i.v. cocaine
Fischman et al., 1985		i.n.	96			Acute tolerance to both cardiovascular and subjective effects

*ARCI = Addiction Research Center Inventory; f.b. = freebase; i.n. = nasal; i.v. = intravenous; p.o. = oral.

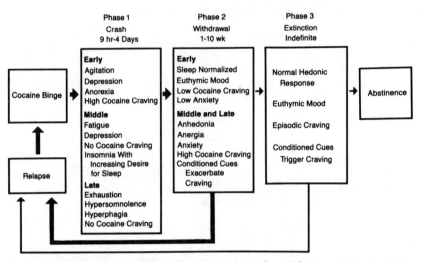

Phase 1	Phase 2	Phase 3
Crash	Withdrawal	Extinction
9 hr-4 Days	1-10 wk	Indefinite

Cocaine Binge

Early
Agitation
Depression
Anorexia
High Cocaine Craving

Middle
Fatigue
Depression
No Cocaine Craving
Insomnia With
  Increasing Desire
  for Sleep

Late
Exhaustion
Hypersomnolence
Hyperphagia
No Cocaine Craving

Early
Sleep Normalized
Euthymic Mood
Low Cocaine Craving
Low Anxiety

Middle and Late
Anhedonia
Anergia
Anxiety
High Cocaine Craving
Conditioned Cues
  Exacerbate
  Craving

Normal Hedonic
Response

Euthymic Mood

Episodic Craving

Conditioned Cues
Trigger Craving

Abstinence

Relapse

Duration and intensity of symptoms vary based on binge characteristics and diagnosis. Binges range from under four hours duration to six or more days. High cocaine craving early in phase 1 continues for up to 20 hours, but usually lasts less than six, and is followed by period of noncraving with similar duration in next subphase (middle-phase 1). Substantial craving then returns only after lag of up to five or more days, during phase 2.

Figure 3.1. Gawin and Kleber's (1984) model of abstinence symptomatology. (Reproduced with permission.)

NEUROPHARMACOLOGY OF COCAINE

The question before us now is this: How can the phenomena of cocaine use in humans be explained at the neurophysiological level? The wide variation of effects as a function of time, dosage, and abstinence suggests a complex series of related neural events. First the effects of cocaine on dopamine (DA), norepinephrine (NE), and serotonin (5-HT) neurotransmitter systems will be reviewed. These have received the most study. Then less-well-studied effects of cocaine on other neuronal systems will be described, including other neurotransmitters, the local anesthetic effect, and the calcium intracellular second messenger system. Most of these data derive from animal studies. A subsequent section will review human clinical and psychopharmacological findings.

Dopaminergic Systems

Many of cocaine's behavioral effects may be attributable to DA systems (see Chapter 2). It is well established that cocaine rapidly blocks the reuptake of DA into dopaminergic nerve terminals (Taylor & Ho, 1978;

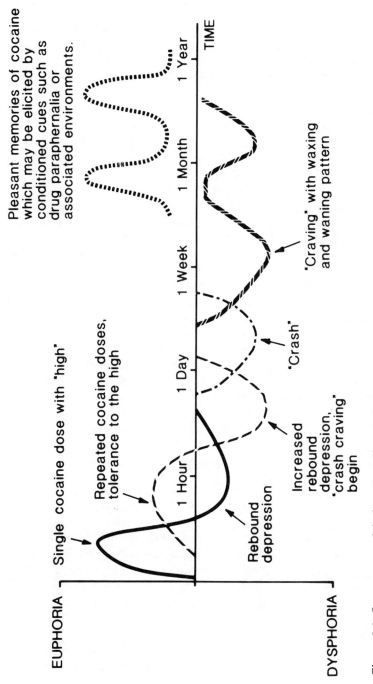

Figure 3.2. Summary model of cocaine effects in humans.

Ross & Renyi, 1966, 1967; Hadfield & Nugent, 1983). Reuptake is the main mechanism by which DA is cleared from the synapse (Cooper et al., 1982). Reuptake blockade by cocaine is presumably responsible for rapid accumulation of DA in the synaptic cleft (Bagchi & Reilly, 1983) and stimulation of DA neurotransmission.

Recently, high-affinity binding sites for tritiated (3H)-cocaine have been identified in the rat corpus striatum. The binding was eliminated by treatment with 6-hydroxydopamine, a selective dopaminergic neurotoxin, suggesting that the binding site is on dopamine nerve terminals in the striatum. Furthermore, drugs, such as nomifensine, which inhibit dopamine reuptake, also inhibited cocaine binding (Kennedy & Hanbauer, 1983). This suggests that the cocaine binding site is indeed closely linked to the reuptake site, although its functional significance remains to be established. If this is indeed a major site of cocaine's action, it suggests a strategy for blocking cocaine's effects, namely, use of other DA reuptake blockers.

Cocaine also causes a dose-related upregulation of postsynaptic DA receptors. This effect has been demonstrated with chronic repeated cocaine administration (Borison et al., 1979; Taylor et al., 1979). Postsynaptic receptors generally upregulate when there is a deficiency of transmitter, such as with "denervation supersensitivity." This suggests that DA depletion develops during chronic cocaine administration. However, Memo et al. measured a 37% increase in 3H-spiroperidol binding in rat caudate and nucleus accumbens one hour after a single 20 mg/kg intraperitoneal injection of cocaine (Memo et al., 1981). They also measured an increase in DA stimulation of adenylate cyclase and in calmodulin. Although this may mean that the depletion effect is very rapid, the authors also suggest that cocaine may interact directly with the postsynaptic receptor complex.

Other evidence suggests that DA depletion results from chronic cocaine intake. Taylor and Ho demonstrated increased activity of tyrosine hydroxylase, the rate-limiting enzyme in the biosynthesis of DA, after repeated cocaine injections in rats (Taylor & Ho, 1977). This is consistent with DA depletion resulting in a compensatory increase in its synthetic enzyme activity. Increased activity might also result from a direct effect of cocaine on tyrosine hydroxylase. In the same experiment, Taylor and Ho demonstrated increased DA turnover suggestive of a tendency toward DA depletion, although they measured only a slight decrease in brain DA concentrations, which was not statistically significant. Their relatively mild dose schedule of 10 mg/kg/day for five consecutive days may explain why more DA depletion was not seen (Taylor & Ho, 1977). A dosage of 10 mg/kg/day is only 70 mg/day in an average-sized man, which is small compared to what many heavy cocaine abusers consume. In another study, DA concentrations in the rat caudate nucleus (a component of the corpus striatum and site of DA nerve terminals originating from the substantia nigra) actually increase to over 50% of baseline within 20 minutes of an intraperitoneal injection of cocaine, 20 mg/kg (Pradhan et al., 1978a). This also suggests increased DA synthesis. Unfortunately, the effects of higher repeated doses of cocaine on DA depletion have not been studied in animals.

To summarize (see Figure 3.3), the acute effect of cocaine on DA neurons is stimulatory via DA reuptake blockade, increased DA synthesis, and upregulation of postsynaptic DA receptors. In contrast to the acute stimulatory effects, it appears likely that chronic cocaine intake leads to DA depletion.

DA pathways in the central nervous system consist of a number of short and intermediate-length tracts within the brain stem and hypothalamus and several long tracts. The longs tracts originate in the substantia nigra and ventral tegmental area and project to the corpus striatum, mainly caudate and putamen (nigrostriatal pathways), limbic structures including the nucleus accumbens (mesolimbic pathways), and limbic cortex including the frontal cortex (mesocortical pathways) (see Figure 3.4) (Cooper et al., 1982).

The mesolimbic and mesocortical DA tracts appear to be an integral part of a reward-mediating system within the brain. This reward system appears to originate with myelinated fibers from the lateral hypothalamus which descend in the median forebrain bundle and terminate in the ventral tegmental area, where they link with the DA tracts. Opiates appear to exert their rewarding effect within the ventral tegmental area, whereas stimulants exert their rewarding effects at the DA nerve terminals (Wise, 1984). Specifically, destruction of the nucleus accumbens, a terminus of mesolimbic DA fibers, has been shown to disrupt intracranial cocaine self-administration by animals, a model of cocaine reinforcement (Roberts et al., 1977, 1979; Zito et al., 1985), although there is a conflicting report (Goeders & Smith, 1984). Rats will self-administer cocaine into the medial prefrontal cortex, a major terminus of the mesocortical DA fibers, suggesting that cocaine stimulation there is rewarding (Goeders & Smith, 1984). Furthermore, dopamine receptor blockade with sulpiride attentuated cocaine self-administration in this paradigm, and specific DA cell destruction with 6-hydroxydopamine eliminated it completely (Goeders & Smith, 1983).

Drug self-administration in animals is important, because it predicts

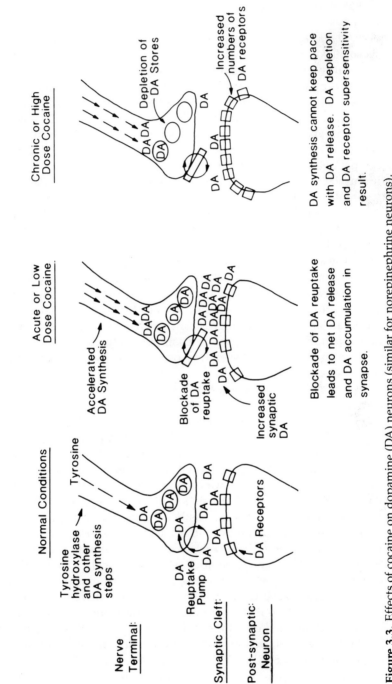

Figure 3.3. Effects of cocaine on dopamine (DA) neurons (similar for norepinephrine neurons).

NERVE
NEURON

Tyrosine
+ hyroxylase

↓

DA

ake

(DA) → neurotransmitter

(DA)

DA — DA update
Blocker

DA receptors

NEURON

① if many many years of migrane
headache, which do not lose intensity
with available pain killers, can
cause an Increase in the # of DA
receptors,

↓ direction
of thought
process

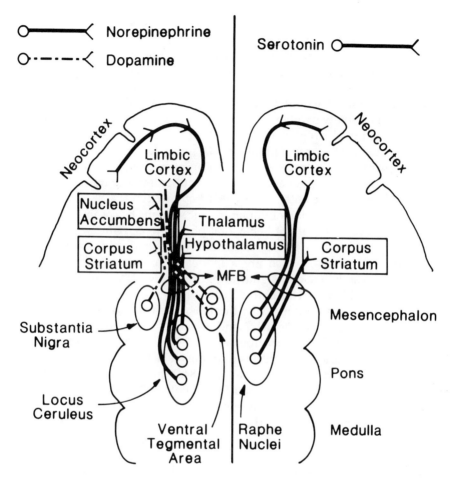

MFB : Median Forebrain Bundle

Figure 3.4. Schematic representation of major CNS, dopamine, norepinephrine, and serotonin pathways likely involved in cocaine behavioral effects.

addictiveness in humans (Johanson, 1984). As with self-administration of cocaine directly to brain sites described above, rats will work for peripheral (intravenous) injections of cocaine. This effect is also diminished by dopamine blockers at high doses (Woolverton & Balster, 1981). Lower doses of dopamine blockers actually increase responding in this paradigm (Roberts & Vickers, 1984; De La Garza & Johanson, 1982). The latter finding seems contradictory, although it can be understood as an attempt to override the blockade.

The results of discriminative stimulus experiments in animals suggest that DA systems mediate cocaine stimulus properties. The subjective effects of drugs can be studied in animals with a paradigm in which the drug is a conditioned stimulus signaling the availability of some other reward. The ability of other drugs to generalize to the conditioned stimulus of the initial drug is an index of similarity between drugs. Also, pharmacological manipulations can be used to study the underlying mechanisms of the drug's stimulus properties. It has been shown that the cocaine stimulus generalizes to other dopamine agonists and is disrupted by dopamine antagonists (see Chapter 2).

In summary, activation of dopaminergic systems by cocaine appears to underlie several important behavioral phenomena, namely, self-administration, which is a model of reward value and addictiveness, and stimulus properties, which are a model of subjective effects such as euphoria. The behavioral significance of putative DA depletion and receptor upregulation with chronic cocaine intake remains to be clearly delineated. Effects observed in humans, such as acute tolerance, rebound depression, the "crash," and "craving," have been attributed to DA depletion and receptor supersensitivity. This has spurred efforts to treat cocaine addiction with desipramine, which downregulates supersensitive receptors (Kleber & Gawin, 1984a), and bromocriptine, which binds and stimulates unoccupied DA receptors (Dackis & Gold, 1985a, b). These methods have been successful in early trials. They will be described in more detail in the section on human neurobiological evidence.

Norepinephrine Systems

Numerous studies have shown that cocaine inhibits the reuptake of NE (Ross & Reny, 1966, 1967; Hawks et al., 1974; Muscholl, 1961; Whitby et al., 1960; Langer & Enero, 1974; Just et al., 1976; Taylor & Ho, 1978). As with DA, this is the most important mechanism for clearing released NE from the synaptic cleft (Cooper et al., 1982). Reuptake blockade presumably leads to accumulation of NE in the synaptic cleft and hence a stimulatory effect on NE systems. The literature is not unanimous on this point. Several studies have failed to demonstrate NE reuptake inhibition (Chanda et al., 1979; Banerjee et al., 1979), although this may simply relate to differences in experimental technique.

Repeated cocaine administration has been shown to deplete brain concentrations of NE. In one study it appears to be a biphasic effect with increased NE brain concentrations over the first 20 minutes after intraperitoneal cocaine injection in the rat followed by diminished NE concentrations over the next 40 minutes (Pradhan et al., 1978a). In another study with rats five consecutive daily injections of 10 mg/kg of cocaine led to a 30% decrease in NE in the hypothalamus and thalamus (Taylor & Ho, 1977), which are targets for noradrenergic fibers originating in the locus ceruleus (Cooper et al., 1982). Analysis of the NE metabolites suggested this was due to increased NE metabolism and turnover (Taylor & Ho, 1977).

As with DA systems, cocaine activates tyrosine hydroxylase, the rate-limiting enzyme in the biosynthesis of NE (Taylor & Ho, 1977; Pradhan, 1983). This again is consistent with a compensatory increase in NE synthesis under conditions of NE depletion. It could also be explained by a direct effect on the enzyme.

Cocaine has been shown to upregulate NE beta receptors. (3H)-Dihydroaprenolol (3H-DHA) binding (an indicator of beta-receptor binding) in rat brain homogenates has been examined as a function of time after cessation of daily cocaine doses of 10 mg/kg for six weeks. One hour after cessation the number of receptor sites was increased by 70% over control. The increase peaked at 140% at 12 hours after cessation. It declined thereafter to 32% at 48 hours and remained steady at a 42% increase at 96 hours after cocaine cessation (Banerjee et al., 1979; Chanda et al., 1979). Cocaine also led to a statistically significant 52% increase in 3H-DHA binding at 12 hours after a single 10 mg/kg dose. Curiously, cocaine failed to block NE reuptake in this setting. There was also an increase in NE-stimulated cyclic AMP accumulation, suggesting that the increase in receptors was functionally significant (Banerjee et al., 1979; Chanda et al., 1979).

In summary (see Figure 3.3), the effects of cocaine on noradrenergic neurons resemble its effects on dopaminergic neurons. Most studies demonstrate that cocaine blocks NE reuptake acutely, although there are contradictory findings. In any case, this results in NE accumulation at the synapse and stimulation of NE neurotransmission. NE depletion develops rapidly. Tyrosine hydroxylase is stimulated, presumably in response to NE depletion. Postsynaptic β-adrenergic receptors are upregulated, also presumably a response to NE depletion. This effect persists for at least days after cessation of chronic cocaine intake.

Central NE neurons originate mainly from the locus ceruleus in the pons. Some axons ascend to innervate all areas of cerebral and cerebellar cortex and specific areas in the thalamus and hypothalamus (see Figure

3.4). The function of these neurons is not clearly established, although much evidence suggests that they modulate global alertness and vigilance (Cooper et al., 1982).

NE neurons are also widely involved in the peripheral autonomic nervous system. There they mediate a variety of effects, such as increased heart rate and contractility, increased peripheral muscle contractility, increased blood glucose, pupillary dilation, piloerection, sweating, and so on, which are associated with behavioral arousal and the "fight or flight" reflex (Gilman et al., 1985).

The behavioral effects of cocaine attributable to central NE pathways are poorly understood. It seems logical that the arousal and vigilance associated with acute cocaine intake would result from cocaine's acute stimulatory effect at central NE synapses. Results of discriminative stimulus studies do suggest that some of cocaine's stimulus properties are NE mediated. However, it is unclear whether these NE stimulus properties are mediated by central or peripheral NE fibers (see Chapter 2). The tachycardia and other signs of peripheral sympathetic arousal induced by cocaine are most suggestive of a peripheral effect, although it is possible that they originate through central NE stimulation. Many of cocaine's acute toxic effects with high doses, including restlessness, tremor, diaphoresis, hypertension, and even cardiac arrhythmias and death, resemble extreme peripheral sympathetic arousal. Propranalol, a β-adrenergic blocker, has been reported to be an effective antidote for acute cocaine poisoning (Rappolt et al., 1977).

The available literature suggests that cocaine self-administration is not NE mediated. For example, Roberts et al. showed that 6-hydroxydopamine-induced destruction of NE fibers ascending to the cortex and hypothalamus had no effect on responding for cocaine. In the same study, lesions of DA fibers to the nucleus accumbens produced a large, persistent reduction in cocaine self-administration (Roberts et al., 1977). Since self-administration is a predictor of addictive potential and presumably reflects a drug's euphoriant and rewarding properties, cocaine-induced NE activation may not contribute to the cocaine euphoria.

The behavioral significance of NE depletion and beta-receptor supersensitivity has not been established. These phenomena occur over the same time course as cocaine tolerance, rebound depression, and the "crash." Gawin and Kleber have noted that beta-receptor supersensitivity is a proposed mechanism of depression. They argue from this that cocaine-induced beta-receptor supersensitivity underlies postcocaine dysphoria and craving. This promotes addiction because of attempts to self-medicate these feelings with more cocaine. This has been their rationale for the treatment of cocaine abuse with desipramine, which downregulates beta receptors (Kleber & Gawin, 1984a). Preliminary results suggest that this treatment is effective (Gawin & Kleber, 1984). These data will be discussed more fully in the upcoming section on human neurobiological evidence.

Serotonin Systems

Cocaine inhibits the reuptake of both serotonin (5-hydroxytryptamine, 5-HT) and its metabolic precursor tryptophan into 5-HT neurons (Ross & Renyi, 1969). As with DA and NE neurons, 5-HT reuptake appears to be a major mechanism for clearance of released transmitter from the synapse (Cooper et al., 1982). This presumably makes more 5-HT available to interact with receptors within the synapse, at least transiently. However, unlike DA and NE neurons, this does not appear to lead to increased turnover of 5-HT. Rather, 5-HT and tryptophan turnover are decreased (Schubert et al., 1970; Friedman et al., 1975). This might result from stimulation of inhibitory presynaptic autoreceptors by augmented synaptic concentrations of 5-HT or some other negative feedback mechanism. However, it appears more likely that tryptophan uptake inhibition explains the decreased 5-HT turnover induced by cocaine. Tryptophan uptake appears to control the activity of tryptophane hydroxlyase (Mandell & Knapp, 1977), which is the rate-limiting enzyme in the synthesis of 5-HT (Cooper et al., 1982). Cocaine appears to inhibit tryptophan hyroxlyase and 5-HT synthesis (Taylor & Ho, 1977; Pradhan, 1983) by means of its inhibition of tryptophan uptake (Knapp & Mandell, 1972; Mandell & Knapp, 1977).

Cocaine also causes rapid depletion of brain levels of 5-HT, which is presumably due to decreased 5-HT synthesis coupled with 5-HT reuptake blockade (Taylor & Ho, 1977; Pradhan et al., 1978b). In contrast, cocaine causes initial increases in NE and DA concentrations, which are then followed by depletion.

Interestingly, high-affinity binding sites for (3H)-cocaine have been discovered in association with 5-HT neurons in the CNS. (3H)-Cocaine binding to these sites is inhibited by other 5-HT uptake inhibitors, such as imipramine, suggesting that the binding site is indeed localized on the reuptake mechanism (Reith et al., 1985). The evidence also suggests that the cocaine and imipramine sites are distinct entities (Reith et al., 1984). Preliminary evidence also shows that a peptide fraction from the supernatant of brain homogenates inhibits cocaine binding at this site, suggesting the existence of a peptide "cocaine inhibitory factor" (Reith et al., 1980). The functional significance of this binding site remains to be established. However, it is tempting to speculate that cocaine mimics the effects of a group of endogenous substances at receptors that regulate the activity of reuptake mechanisms.

Although 5-HT receptor adaptation during chronic cocaine intake analogous to that seen with NE and DA systems seems likely, this has not been studied.

In summary (see Figure 3.5), the net effect of cocaine on 5-HT neurons appears to be largely inhibitory. Both 5-HT synthesis and turnover are reduced, and 5-HT concentrations are depleted. This appears to be a monophasic effect, in contrast to NE and DA neurons, which display a biphasic response to cocaine—initial stimulation followed by depletion and inhibition.

5-HT neurons in the CNS originate in the raphe regions of the pons and upper brain stem. The caudal cell clusters mainly project axons down into the medulla and spinal cord. The rostral cell clusters course through the median forebrain bundle and provide extensive innervation to the diencephalon and telencephalon, including the corpus striatum, caudate nucleus, and cerebral cortex (see Figure 3.4) (Cooper et al., 1982). The behavioral and physiological functions of central 5-HT circuits are less clearly understood even than the functions of NE and DA circuits. Stimulation of central 5-HT fibers usually has inhibitory effects, and early studies with LSD suggested that LSD exerts its hallucinogenic and psychotomimetic effects by interfering with the inhibitory effects of 5-HT. However, recent work has suggested that LSD effects are more obscure and complicated (Cooper et al., 1982).

It is reasonable to hypothesize that the stimulating effects of cocaine may result in part from 5-HT inhibition. Chemical or physical lesioning of 5-HT raphe neurons has been shown to augment motor activity induced by cocaine (Scheel-Kruger et al., 1975). Pretreatment with methysergide, a 5-HT antagonist, has been shown to augment cocaine-induced increases in some aspects of motor activity during a conditioned shock avoidance task (Huang & Wilson, 1984). Methergoline, another 5-HT antagonist, has also been shown to enhance some aspects of cocaine-induced motor activity (Scheel-Kruger et al., 1975). In another study, injections of 5-hydroxytryptophan, a metabolic precursor of 5-HT which would presumably increase 5-HT synthesis and availability, decreased cocaine-induced spontaneous motor activity and stereotypy and decreased brain DA levels (Pradhan et al., 1978b). These results support the notion that 5-HT inactivation by cocaine contributes to its motor-stimulating properties. The effects of manipulations of 5-HT neurons on other

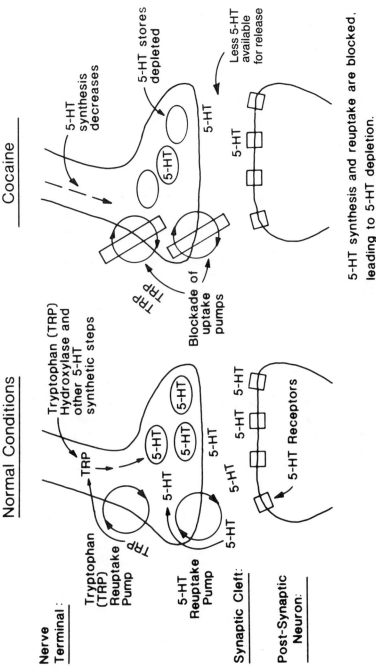

Figure 3.5. Effects of cocaine on serotonin (5-HT) neurons.

behavioral paradigms, such as cocaine self-administration or discriminative stimulus properties, have not been studied.

Lithium has been shown in rats to reverse the decline in tryptophan uptake and 5-HT synthesis caused by cocaine (Mandell & Knapp, 1979) and to antagonize motor effects of cocaine (Post et al., 1984). In humans, lithium has been reported in case studies to reduce cocaine euphoria (Cronson & Flemenbaum, 1978), although a controlled study failed to confirm this (Resnick et al., 1977b). Imipramine has also been reported to reduce cocaine euphoria in humans, both in the clinical setting (Rosecan, 1983) and in a small placebo-controlled laboratory challenge (Rosecan & Klein, 1986). Trazodone has also been shown in a laboratory setting to reduce physiological and possibly subjective effects of cocaine in humans (Rowbotham et al., 1984). Imipramine and trazodone are both serotonergic antidepressants which may work by normalizing activity in 5-HT systems. Also, as discussed above, imipramine may inhibit binding of cocaine to its putative binding site on 5-HT neurons (Reith et al., 1985). These clinical findings suggest that some of cocaine's euphoriant and rewarding properties may be mediated by 5-HT depletion. This will be discussed further in the upcoming section on human neurobiological evidence.

Other Neurobiological Systems

The effects of cocaine on NE, DA, and 5-HT systems have received the most study. However, there is evidence that cocaine interacts with several other neurobiological systems. Some of these may be secondary effects due to biochemical or neuronal interconnections with systems primarily effected by cocaine. Some may be direct cocaine effects. Also, little is known about interconnections between neuronal systems. A brief cataloguing of these less studied systems will highlight the potential complexity of cocaine effects. This will also suggest other psychopharmacological approaches to cocaine abuse.

Local anesthetic effects

Cocaine has been used as a local anesthetic since the nineteenth century. The basis of this effect appears to be sodium channel blockade, interfering with impulse propagation down axons (Matthews & Collins, 1983). It is reasonable to ask whether the local anesthetic effects contribute to cocaine's central stimulating and rewarding effects, perhaps by inhibiting impulse flow through inhibitory systems. Other local anesthetics, procaine and lidocaine, have been shown to partially share stimulus properties with cocaine (De La Garza & Johanson, 1983). Procaine is self-administered by monkeys (Ford & Balster, 1977), although monkeys' preferences were shown to be much stronger for cocaine in another study (Johanson & Aigner, 1981). Also, humans may confuse procaine or lidocaine at high doses with cocaine at low doses (Van Dyck et al., 1982; Fischman & Schuster, 1983a, b). Thus other local anesthetics may have mildly stimulating and rewarding properties. However, the contribution of local anesthetic effects to cocaine's central effects has yet to be established.

Post et al., proposed that cocaine's local anesthetic effects contribute to behavioral sensitization, because lidocaine also produces behavioral sensitization. Behavioral sensitization refers to progressive increases in motor activity with repeated identical daily doses of cocaine. It has been suggested as a model of effects of chronic cocaine intake (Post et al., 1983). Post et al. have also suggested that the local anesthetic effects of cocaine explain its tendency to cause seizures after repeated doses, once again on the basis that repeated doses of lidocaine lead to seizures (Post et al., 1983).

Endorphins and other polypeptides

As discussed in Chapter 2, opiate agonists share stimulus properties with cocaine. This is probably based on actions at different sites along the mesolimbic and mesocortical DA pathways thought to mediate reward. Opiates act on the cell bodies in the ventral tegmental area, whereas cocaine acts at the nerve terminals (Wise, 1984). Surprisingly, naloxone, an opiate antagonist, has been shown to potentiate the stimulating and euphoriant effects of cocaine in humans (Byck et al., 1982). It is also of interest that some human addicts prefer a combination of heroin and cocaine to either one alone, suggesting some form of synergy between their rewarding effects.

There are at least a dozen known neuroactive peptides, and there are undoubtedly many more as yet undiscovered (Cooper et al., 1982). Any of these might interact significantly with cocaine. Reith et al.'s report of a peptide fraction from brain homogenates that inhibits binding of cocaine to its high-affinity binding site is of special interest. This requires replication and further study (Reith et al., 1980). Post et al. have shown that a strain of vasopressin-deficient rats fails to develop cocaine-induced behavioral sensitization (Post et al., 1982). Vasopressin is a neuropeptide that has been shown to play a role in learning and memory. Post and

Contel suggest that learning and memory processes, mediated in part by vasopressin, may play a role in cocaine effects (Post & Contel, 1983). Cues such as the sight of paraphernalia or the sensation of dental local anesthesia are known to elicit cocaine craving in human abusers, even after months or years of abstinence. This also suggests an important conditioning component in chronic cocaine effects.

γ-Aminobutyric acid (GABA)

GABA is an inhibitory neurotransmitter with wide distribution in the CNS (Cooper et al., 1982). Valium appears to exert its sedative and anxiolytic effects by potentiating GABA (Gilman et al., 1985). Gale has shown that chronic cocaine administration to rats increases GABA synthesis and turnover and decreases (3H)-GABA binding in the corpus striatum. These effects were not altered by the DA blocking agent droperidol, suggesting that they are independent of DAergic innervation. Chronic cocaine administration had no effects on GABA turnover or binding in other brain areas, suggesting that these effects relate to specific neuronal interconnections within the striatum rather than a direct effect of cocaine on GABA neurons (Gale, 1984). Valium has been shown to block lidocaine-induced behavioral sensitization in animals (Post & Contel, 1983). Clinical experience has shown that some cocaine abusers like to take valium with cocaine. This suggests that there may be some synergy between cocaine and GABA, although it may also represent nonspecific sedative effects sought by abusers to "come down."

Acetylcholine (ACh)

Cocaine is structurally similar to ACh antagonists such as atropine, yet its interactions with cholinergic systems have received little attention. Cocaine has been shown to stimulate choline transport (Carrol & Butterbaugh, 1975) and to acutely increase ACh levels in the caudate nucleus (Pradhan et al., 1978a). Cocaine has been shown to inhibit ACh-induced ion flux in membrane vesicles from the electric organ of the electric fish *Electrophorus electricus* (Karpen et al., 1982). The cholinergic antagonist scopolamine has been shown to increase certain aspects of cocaine-induced motor activity (Scheel-Kruger et al., 1975). Physostigmine, an anticholinesterase and potentiator of ACh, has been shown to reduce cocaine self-administration in monkeys (De La Garza & Johanson, 1982). Physostigmine has also been shown to inhibit cocaine-induced seizures in cats (Castellani et al., 1983). In the clinical setting, physostigmine has been shown to reduce symptoms of mania, which bears some similarity to acute cocaine intoxication. Taken together, this evidence suggests that some of the stimulating and rewarding properties of cocaine may result from inhibition of ACh systems. It remains unclear whether this represents a direct effect of cocaine on ACh neurons or an indirect effect based on interconnections between ACh neurons and systems primarily affected by cocaine.

Calcium

Calcium is a fundamental component of messenger systems that translate extracellular events, such as an action potential or binding of a transmitter to a receptor, into intracellular effects. The external event promotes calcium influx. Calcium binds to calmodulin, which activates protein kinases, which in turn phosphorylate intracellular proteins that carry out intracellular effects. The calcium-calmodulin system appears to be involved in neurotransmission both presynaptically, where it mediates the action-potential-induced influx of calcium, and postsynaptically, where it mediates between transmitter binding to receptors and intracellular effects (Rasmussen, 1986a,b).

Several experiments suggest that cocaine potentiates the contraction of rat and guinea pig vas deferens by increasing the influx of calcium into smooth muscle cells (Hisayama et al., 1981; Araki & Gomi, 1982; Araki et al., 1982a). This effect was blocked by reserpine (Araki & Gomi, 1982) and by the α-adrenergic receptor antagonist dibenamine (Araki et al., 1982b), suggesting that it is mediated by cocaine's catecholaminergic properties.

Memo et al. studied DA receptor supersensitivity induced by cocaine in the rat caudate nucleus (Memo et al., 1981). They measured DA receptor supersensitivity and increased membrane-bound calmodulin after a single dose of cocaine. They cite evidence that the calcium-calmodulin system is involved in the transduction of DA receptor binding into intracellular effects (Gnegy et al., 1977) and speculate that cocaine may interact directly with the postsynaptic membrane, activating the calcium-calmodulin system and inducing receptor supersensitivity (Memo et al., 1981). However, this might also be an indirect effect.

In the clinical setting, verapamil, a calcium channel blocker, has been found to reduce symptoms of mania (Dubovsky et al., 1985), which superficially resembles cocaine intoxication. Another calcium channel blocker, nitrendipine, has been shown to dramatically reduce the cardiac toxicity of cocaine in rats (Nahas, 1985). This may be a nonspecific antiadrenergic effect, although it might also reflect a more specific interaction between cocaine and membrane calcium channels.

Phenylethylamine (PEA)

PEA is an endogenous amine present in the CNS which is synthesized along an alternate metabolic pathway from the catecholamine precursor phenylalanine. It is actively taken up by brain tissue. It is also the preferred substrate for type B monoamine oxidase (MAO-B). MAO-inhibitor (MAO-I) antidepressants markedly elevate brain PEA levels. PEA and its metabolic end product phenylacetic acid (PAA) have been shown to be low in various body fluids of depressed patients. This has led to the hypothesis that low PEA is a cause of depression which is corrected by MAO-I antidepressants (Sabelli et al., 1986).

PEA has been shown to have behavioral effects similar to those of stimulants (Sabelli et al., 1986) and is self-administered by dogs (Shannon & Degregorio, 1982). Also, specific MAO-B inhibitors, such as deprenyl (for which PEA is the preferred substrate), share stimulus properties with cocaine, but the MAO-A inhibitor clogyline does not. This suggests that PEA might be an endogenous cocaine analog or might mediate cocaine effects (Colpaert et al., 1980).

HUMAN NEUROBIOLOGY OF COCAINE

In order to extrapolate from the animal data reviewed above to humans, it is important to seek evidence from the clinical setting that provides insight into the neurobiological substrate for cocaine abuse in humans. Three types of relevant evidence are available: (1) neuroendocrine measurements; (2) the cooccurrence of other psychiatric disorders with cocaine abuse; and (3) the impact of psychopharmacological interventions on cocaine abuse.

Neuroendocrine Measurements

Although it is difficult to directly measure neural events noninvasively, a useful alternative for clinical psychiatric research has been measurement of hormones and other neurohumors in peripheral blood. In particular, hormones secreted by the anterior pituitary gland, such as prolactin (PL), growth hormone (GH), thyroid-stimulating hormone (TSH), and adrenocorticotropic hormone (ACTH), are controlled by peptides released from the hypothalamus, which are in turn regulated by central neurotransmitters such as NA, NE, and 5-HT. Thus, peripheral levels of pituitary hormones provide a "neuroendocrine window" into the activity of DA, NE, and 5-HT systems in the CNS. A major problem with this approach is that the hypothalamic pituitary axis is subject to multiple controlling influences which are difficult to understand and separate. This makes it more difficult to assess specific neurotransmitter systems based on neuroendocrine data (Brown & Seggie, 1980).

Dackis and colleagues studied blood levels of PL in 20 cocaine abusers. PL levels were drawn within 72 hours of hospitalization while serum cocaine levels were still positive. Fifteen of 20 patients had elevated PL levels (using 20 ng/ml as the upper limit of normal). The mean PL level in the patient group was 35.5 ng/ml. Since it has been clearly established that PL secretion is inhibited by DA, the authors conclude that the results suggest DA depletion. However, they acknowledge that control of PL secretion is complex, so that the results might reflect disruptions in other systems such as 5-HT as well (Dackis et al., 1984.)

Gawin and Kleber studied PL blood levels in 21 outpatient cocaine abusers. PL levels were drawn after four to 10 days of abstinence after "crash" symptoms such as oversleeping had normalized and while patients were experiencing significant "craving." Seven of 21 patients had low PL levels (using 5 ng/ml as the lower limit of normal), and the highest PL level measured was 10.6. The authors relate this finding to DA receptor supersensitivity resulting in DA system overactivity (Gawin & Kleber, 1985).

The most obvious explanation for this discrepancy is the different timing of PL levels. Dackis et al.'s high PL levels were drawn within three days of admission in patients who still had positive serum cocaine levels (Dackis et al., 1984). These patients had therefore probably been abstinent only two or three days at most and were probably still experiencing the acute cocaine crash. In contrast, Gawin and Kleber's low PL levels were drawn after four to ten days of abstinence when the crash had resolved and all patients were experiencing craving (Gawin & Kleber, 1985). The animal data reviewed previously suggest that DA stores are depleted by chronic cocaine use, while DA receptors are upregulated. If DA stores are repleted by the end of the crash phase, while DA receptors remain upregulated, this would lead to functional DA overactivity in the post crash phase (Figure 3.6). This would explain the shift from high PL during crash to low PL after crash. This is instructive in several respects. It suggests a general mechanism for the shifting nature of cocaine abstinence symptomatology, namely, different rates of normalization for different systems dysregulated by cocaine. It also points out that control of

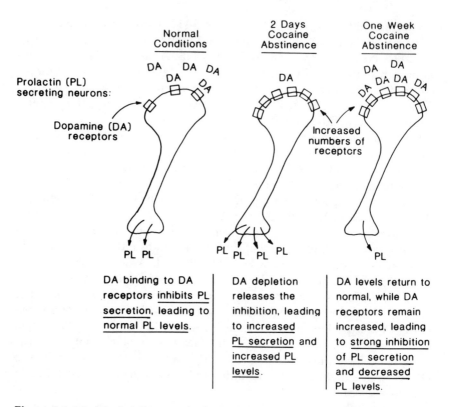

Figure 3.6. Model of shifting prolactin (PL) levels during early abstinence from cocaine.

timing is extremely important in neurobiological studies of cocaine abuse.

In addition to PL levels, Gawin and Kleber simultaneously obtained GH levels and a 1-mg dexamethasone suppression test (DST). Twenty percent of the sample had elevated GH. The authors cite evidence that DA and NE stimulate GH release and interpret their findings as consistent with DA and NE receptor upregulation and functional overactivity. This is also consistent with the interpretation of their PL findings. Forty-two percent of the sample had abnormal DST, further suggestive of derangement of the central NE system. All abnormal serum levels and

DSTs were repeated after four weeks of abstinence, and all had returned to normal. The significance of the follow-up data is clouded, since some of the patients had been treated with either lithium or desipramine. However, the data do suggest that these were mainly cocaine-induced abnormalities which disappeared gradually with time in abstinence (Gawin & Kleber, 1985).

Dackis and colleagues studied the TSH response to a standard dose of TRH (thyrotropin-releasing hormone, the hypothalamic factor responsible for stimulating TSH release) in 17 cocaine abusers within one week of hospitalization. All 17 were free of other substance abuse disorders or of major affective illness. Eight of 17 patients (47%) had an abnormally low TSH response to TRH. The authors cite evidence that TRH release is stimulated by NE and DA. They suggest that their findings are consistent with NE and DA overactivity during cocaine abuse. This would result in chronically elevated TRH levels, which would downregulate TRH receptors on TSH-producing cells in the anterior pituitary. With downregulated TRH receptors, these cells would mount a blunted TSH response to TRH (Dackis et al., 1985).

Another indirect approach to the study of central neurotransmitters is to study the urinary excretion of transmitter metabolites. This method is limited by the fact that a significant percentage of such metabolites are produced peripherally and do not reflect the CNS. Tennant found significantly reduced urinary excretion of MHPG (a principal metabolite of central NE) in a group of eight chronic cocaine users. All had used cocaine within 12 hours of the urine collections. This finding is consistent with central NE depletion resulting from chronic cocaine abuse (Tennant, 1985).

Another biological measure that has been useful as a "window" into CNS functioning is sleep electroencephalogram (EEG) monitoring of the distribution and quantity of rapid-eye-movement (REM) sleep. A recent theory with considerable supporting evidence holds that REM sleep is increased by cholinergic stimulation and inhibited by NE and 5-HT (McCarley, 1982). Post and colleagues administered oral cocaine to a small group of depressed inpatients (not cocaine abusers). Doses were gradually increased up to 100 mg twice per day over an average trial length of 10 days. Sleep EEG studies on a subgroup of these patients showed a dose-related decrease in REM sleep and in total sleep time. This is consistent with low ACh and high NE and is not consistent with 5-HT depletion. REM rebound was also observed after cessation of daily cocaine (Post et al., 1974), which is consistent with depleted NE and 5-HT. Sleep EEG has not been studied in cocaine abusers.

In summary, the results of these biological studies are generally consistent with the animal data. They suggest DA and NE activation by cocaine, depletion with chronic use and early in abstinence, and possibly a rebound to a state of functional overactivity later in abstinence, which coincides with the shift in abstinence symptomatology from crash to craving. More research is needed to explore variables such as cocaine dose and timing effects and to apply other relevant biological tests. This approach seems especially promising in attempts to understand cocaine-induced phenomena, such as the crash and craving, which do not have clear counterparts in animal models.

Psychiatric Diagnosis in Cocaine Abuse

Several small diagnostic case series have shown a high incidence of affective disorders among cocaine abusers. Two studies where diagnoses were obtained systematically with structured interviews in consecutive series of patients—one of 30 inpatients (Weiss et al., 1983) and another of 30 outpatients (Gawin & Kleber, 1986)—yielded similar findings. Twenty percent of the samples had disorders in the bipolar spectrum, mainly milder hypomanic and cyclothymic forms. Thirty percent had disorders in the unipolar spectrum, mainly major depression and dysthymia. These data are problematic because cocaine causes states resembling both hypomania and depression. Thus, despite a carefully administered structured interview, it may be difficult to differentiate affective disturbances secondary to cocaine from those which are primary and autonomous.

Methodological problems aside, this pattern seems intuitively likely on the grounds that the cocaine euphoria would be attractive to persons as "self-medication" for an underlying depression or as an attempt to augment hypomanic states. Although it is widely accepted that most affective disorders stem from some underlying biological vulnerability, the specific mechanisms are poorly understood. However, the diagnostic data on affective disorders in cocaine abuse at least suggest a common biological vulnerability. Thus, future research on the neurobiology of affective disorders may enhance our understanding of cocaine abuse, and vice versa. Also, the existence of distinct groups of cocaine abusers with different coexisting psychiatric disorders suggests that there is biological heterogeneity among cocaine abusers. Identification of biologically homogeneous subgroups within a disorder is probably essential for successful research efforts in biological psychiatry (Buchsbaum & Rieder, 1979).

Several authors have offered hypotheses on neurobiological links between cocaine abuse and affective disorders. Gawin and Kleber note that upregulation of β-adrenergic receptors in the CNS has been proposed as a mechanism of depression, while the efficacy of tricyclic antidepressants such as desipramine has been ascribed to their capacity to downregulate beta receptors. Gawin and Kleber note the evidence that cocaine also upregulates beta receptors and state this as a rationale for the treatment of cocaine abuse with desipramine (Kleber & Gawin, 1984a). Implicit in this reasoning is the hypothesis that a tendency toward pathological upregulation of beta receptors is a vulnerability common to both depression and cocaine abuse.

Mandell and Knapp suggest that dysregulation of 5-HT systems underlies bipolar affective disorders and that lithium acts by correcting this dysregulation. These authors also present evidence that cocaine depletes 5-HT by inhibiting tryptophan uptake and 5-HT synthesis, whereas lithium promotes tryptophan uptake and 5-HT synthesis antagonizing the cocaine effect (Mandell & Knapp, 1979). This has been proposed as a rationale for the use of lithium in the treatment of cocaine abuse (Kleber & Gawin, 1984a). This suggests the hypothesis that a tendency toward pathological dysregulation of 5-HT systems is a vulnerability common to both bipolar disorders and cocaine abuse.

A subtype of unipolar depression, termed "atypical depression" (AD), has been delineated by the work of Klein, Quitkin, and others (Liebowitz et al., 1984). AD consists of reactive mood while depressed and at least two of four vegetative features—oversleeping, overeating, severe lethargy, and pathological rejection sensitivity. Rejection sensitivity is defined as depressive reactions to criticism or rejection from significant others which are exaggerated and result in functional impairment: for example, a man jilted in romance who subsequently avoids dating for several years because of fear of rejection. Considerable evidence shows that AD responds selectively to MAO-I antidepressants. This suggests that AD is a biologically homogeneous subgroup within the larger universe of unipolar depression. Anecdotal evidence holds that ADs frequently abuse stimulants in an attempt to self-medicate. Also, the crash phase after a period of heavy cocaine abuse includes lethargy, overeating, and oversleeping and thus resembles AD. This had led Klein to hypothesize that ADs have a deficiency in an endogenous stimulant neurohumor, possible PEA (Klein, 1986).

We studied in detail a consecutive series of eight cocaine abusers in treatment in our outpatient clinic at Columbia–Presbyterian Medical Center, New York City. Three of eight had histories of depression with

significant rejection sensitivity (Nunes, 1985). We are currently conducting a formal diagnostic study, including a structured interview designed
to diagnose AD, on a consecutive series of cocaine abusers seeking outpatient treatment. Preliminary results on the first 20 patients show that
seven of 20 meet full criteria for AD on a lifetime basis (Nunes et al.,
1986). Thus AD may represent another biologically homogenous subgroup within cocaine abuse.

Several sources suggest that a small percentage of cocaine abusers has
residual attention deficit disorder (Gawin & Kleber, 1986; Khantzian,
1983; Khantzian et al., 1984). Also, preliminary analysis of our formal
diagnostic study shows a small percentage meeting criteria for social
phobia of mild to moderate severity (Nunes et al., 1986). These also may
represent subgroups with distinct biological vulnerabilities to cocaine
abuse.

In summary, the diagnostic findings suggest that cocaine abuse is heterogeneous with several subgroups, including hypomanics and cy-
clothymics, unipolar depressives, ADs, persons with attention deficit
disorder, those with social phobia, and finally those without a concurrent psychiatric diagnosis (Figure 3.7). Clearly, more diagnostic studies
with larger samples are needed. Although the biological implications
remain largely speculative, this approach has heuristic value. It suggests
a linkage between the biological basis of cocaine abuse and other psychiatric disorders.

Psychopharmacological Interventions in Cocaine Abuse

The success or failure of a psychopharmacological intervention can be
looked upon as a biological marker or as a test of a pathophysiological
hypothesis. Since the modes of action of most psychopharmacological
drugs are incompletely understood, a successful intervention can yield
only limited information about specific biological mechanisms of a disease. However, as with the neuroendocrine method, this does provide a
way of examining hypotheses about underlying mechanisms.

Moreover, a major motive for attempting to understand the neurobiology of cocaine abuse is to help suggest effective psychopharmacological
interventions. The findings reviewed in this chapter thus far suggest a
number of possible psychopharmacological interventions. There are two
types of rationale. The first is appropriate medication treatment of a
concurrent psychiatric disorder for which the cocaine abuse is "self-
medication." An example would be use of antidepressant medication for
cocaine abuse with concurrent depression. Resolution of both depres-

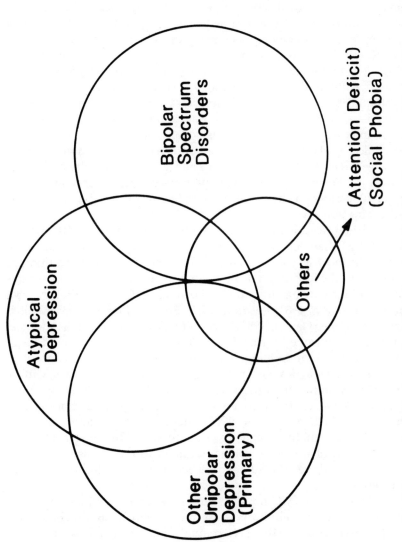

Figure 3.7. Universe of cocaine abusers including those without other diagnosis and those with secondary depression.

sion and cocaine abuse would support the notion that the depression contributed to the pathophysiology of the cocaine abuse. The second rationale is use of a medication to reverse neurophysiological derangements presumed to underlie cocaine abuse. An example would be use of an antidepressant to downregulate receptors supersensitized by cocaine abuse. Resolution of cocaine abuse and/or specific symptoms such as craving would support the notion that supersensitive receptors contribute significantly to the pathophysiology of cocaine abuse.

Psychopharmacological interventions for cocaine abuse that have been attempted and reported in the literature are summarized in Table 3.3. Most of these interventions have been tested only in individual cases or in open clinical trials and thus require confirmation from more rigorous clinical research. The following discussion will focus on the pathophysiological implications of the psychopharmacological intervention data. Chapter 10 focuses on clinical recommendations for psychopharmacology in cocaine abuse.

Three antidepressants, desipramine (DMI), imipramine (IMI), and trazodone (TRZ), have been used for the treatment of cocaine abuse. (A fourth agent, nortriptyline, has also been used, but published findings are not yet available.) All three agents have been reported in open trials to lower cocaine craving and promote abstinence (Gawin & Kleber, 1984; Tennant & Rawson, 1983; Rosecan, 1983; Small & Purcell, 1985). This is supported by one (Gawin, 1985) of two (Tennant & Tarver, 1984) double-blind placebo-controlled trials with desipramine. This effect could result from treatment of underlying depression, supporting the concept of depression as a biological factor driving cocaine abuse. However, clinical impressions from the open trials (Gawin & Kleber, 1984; Rosecan, 1983) and preliminary results from an ongoing double-blind placebo-controlled trial with DMI (Gawin, 1985) suggest that antidepressants are helpful with or without a diagnosis of depression. This suggests that the antidepressants also reverse some cocaine-induced imbalance in brain physiology that drives the addiction, such as upregulated postsynaptic beta receptors.

It is of interest that IMI and TRZ, both potent 5-HT reuptake blockers, may block the cocaine euphoria (Rosecan & Klein, 1986; Rowbotham et al., 1984). In contrast, DMI, an NE reuptake blocker with less effect on 5-HT systems, appears not to block cocaine euphoria. As reviewed previously, cocaine depletes 5-HT. IMI and TRZ may oppose this and in so doing attenuate cocaine euphoria. This suggests a significant serotonergic contribution to cocaine euphoria in humans. Also, we have reviewed evidence that cocaine binding at 5-HT neurons is inhibited by

Table 3.3

Psychopharmacological Interventions in Cocaine Abuse

Medication	Rationales	Findings: Craving abstinence	Findings: Blocks euphoria	Comments
Desipramine	1. Treat underlying depression 2. Downregulate beta receptors 3. Interfere with cocaine binding	+	−	Supported by open clinical trials and 1 of 2 placebo-controlled trials
Imipramine	1. Treat underlying depression 2. Regulate 5-HT systems 3. Interfere with cocaine binding	+	+	Open clinical trials; blocking shown in one small placebo-controlled laboratory cocaine challenge
Trazodone	1. Treat underlying depression 2. Regulate 5-HT systems	+	?	Case reports; blocking of some cocaine effects in laboratory challenge
Lithium	1. Treat underlying bipolar disorder 2. Reverse cocaine effects on 5-HT systems	+	?	Cases, open clinical trials; blocking not confirmed by laboratory challenge; efficacy limited to bipolar patients?
Stimulants Methylphenidate Pemoline	1. Treat underlying ADD 2. Replace cocaine with more benign stimulant	+	−	Cases, open clinical trials; effect appears limited to ADD patients
Amino Acids Tryptophan	1. Promote 5-HT synthesis, combat depletion	?	−	Open clinical trials; data unclear
Tyrosine	1. Promote NE, DA synthesis, combat depletion	?	−	Open clinical trials; data unclear
Bromocriptine	1. Occupy supersensitive DA receptors	+	−	Small placebo-controlled trial

ADD = attention deficit disorder.

other 5-HT reuptake blockers, including IMI. This further raises the possibility that cocaine binding at 5-HT neurons contributes to cocaine euphoria, since both binding and euphoria may be blocked by IMI.

Lithium has been used to treat cocaine abuse in cases and open clinical trials that suggest that it lowers craving and promotes abstinence (Gawin & Kleber, 1984; Cronson & Flemenbaum, 1978). The evidence suggests that this effect holds only in patients with a concurrent bipolar spectrum disorder (Gawin & Kleber, 1984). Although more definitive studies are needed, this supports the notion that a subgroup of cocaine abusers has an underlying bipolar disorder that drives their addiction.

Clinical case reports have suggested that lithium blocks the cocaine euphoria (Cronson & Flemenbaum, 1978). This supports the notion of pharmacological antagonism of cocaine by lithium, perhaps via the serotonergic mechanism suggested by Knapp and Mandell (Mandell & Knapp, 1979). However, a small controlled study failed to confirm this effect (Resnick et al., 1977b).

Case reports and open clinical trials suggest that methylphenidate (MPH) (Khantzian, 1983; Khantzian et al., 1984) and magnesium pemoline (Weiss et al., 1985) reduce cocaine craving and promote abstinence in cocaine abusers with residual attention deficit disorder (ADD). An open trial found MPH ineffective in non-ADD cocaine abusers (Gawin et al., 1985). This supports the notion that a small subgroup of cocaine abusers has an underlying ADD that drives the addiction.

Tyrosine (Gold et al., 1983; Rosecan, 1983), a metabolic precursor of NE and DA, and typtophan (Rosecan, 1983), a metabolic precursor of 5-HT, have been administered to cocaine abusers. The rationale for this is promotion of synthesis of NE, DA, and 5-HT in order to overcome putative cocaine-induced depletion. The evidence for clinical efficacy is suggestive but weak, and more definitive studies are needed.

Bromocryptine, a DA agonist, has been shown to dramatically reduce craving in a small placebo-controlled study with inpatients experiencing severe craving (Dackis & Gold, 1985a). This supports the notion that cocaine craving is produced by supersensitive DA receptors unoccupied in the face of depleted DA stores. Bromocriptine occupies these vacant sites as an agonist and thus presumably reduces craving (Dackis & Gold, 1985b).

In addition to the above, our review of cocaine neurobiology suggests several other psychopharmacological interventions that have yet to be tried or reported (see Table 3.4). For example, a combination of bromocriptine and imipramine might be tried with the rationale that it would simultaneously antagonize cocaine effects of DA, NE, and 5-HT systems.

Table 3.4

Other Possible Psychopharmacological Interventions for Cocaine Abuse

Medication	Craving	Blocks euphoria	Rationales
	Predicted Effects:		
Imipramine plus bromocriptine	+	+	1. Regulate both DA and 5-HT systems
Monoamine oxidase inhibitors	+	−	1. Treat underlying AD 2. Counteract PEA deficit
Nomifensine (currently unavailable)	+	+	1. Treat underlying depression 2. Prevent cocaine binding to reuptake site on DA neurons
Phenylalanine	+	−	1. Counteract PEA deficit 2. Counteract DA or NE deficit
Calcium channel blockers	−	+	1. Nonspecific antiadrenergic effects 2. Antagonize calcium-mediated cocaine effects
Physostigmine	?	+	1. Counteract cocaine antagonism of ACh
Lecithin	?	+	1. Counteract cocaine antagonism of ACh

DA = dopamine; 5-HT = serotonin; AD = atypical depression; PEA = phenylethylamine; NE = norepinephrine; ACh = acetylcholine.

MAO-I might be effective in cocaine abuse, based on several rationales. We have discussed preliminary evidence that some cocaine abusers have "atypical depression" (AD) (Nunes et al., 1986), a subtype of depression that is selectively MAO-I responsive (Liebowitz et al., 1984). We have also discussed the possibility that a PEA deficit might be involved in the pathophysiology of cocaine abuse (PEA deficiency has also been proposed as the basis of AD [Klein, 1986]). MAO-Is raise brain PEA levels. Unfortunately, cocaine taken with an MAO-I could result in a dangerous hyptertensive crisis. Therefore, this approach would have to be undertaken with extreme caution and careful forethought.

Another intervention suggested by the PEA deficiency hypothesis is phenylalanine, which is the metabolic precursor of PEA.

Evidence for the role of calcium in cocaine neuropharmacology has been reviewed above. This suggests that calcium channel antagonist drugs such as verapamil or nifedipine might be useful for blockade of the cocaine euphoria. Again, careful forethought would need to be exercised in regard to possible interactions between these drugs and cocaine in the clinical setting.

Evidence has been presented above that ACh systems may contribute to the pathophysiology of cocaine abuse. Specifically, cocaine may lead to ACh deficiency, and cholinergic agonists appear to lessen some cocaine-induced behaviors in laboratory animals that are enhanced by ACh antagonists. This suggests that anticholinesterase drugs such as physostigmine might be useful in cocaine abuse. Once again, careful forethought would need to be exercised regarding possible interactions with cocaine in the clinical setting. Alternatively, lecithin, a dietary precursor of ACh, might be tried.

In summary, the findings on psychopharmacological treatment of cocaine abuse must be considered tentative, based as they are largely on open trials and cases. However, a number of the psychopharmacological interventions do appear to show promise. This suggests the validity of the corresponding putative mechanisms of cocaine addiction. Also, the fact that some interventions appear useful only for specific diagnostic groups supports the general notion, raised by the diagnostic data, of biological heterogeneity within cocaine addiction. That is, cocaine addiction may result from a variety of distinct biological mechanisms, which require distinct treatment interventions. It will be important in future biological and treatment research to distinguish subtypes of cocaine addiction and to study each in isolation.

CONCLUSIONS AND FUTURE DIRECTIONS

This chapter has covered a wide variety of evidence bearing on the neurophysiological mechanisms of cocaine effects and cocaine addiction. Several major hypotheses have emerged.

The *DA hypothesis* (Dackis & Gold, 1985b) enjoys perhaps the strongest support from the evidence. According to this formulation, cocaine acutely enhances DA neurotransmission by blocking DA reuptake and increasing DA synthesis. This stimulatory effect on mesocortical and mesolimbic DA tracts results in the highly pleasant and rewarding cocaine euphoria. Repeated cocaine use rapidly leads to presynaptic DA depletion and postsynaptic DA receptor supersensitivity, which results in tolerance, dysphoria, and craving. Addiction results from the drive to repeatedly experience the euphoria and/or reduce the dysphoric effects. This is supported by a variety of animal studies and findings in humans, including high prolactin levels after heavy cocaine use (consistent with DA depletion) and successful reduction of craving with bromocriptine (a DA agonist) and desipramine (possibly a mild DA agonist based on DA reuptake blockade, which may also inhibit cocaine binding at the DA reuptake site). The model fails to explain a number of findings, including the following:

1) Neuroleptic DA blockers (except in high doses) increase cocaine self-administration in animals.
2) PL levels are low (consistent with DA system overactivity) one week after cessation of heavy cocaine use but craving and other dysphoric states may persist.
3) The bromocriptine treatment does not itself produce euphoria.

The *NE hypothesis* holds that cocaine acutely enhances NE neurotransmission via reuptake blockade and increased NE synthesis and that this contributes to cocaine euphoria. NE depletion and beta-receptor supersensitivity rapidly develop, contributing to craving and other dysphoric effects of cocaine abuse. Although these physiological changes are supported by a variety of animal studies and human neuroendocrine data, their behavioral significance is less clear. Animal self-administration studies fail to confirm a role for NE in cocaine's rewarding properties, although it is possible that humans find the NE enhancement reinforcing. Instead, NE enhancement may underlie the acute toxic effects of cocaine. The successful use of desipramine (norepinephrine reuptake blocker that downregulates beta receptors) to reduce cocaine craving in preliminary clinical trials provides the strongest evidence for a link between beta-receptor supersensitivity and the craving and dysphoria of chronic cocaine use.

According to the *5-HT hypothesis*, cocaine rapidly depletes 5-HT by blocking 5-HT reuptake and reducing 5-HT synthesis (via blockade of tryptophan uptake). These physiological changes have been relatively well documented in animals. This reduces presumed inhibitory influences of 5-HT promoting cocaine's stimulatory effects and thus contributing the euphoriagenic and possibly also the acute toxic effects of cocaine. This formulation has received little testing in animal models. The strongest confirmatory evidence comes from clinical studies showing that serotonergic medications such as imipramine and lithium attenuate cocaine euphoria, reduce craving, and promote abstinence. However, these data are very preliminary and require replication. Also, it is diffi-cult to explain how an essentially monophasic 5-HT depletion effect could account for the biphasic aspects of cocaine effects (euphoria fol-lowed by dysphoria).

The *self-medication hypothesis* holds that cocaine abusers suffer from one of several underlying mood disorders. Cocaine temporarily relieves their suffering, but then exacerbates it, locking them into a cycle of repeated use and addiction. For example, some cocaine abusers may be depressives who obtain a temporary mood lift from cocaine followed by enhanced dysphoria. The mood disorders may result from tendencies toward dopaminergic, noradrenergic, serotonergic, or other dysregula-tions which are exacerbated by cocaine. Preliminary diagnostic studies have documented the presence of unipolar depression, atypical depres-sion, and low-grade bipolar disorders in a large percentage of cocaine abusers. These need to be replicated and combined with neuroendocrine and psychopharmacological studies in order to examine the underlying biological mechanisms. This model suggests the important notion that cocaine abusers may be biologically heterogeneous, with different sub-groups requiring specific treatment approaches.

The evidence presented in this chapter permits the formulation of a number of other hypotheses of cocaine addiction. For example, an *ACh hypothesis* would hold that cocaine antagonizes ACh and that treatments that enhance ACh would be effective. A *calcium-hypothesis* would hold that cocaine enhances calcium transport, and that this could be antago-nized by calcium channel blockers. A *PEA hypothesis* would hold that cocaine depletes PEA or mimics PEA in individuals with a PEA deficien-cy. A *peptide hypothesis* would hold that cocaine mimics the action of a class of endogenous peptides that regulate reuptake mechanisms. All of these stand on the barest of evidence and need further testing.

A general drawback of these models is that they are all of the "rheo-static" or "glandular" variety. They posit an excess or deficiency of one or another neurotransmitter or effector. Klein and colleagues (Klein et al., 1980) and others (Siever & Davis, 1985) argue that "thermostatic" or systems models may be more successful in explaining neuropsychiatric disorders. Such models account for the interplay of feedback between a number of interconnected neural systems. For example, it is possible to formulate a *dopamine-serotonin balance hypothesis* of cocaine addiction whereby a normal balance of 5-HT inhibitory control over DA is disrupt-ed by cocaine. Unfortunately, relatively little is known about the inter-connections between neural systems that would form the basis for such models.

The Incan myth discussed at the outset held that the coca plant sprang from the blood of a beautiful, but adulterous woman who was executed for her crimes. It was to be chewed by men to remind them of her (Petersen, 1977), and presumably of the dire consequences of hubris and sexual adventurism. Perhaps cocaine should similarly warn neurobiologists and clinicians against scientific hubris. The evidence presented in this chapter amounts to a number of interesting leads into the mechanism of action of cocaine. However, the complexity of the problem is also evident. No definitive model of cocaine neurobiology can yet be offered. It is hoped that this chapter provides a foundation for the formulation and testing of neurobiological and psychopharmacological hypotheses of cocaine addiction.

REFERENCES

Anden NE, Dahlstrom A, Fuxe K, et al: Ascending monoamine neurons to telencephalon and diencephalon. Acta Phsyiol Scand 67:313, 1966.

Araki K, Gomi Y: Pharmacological studies on supersensitization. VIII. Dissociation of induction of supersensitivity from presynaptic action of cocaine on isolated vas deferens of guinea pig. J Pharmacobiodyn 5:796–802, 1982.

Araki K, Muramatsu M, Gomi Y: Pharmacological studies on supersensitization. VI. Effect of cocaine on the utilization of calcium in acetylcholine-induced contraction of isolated vas deferens of guinea pig. J Pharmacobiodyn 5:693–698, 1982a.

Araki K, Muramatsu M, Kontani H, Gomi Y: Pharmacological studies on supersensitization. VII. Inhibitory effect of dibenamine on cocaine-induced supersensitivity of isolated vas deferens of guinea pig. J Pharmacobiodyn 5:789–795, 1982b.

Bagchi SP, Reilly MA: Intraneuronal dopaminergic action of cocaine and some of its metabolites and analogs. Neuropharmacology 22:1289–1295, 1983.

Banerjee SP, Sharma VK, Kung-Cheung LS, Chanda SK, Riggi SJ: Cocaine and D-amphetamine induce changes in central beta-adrenoceptor sensitivity: effects of acute and chronic drug treatment. Brain Res 175:119–130, 1979.

Borison, RL, Hitri A, Klawans HL, Diamond BI: A New Animal Model for Schizophrenia: Behavioral and Receptor Binding Studies, in Usdin E, Kopin IJ, Barchas J, eds, Catecholamines: Basic and Clinical Frontiers, New York, Pergamon Press, 1979, pp 719–721.

Bose C: Cocaine poisoning. Br Med J 1:16–17, 1913, in Cocaine—Summaries of Psychosocial Research, Rockville, MD, NIDA, 1976, pp 68–69.

Bose KC: Cocaine intoxication and its demoralizing effects. Br Med J 1:1020–1022, 1902, in Cocaine—Summaries of Psychosocial Research, Rockville, MD, National Institute of Drug Abuse (NIDA), 1976, pp 66–67.

Brown GM, Seggie J: Neuroendocrine mechanisms and their implications for psychiatric research. Psychiatr Clin North Am 3:205–221, 1980.

Buchsbaum MS, Rieder RO: Biologic heterogeneity and psychiatric research; platelet MAO activity as a case study. Arch Gen Psychiatry 36:1163–1169, 1979.

Buck AA, Sasaki TT, Hewitt JJ, Macrae AA: Coca chewing and health: an epidemiologic study among residents of a Peruvian village. Am J Epidemiol 88:159–177, 1968, in Cocaine—Summaries of Psychosocial Research, Rockville, MD, NIDA, 1976, pp 96–99.

Byck R, Ruskis A, Ungerer J, Jatlow P: Naloxone potentiates cocaine effect in man. Psychopharmacol Bull 18:214–215, 1982.

Carrol P, Butterbaugh G: High affinity choline transport in guinea pig brain and the effect of norepinephrine. J Neurochem 24:917–924, 1975.

Castellani S, Ellinwood EH, Kilbey MM, Petrie WM: Cholinergic effects on arousal and cocaine-induced olfactory-amygdala spindling and seizures in cats. Physiol Behav 31:461–466, 1983.

Chanda SK, Sharma VK, Banerjee SP: Beta-adrenoceptor sensitivity following psychotropic drug treatment, in Usdin E, Ed: Catecholamines: Basic and Clinical Frontiers, New York, Pergamon Press, 1979, pp 586–588.

Chopra IC, Chopra RN: The cocaine problem in India. Bull Narcotics 10:12–24, 1958, in Cocaine—Summaries of Psychosocial Research, Rockville, MD, NIDA, 1976a, pp 85–87.

Chopra RN, Chopra GS: Cocaine habit in India. Indian J Med Res 18:1013–1046, 1930/1931, in Cocaine—Summaries of Psychosocial Research, Rockville, MD, NIDA, 1976b, pp 76–78.

Coleman DL, Ross TF, Naughton JL: Myocardial ischemia and infarction related to recreational cocaine use. West J Med 136:444–446, 1982.

Colpaert FC, Niemegeers CJ, Janssen PA: Evidence that a preferred substrate for type B monoamine oxidase mediates stimulus properties of MAO inhibitors: a possible role for beta-phenylethylamine in the cocaine cue. Pharmacol Biochem Behav 13:513–517, 1980.

Cooper JR, Bloom FE, Roth RH: The Biochemical Basis of Neuropharmacology, New York, Oxford, Oxford University Press, 1982.

Cronson AJ, Flemenbaum A: Antagonism of cocaine highs by lithium. Am J Psychiatry 135:856–857, 1978.

Dackis CA, Gold MS: Bromocriptine as a treatment for cocaine abuse. Lancet 2:1151–1152, 1985a.

Dackis CA, Gold MS: New concepts in cocaine addiction: the dopamine depletion hypothesis. Neurosci Biobehav Rev 9:469–477, 1985b.

Dackis CA, Gold MS, Estroff TW, Sweeney DR: Hyperprolactinemia in cocaine abuse. Soc Neurosci Abstr 10:1099, 1984.

Dackis CA, Estroff TW, Sweeney DR, Pottash ALC, Gold MS: Specificity of the TRH test for major depression in patients with serious cocaine abuse. Am J Psychiatry 142:1097–1099, 1985.

De La Garza R, Johanson CE: Effects of haloperidol and physostigmine on self-administration of local anesthetics. Pharmacol Biochem Behav 17:1295–1299, 1982.

De La Garza RD, Johanson, CE: The discriminative stimulus properties of cocaine in the rhesus monkey. Pharmacol Biochem Behav 19:145–148, 1983.

Dubovsky SL, Franks RD, Schrier D: Phenelzine-induced hypomania: effect of verapamil. Biol Psychiatry 20:1009–1014, 1985.

Fischman MW, Schuster CR: Cocaine effects in sleep-deprived humans. Psychopharmacology 72:1–8, 1980.

Fischman MW, Schuster CR: A comparison of the subjective and cardiovascular effects of cocaine and lidocaine in humans. Pharmacol Biochem Behav 18:123–127, 1983a.

Fischman MW, Schuster CR: A comparison of the subjective and cardiovascular effects of cocaine and procaine in humans. Pharmacol Biochem Behav 18:711–716, 1983b.

Fischman MW, Schuster CR, Resnekov L, et al: Cardiovascular and subjective effects of intravenous cocaine administration in humans. Arch Gen Psychiatry 33:983–989, 1976.

Fischman MW, Schuster CR, Javaid J, Hatano Y, Davis J: Acute tolerance development to the cardiovascular and subjective effects of cocaine. J Pharmacol Exp Ther 235:677–682, 1985.

Ford RD, Balster RL: Reinforcing properties of intravenous procaine in rhesus monkeys. Pharmacol Biochem Behav 6:289–296, 1977.

Freud S: Über Coca. Therapie. 2:289–314, 1884, in Byck R, ed: Cocaine Papers by Sigmund Freud, New York, Stonehill, 1974, pp 47–73.

Freud S: On the general effect of cocaine. Med-chir Centralbl 32:374–375, 1885, in Byck R, ed: Cocaine Papers by Sigmund Freud, New York, Stonehill Publishing, 1974, pp 111–118.

Freud S: Craving for and fear of cocaine. Wein Med Wochenschr 28:929–932, 1887, in Byck

R, ed: Cocaine Papers by Sigmund Freud, New York, Stonehill Publishing, 1974, pp 169–176.

Friedman E, Gershon S, Rotrosen J: Effects of acute cocaine treatment on the turnover of 5-hydroxytryptamine in the rat brain. Br J Pharmacol 54:61–64, 1975.

Gale K: Catecholamine-independent behavioral and neurochemical effects of cocaine in rats. NIDA Res Monogr Ser 54:323–332, 1984.

Gawin FH: Paper presented at the American College of Neuropsychopharmacology, December 1985.

Gawin FH, Kleber HD: Cocaine abuse treatment: open pilot trial with desipramine and lithium carbonate. Arch Gen Psychiatry 41:903–909, 1984.

Gawin FH, Kleber HD: Neuroendocrine findings in chronic cocaine abusers: a preliminary report. Br J Psychiatry 147:569–573, 1985.

Gawin FH, Kleber HD: Abstinence symptomatology and psychiatric diagnosis in cocaine abusers: clinical observations. Arch Gen Psychiatry 43:107–113, 1986a.

Gawin F, Riordan C, Kleber H: Methylphenidate treatment of cocaine abusers without attention deficit disorder: a negative report. Am J Drug Alcohol Abuse 11:193–197, 1985.

Gilman AG, Goodman LS, Rall TW, Murad F: The Pharmacologic Basis of Therapeutics, 7th ed, New York, Macmillan, 1985.

Gnegy ME, Uzunov P, Costa E: Participation of an endogenous Ca2+ binding protein activator in the development of drug induced supersensitivity of striatal dopamine receptors. J Pharmacol Exp Ther 202:558–564, 1977.

Goeders NE, Smith JE: Cortical dopaminergic involvement in cocaine reinforcement. Science 221:773–775, 1983.

Goeders NE, Smith JE: 6-(OH)-Dopamine lesions of medial prefrontal cortex on intracranial cocaine self-administration. Soc Neurosci Abstr 10:1206, 1984.

Gold MS, Pottash HL, Annitto WJ, Verebey K, Sweeney DR: Cocaine withdrawal: efficacy of tyrosine (abstract). Soc Neurosci 157:1983.

Gordon A. Insanities caused by acute and chronic intoxication with opium and cocaine. A study of 171 cases. JAMA 51:97–101, 1908, in Cocaine—Summaries of Psychosocial Research, Rockville, MD, NIDA, 1976, pp 68–69.

Hadfield MG, Nugent EA: Cocaine: comparative effect on dopamine uptake in extrapyramidal and limbic systems. Biochem Pharmacol 32:744–746, 1983.

Hammond WA: A volunteer paper. Trans Med Soc Virginia, November 1887, pp 212–226, in Byck R, ed: Cocaine Papers by Sigmund Freud, New York, Stonehill Publishing, 1974, pp 177–193.

Hawks RL, Kopin IJ, Colburn RW, Thoa NB: Norcocaine: a pharmacologically active metabolite of cocaine found in brain. Life Sci 15:2189–2195, 1974.

Hisayama T, Takayanagi I, Kasuya Y: Effects of cocaine on Ca-mobility in microsomal fraction from rat vas deferens. Jpn J Pharmacol 31:1–6, 1981.

Huang D, Wilson MC: The effects of DL-cathinone, D-amphetamine and cocaine on avoidance responding in rats and their interactions with haloperidol and methysergide. Pharmacol Biochem Behav 20:721–729, 1984.

Javaid JI, Fischman MW, Schuster CR, Dekirmenjian H, Davis JM: Cocaine plasma concentration: relation to physiological and subjective effects in humans. Science 202:227–228, 1978.

Johanson CE: Assessment of the dependence potential of cocaine in animals. NIDA Monogr 50:54–71, 1984.

Johanson CE, Aigner T: Comparison of the reinforcing properties of cocaine and procaine in rhesus monkeys. Pharmacol Biochem Behav 15:49–53, 1981.

Jonsson S, O'Meara M, Young JB: Acute cocaine poisoning. Importance of treating seizures and acidosis. Am J Med 75:1061–1064, 1983.

Just WW, Grafenburg L, Thel S, Werner G: Comparative metabolic, autoradiographic and pharmacologic studies of cocaine and its metabolite norcocaine. Naunyn-Schmiedeberg's Arch Pharmacol 293:221, 1976.

Karpen JW, Aoshima H, Abood LG, Hess GP: Cocaine and phencyclidine inhibition of the acetylcholine receptor: analysis of the mechanisms of action based on measurements of ion, flux in the millisecond-to-minute time region. Proc Natl Acad Sci USA 79:2509-2513, 1982.

Kennedy LT, Hanbauer I: Sodium-sensitive cocaine binding to rat striatal membrane: possible relationship to dopamine uptake sites. J Neurochem 41:172-178, 1983.

Khantzian EJ: Cocaine dependence, an extreme case and marked improvement with methyphenidate treatment. Am J Psychiatry 140:784-785, 1983.

Khantzian EJ, Gawin FH, Riordan C, Kleber HD: Methylphenidate treatment in cocaine abuse—a preliminary report. J Substance Abuse Treat 1:107-112, 1984.

Kleber, HD, Gawin FH: Cocaine abuse: a review of current and experimental treatments. NIDA monogr 50:111-129, 1984a.

Kleber HD, Gawin FH: The spectrum of cocaine abuse and its treatment. J Clin Psychiatry 45:18-23, 1984b.

Klein DF: Personal communication to E Nunes, 1986.

Klein DF, Gittelman R, Quitkin F, Rifkin A: Theoretical inferences concerning clinical groupings and psychotropic drugs, in Diagnosis and Drug Treatment of Psychiatric Disorders, 2nd ed, Baltimore and London, Williams & Wilkins, 1980, pp 793-818.

Knapp S, Mandell AJ: Narcotic drugs: effects on the serotonin biosynthetic systems of the brain. Science 177:1209-1211, 1972.

Langer SZ, Enero MA: The potentiation of responses to adrenergic nerve stimulation in the presence of cocaine: its relationship to the metabolic fate of released norepinephrine. J Pharmacol Exp Ther 191:431-443, 1974.

Liebowitz MR, Quitkin FM, Stewart JW, et al: Phenelzine versus imipramine in atypical depression: a preliminary report. Arch Gen Psychiatry 41:669-677, 1984.

Lindemann E, Malamud W: Experimental analysis of the psychopathological effects of intoxicating drugs. Am J Psychiatry, 90:853-881, 1933/1934, in Cocaine—Summaries of Psychosocial Research, Rockville, MD, NIDA, 1976, pp 79-81.

Mandell AJ, Knapp S: Regulation of serotonin biosynthesis in brain: role of the high affinity uptake of tryptophan into serotonergic neurons. Fed Proc 36:2142-2148, 1977.

Mandell AJ, Knapp S: Asymmetry and mood, emergent properties of serotonin regulation; a proposed mechanism of action of lithium. Arch Gen Psychiatry 36:909-916, 1979.

Matthews JC, Collins A: Interactions of cocaine and cocaine congeners with sodium channels. Biochem Pharmacol 32:455-460, 1983.

McCarley R: REM sleep and depression: common neurobiological control mechanisms. Am J Psychiatry 139:565, 1982.

Memo M, Pradhan S, Hanbauer I: Cocaine-induced supersensitivity of striatal dopamine receptors: role of endogenous calmodulin. Neuropharmacology 20:1145-1150, 1981.

Muscholl E: Effect of cocaine and related drugs on the uptake of noradrenaline by heart and spleen. Br J Pharmacol 16:352-359, 1961.

Myers JA, Earnest MP: Generalized seizures and cocaine abuse. Neurology (New York) 34:675-676, 1984.

Nahas G: A calcium channel blocker as antidote to the cardiac effects of cocaine intoxication. N Engl J Med 313:519-520, 1985.

Nanji AA, Filipenko JD: Asystole and ventricular fibrillation associated with cocaine intoxication. Chest 85:132-133, 1984.

Negrete JC, Murphy HBM: Psychological deficits in chewers of coca leaf. Bull Narcotics 19: 11-17, 1967, in Cocaine—Summaries of Psychosocial Research, Rockville, MD, NIDA, 1976, pp 93-95.

NIDA: Cocaine—Summaries of Psychosocial Research, Rockville, MD, National Institute of Drug Abuse (NIDA), 1976.

Nunes E: Treatment of cocaine abuse: a case series and review of the literature. Paper presented at the Taylor Manor Psychiatric Symposium, Ellicott City, MD, Sept. 28, 1985.

Nunes E, Quitkin F, Rosecan J: Psychiatric diagnosis in cocaine abuse: evidence for biological heterogeneity. Paper presented at British Association of Psychopharmacology, Summer Meeting, Cambridge, England, July 14, 1986.

Ortiz VZ: Modificaciones psicologicas y fisiologicas producidas por la coca y la cocaina en los coqueros. Rev Med Exp 3:132–161, 1944.

Owens WD: Signs and Symptoms presented by those addicted to cocaine. JAMA 58:329–330, 1912, in Cocaine—Summaries of Psychosocial Research, Rockville, MD, NIDA, 1976, pp 74–75.

Perez-Reyes M, DiGuiseppi S, Ondrusek G, Jeffcoat AR, Cook CE: Free-base cocaine smoking. Clin Pharmacol Ther 32:459–465, 1982.

Petersen RC: History of cocaine. NIDA Res Monogr Ser 13:17–34, 1977.

Post RM, Contel NR: Human and animal studies of cocaine: implications for development of behavioral pathology, in Creese I, ed.: Stimulants: Neurochemical, Behavioral, and Clinical Perspectives, New York, Raven Press, 1983, pp 169–203.

Post RM, Kotin J, Goodwin FK: The effects of cocaine on depressed patients. Am J Psychiatry 131:511–517, 1974.

Post RM, Contel NR, Gold PW: Impaired behavioral sensitization to cocaine in vasopressin deficient rats. Live Sci 31:2745–2750, 1982.

Post RM, Weiss RB, Pert A: Differential effects of carbamazepine and lithium on sensitization and kindling. Prog Neuro-Psychopharmacol Biol Psychiatry 8:425–434, 1984.

Pradhan S: Effect of cocaine on rat brain enzymes. Arch Int Pharmacodyn 226:221–228, 1983.

Pradhan S, Roy SN, Pradhan SN: Correlation of behavioral and neurochemical effects of acute administration of cocaine in rats. Life Sci 22:1737–1744, 1978a.

Pradhan SN, Battatchargya AK, Pradhan S: Serotonergic manipulation of the behavioral effects of cocaine in rats. Commun Psychopharmacol 2:481–486, 1978b.

Rappolt RT, Gay GR, Inaba DS: Propranalol: a specific antagonist to cocaine. Clin Toxicol 10:265–271, 1977.

Rasmussen H: The calcium messenger system, I. N Engl J Med 314:1094–1101, 1986a.

Rasmussen H: The calcium messenger system. II. N Engl J Med 314:1164–1170, 1986b.

Reith MEA, Sershen H, Lajtha A: Endogenous peptide(s) inhibiting (3H)cocaine binding in mouse brain. Neurochem Res 5:1291–1299, 1980.

Reith MEA, Allen DL, Sershen H, Lajtha A: Similarities and differences between high-affinity binding sites for cocaine and imipramine in mouse cerebral cortex. J Neurochem 43:249–255, 1984.

Reith MEA, Meisler BE, Sershen H, Lajtha A: Sodium-independent binding of (3H)cocaine in mouse striatum is serotonin related. Brain Res 342:145–148, 1985.

Resnick RB, Kestenbaum RS, Schwartz LK: Acute systemic effects of cocaine in man: a controlled study by intranasal and intravenous routes. Science 195:696–698, 1977a.

Resnick RB, Washton AM, LaPlaca RW, Stone-Washton N: Lithium carbonate as a potential treatment for compulsive cocaine use: a preliminary report. Read before the 32nd Annual Convention and Scientific Meeting of the Society of Biological Psychiatry, Toronto, April 28, 1977b, cited in Gawin & Kleber, 1984.

Roberts DC, Vickers G: Atypical neuroleptics increase self-administration of cocaine: an evaluation of a behavioral screen for antipsychotic activity. Psychopharmacology (Berlin) 82:135–139, 1984.

Roberts DC, Corcoran ME, Fibiger HC: On the role of ascending catecholaminergic systems in intravenous self-administration of cocaine. Pharmacol Biochem Behav 6:615–620, 1977.

Roberts DCS, Koob GF, Klonoff P: Extinction and recovery of cocaine self-administration following 6-(OH)-dopamine lesions of the nucleus accumbens. Pharmacol Biochem Behav 12:781–787, 1979.

Rosecan JS: The treatment of cocaine abuse with imipramine, L-tyrosine, and L-tryptophan. Paper presented at the VII World Congress of Psychiatry, Vienna, July 14, 1983.

Rosecan JS, Klein DF: Imipramine blockade of cocaine euphoria with double-blind challenge. Presented at the 139th Annual Meeting of the American Psychiatric Association, Washington DC, May 10–16, 1986.

Ross SB, Renyi AL: Uptake of some tritiated amines by mouse brain cortex slices in vitro.

Acta Pharmacol Toxicol 24:297–309, 1966.

Ross SB, Renyi AL: Inhibition of the uptake of tritiated catecholamines by antidepressant and related agents. Eur J Pharmacol 2:181–186, 1967.

Ross SB, Renyi AL: Inhibition of the uptake of 5-hydroxytryptamine in brain tissue. Eur J Pharmacol 7:270–277, 1969.

Rowbotham MC, Jones RT, Benowitz NL, Jacob P: Trazadone—oral cocaine interactions. Arch Gen Psychiatry 41:895–899, 1984.

Sabelli HC, Fawcett J, Gusovsky F, et al: Clinical studies on the phenylethylamine hypothesis of affective disorder: urine and blood phenylacetic acid and phenylalanine dietary supplements. J Clin Psychiatry 47:66–70, 1986.

Schachne JS, Roberts BH, Thompson PD: Coronary artery spasm and myocardial infarction associated with cocaine use (letter). N Engl J Med 75:1061–1064, 1983.

Scheel-Kruger J, Baestrup C, Nielson M, Golembrowska K, Mogilnicka E: Cocaine: discussion on the role of dopamine in the biochemical mechanism of action, in Ellinwood EH, Kilbey MM, eds: Cocaine and Other Stimulants, New York, London, Plenum Press, 1975, pp 373–407.

Schubert J, Fryo B, Nyback H, Sedvall G: Effects of cocaine and amphetamine on the metabolism of tryptophan and 5-hydroxytryptamine in mouse brain in vivo. J Pharm Pharmacol 22:860–862, 1970.

Shannon HE, Degregorio CM: Self-administration of the endogenous trace amines beta-phenylethylamine, N-methyl phenylethylamine and phenylethanolamine in dogs. J Pharmacol Exp Ther 222:52–60, 1982.

Siever LJ, Davis KL: Overview: toward a dysregulation hypothesis of depression. Am J Psychiatry 142:1017–1031, 1985.

Small GW, Purcell JJ: Trazadone and cocaine abuse. Arch Gen Psychiatry 42:524, 1985.

Smith DE: Diagnostic, treatment, and aftercare approaches to cocaine abuse. J Subst Abuse Treat 1:5–9, 1984.

Taylor D, Ho BT: Neurochemical effects of cocaine following acute and repeated injection. J Neurosci Res 3:95–101, 1977.

Taylor D, Ho BT: Comparison of inhibition of monoamine uptake by cocaine, methylphenidate and amphetamine. Res Commun Chem Pathol Pharmacol 21:67–75, 1978.

Taylor DL, Beng TH, Fagan JD: Increased dopamine receptor binding in rat brain by repeated cocaine injections. Commun Psychopharmacol 3:137–142, 1979.

Tennant FS: Effect of cocaine dependence on plasma phenylalanine and tyrosine levels and on urinary MHPG excretion. Am J Psychiatry 142:1200–1201, 1985.

Tennant FS, Rawson RA: Cocaine and amphetamine dependence treated with desipramine. NIDA Res Monogr Ser 43:351–355, 1983.

Tennant FS, Tarver AL: Double-blind comparison of desipramine and placebo in withdrawal from cocaine dependence. NIDA Res Monogr Ser 55:159–163, 1984.

Van Dyck C, Ungerer J, Jatlow P, Barash P, Byck R: Intranasal cocaine: dose relationships of psychological effects and plasma levels. Int J Psychiatry Med 12:1–13, 1982.

Weiss, RD, Mirin SM, Michael JL: Psychopathology in chronic cocaine abusers. Paper presented at American Psychiatric Association, Annual Meeting, New York, May 1983.

Weiss RD, Pope HG, Mirin SM: Treatment of chronic cocaine abuse and attention deficit disorder, residual type, with magnesium pemoline. Drug Alcohol Depend 15:69–72, 1985.

Whitby LG, Hertting G, Axelrod J: Effect of cocaine on the disposition of noradrenaline labelled with tritium. Nature 187:604–605, 1960.

Wise RA: Neural mechanisms of the reinforcing action of cocaine. NIDA Res Monogr Ser 50:15–33, 1984.

Woolverton WL, Balster RL: Effects of antipsychotic compounds in rhesus monkeys given a choice between cocaine and food. Drug Alcohol Depend 8:69–78, 1981.

Zito KA, Vickers G, Roberts DC: Disruption of cocaine and heroin self-administration following kainic acid lesions of the nucleus accumbens. Pharmacol Biochem Behav 23:1029–1036, 1985.

III

Treatment Issues

Chapter 4

Overview of Cocaine Abuse Treatment

Henry I. Spitz, M.D.,
and Jeffrey S. Rosecan, M.D.

The treatment of the cocaine-abusing patient presents a challenge to the clinician. Many variables must be taken into account in order to provide effective and comprehensive management of the problem. Prominent in this regard are treatment planning decisions which encompass individual, intrapsychic, environmental, familial, and pharmacological considerations.

To date, no definitive treatment for cocaine abuse exists about which there is general consensus in the literature. There are, however, many promising and some well-documented efforts that address central concerns related to the resolution of cocaine abuse problems. This chapter will provide an overview of the psychological and biological treatment strategies currently available to the practitioner.

CLINICAL CONSIDERATIONS

Definition of the Problem

Prior to embarking on a treatment plan, the clinician must be clear about the nature of the condition to be treated, its severity, and the optimal timing of the treatment intervention. A natural starting point for this process centers on obtaining clarity in the definition of the disorder. The essential feature of cocaine abuse has been characterized by the *Diagnostic and Statistical Manual* (DSM-III) of the American Psychiatric Association (1980) as: "a pathological pattern of use for at least one month that causes impairment in social or occupational functioning." Additionally, elements such as repetitive use, daytime intoxication, and episodes of cocaine overdosage are regarded as central to the definition of the disorder. Negative intrusion into the work, friendship, familial, or legal spheres is also a prominent sequela of excessive cocaine use. Duration of disturbance of a prolonged period, months or years, is a frequent accompanying finding.

Kleber (1974) initially defined drug abuse in general as "the nonprescription use of psychoactive chemicals by an individual to alter his/her psychological state in a situation in which the individual or society incurs some harm." Later, Kleber and Gawin (1984a) applied this definition to cocaine use in particular and broadened it to help define those cocaine users who were in need of treatment. They suggested that any cocaine user who finds that he/she cannot stop or significantly cut back his/her drug use, in spite of the presence of problems arising from the use, meets the criteria for a person needing outside intervention.

Grinspoon and Bakalar (1985) have reviewed the problems inherent in trying to formulate an acceptable definition of cocaine abuse. They cite the World Health Organization definition of "drug dependence of the cocaine type" as representative of the type of broad definition which, while attempting to be comprehensive in scope, leaves itself open to criticism from scientific, social, research, and other groups.

The WHO defines cocaine dependence as

> a state arising from repeated administration of cocaine or an agent with cocaine-like properties, on a periodic or continuous basis. Its characteristics include:
>
> 1) An overpowering desire or need to continue taking the drug and to obtain it by any means;
>
> 2) Absence of tolerance to the effects of the drug during continued administration; in the more frequent periodic use, the drug may be taken at short intervals, resulting in the build up of an intense toxic reaction;
>
> 3) A psychic dependence on the effects of the drug related to a subjective and individual appreciation of these effects; and
>
> 4) Absence of physical dependence and hence absence of an ab-

stinence syndrome on abrupt withdrawal; withdrawal is attended by a psychic disturbance manifested by craving for the drug. (p. 185)

One problem hindering the process of creating an acceptable definition of cocaine abuse rests with the difficulties involved in automatically transferring notions used for other abused substances, opioids, barbiturates, and alcohol, directly to cocaine use. A well-known example of this dilemma is found in the debate about the presence of a true withdrawal state, a condition deemed essential for historical definitions of drugs of addiction, and whether or not it exists in the classical sense for cocaine.

The current animal and human research literature does not describe withdrawal syndromes in the traditional sense, yet other properties of cocaine use, most importantly the postcocaine "crash" period and its physiological and psychological concomitants, suggest that cocaine actively exerts effects of a powerful sort similar to those of other drugs of addiction. Supporting data for the abuse potential of cocaine are also found in research and clinical studies that report the power and intensity of the craving for cocaine found in human and animal users.

It appears at this time that consensus exists regarding cocaine's potency, abuse potential, and appeal for the user and that the dispute surrounding the definition of the disorder lies less with disagreement about the properties of the drug per se and more with the quest to find appropriate, acceptable, and current modes of classification for the varied psychological and physiological states found among cocaine users.

Concepts of tolerance, dependence, withdrawal, and addiction are being reevaluated in light of the rapidly emerging research and clinical experience with cocaine. The present plans for revision of the criteria for cocaine abuse in the DSM-III-R (revised edition) typify an effort to update antiquated substance abuse constructs into clinically utilitarian definitions based on concepts of drug dependence highlighting the salient phenomenological and behavioral manifestations of excessive psychoactive substance use.

In summary, all current definitions of cocaine abuse are broad enough to include a heterogeneous mixture of cocaine abusers. The task of translating any definition into clinically useful form is aided considerably by the addition of at least two other critical dimensions of cocaine use. Clinical experience suggests that an understanding of the route of administration of cocaine and of the pattern of cocaine use aids the clinician in designing a treatment plan for an individual with a cocaine problem.

Cocaine Usage Issues

Although much has been written about the route of cocaine administration and its relationship to the development of subsequent dependence on the drug, Kleber and Gawin (1984b) aptly note that "severe
cocaine abuse can develop with any route of administration."

Forms of cocaine use

The most popular use of cocaine occurs by intranasal "snorting" or
sniffing cocaine powder, thereby bringing it into contact with the highly
vascular mucous membranes that line the nasopharynx. Absorption of
cocaine by this route of administration produces its effects rapidly, but
they ebb in a relatively short time, making repeated administration of the
drug necessary to sustain or recreate its effects. Long-term usage by this
route results in significant irritation and/or damage to the internal structure of the nose and often prompts the cocaine user to search for alternative methods of taking the drug into his system.

"Freebasing," another commonly encountered method by which cocaine is abused, is inhalation of the vapors produced by heating the
cocaine hydrochloride salt and thereby releasing the more powerful free
cocaine base. The latter is smoked in a water pipe and produces rapid
and intense physiological effects which more closely parallel the effects
of intravenous, rather than intranasal, cocaine administration. "Crack," a
form of powerful cocaine that can be smoked directly without the elabo-
rate preparations necessary for freebasing, is rapidly increasing as a form
of cocaine use. Adults as well as adolescents use crack, but its ready
availability and reduced cost make it appealing to an adolescent population within which its use is spreading dramatically.

Freebasing cocaine carries with it the risk of intense craving for the
drug, thereby contributing to the problem of escalating use or "binging"
by cocaine users. Most authorities agree that freebasing methods often
lead to a progressive problem of intensified compulsive cocaine use accompanied by negative individual and interpersonal consequences.
Physical hazards, including lung irritation and potential damage, are
associated with freebasing methods. Intravenous cocaine use is a less
common, but significant form of cocaine administration. Often cocaine is
combined with heroin ("speedballing") in an attempt to offset some of
the deleterious consequences of crashing from cocaine. The physiological and psychological effects of intravenous cocaine use are immediate
and powerful. Changes in cardiovascular function, as well as reports of

euphoria, elation, and an intense "rush," are frequently reported phenomena.

Generally, the heightened sensations following cocaine injection are short-lived (minutes), and if cocaine is not readministered, an intense crash, characterized by dysphoria, irritability, gastrointestinal symptoms, and other unpleasant experiences, ensues. The generic risks of intravenous injection of any impure foreign substance apply to street cocaine as well. Endocarditis, hepatitis, AIDS, and local infection are prominent examples of health problems linked to intravenous cocaine use.

Although cocaine may be ingested orally or applied topically, these are less common forms of drug use and usually are employed for reasons other than "getting high." The local anesthetic effect of cocaine may result in topical genital application as part of the sexual repertoire of some cocaine users.

Patterns of use

Cocaine may be used in varied forms to achieve a variety of goals. In addition to understanding the properties of the drug and its physiological effects, it is helpful to appreciate the problem of use employed by any individual cocaine user.

Resnick and Resnick (1984) and Siegel (1982) proposed clinically useful classification schemes for determining the degree to which an individual uses or abuses cocaine. Adapting the categories proposed by the National Commission on Marijuana and Drug Abuse, they were able to delineate five major cocaine use patterns: experimental, recreational, circumstantial, intensified, and compulsive.

Experimental cocaine use is, as the name implies, a periodic use pattern and is not necessarily limited to cocaine. Adolescents, for example, who are notorious for experimentation with psychoactive drugs of all kinds, may use cocaine as part of the process of polysubstance drug use over time.

Recreational users outnumber all other types of cocaine users. They parallel social drinkers and are in control of their consumption of cocaine. Drug-taking behavior is limited and rarely progresses to heavier use. The major reasons for cocaine use in this group are as a social lubricant and for the direct stimulant properties of the drug itself.

Patterns of circumstantial use involve taking cocaine only under certain conditions or in a particular context and not at times other than these. A Vietnam veteran described circumstantial cocaine use limited to combat experiences only.

Intensified cocaine use has a regular pattern of intranasal use on a daily basis in amounts that usually do not result in altered consciousness, or impaired work or social function.

When cocaine use reaches the point that the drug becomes the organizing concept in one's life, the pattern is considered to be compulsive in nature. Negative spillover into social, vocational, physical, and psychological spheres is prominent. The amount of cocaine used, its frequency and duration of use, and the concomitant expense incurred all are increased to a point beyond which the individual can effectively manage.

Psychological diagnostic issues

A third dimension in the comprehensive evaluation of the cocaine user is the issue of psychiatric diagnosis. Since formal issues of DSM-III diagnosis will be discussed in Chapter 5, at this point some clinically relevant aspects of diagnosis as they relate to treatment planning for the cocaine abuser will be highlighted.

Khantzian (1985a,b) is a proponent of the self-medication hypothesis of cocaine use. His thesis is that the use of cocaine as the drug of choice by drug-dependent individuals is "the result of an interaction between the psychopharmacologic action of the drug and the dominant, powerful feelings with which they struggle." In his view, the interest in cocaine on the part of drug-dependent cocaine users is no mere accident but, rather, rests largely on the properties of cocaine that "relieve distress associated with depression, hypomania and hyperactivity."

The self-medication hypothesis suggests that cocaine-dependent individuals are trying to achieve a state of emotional balance with mood normalization, increased energy and activity levels, and reduction of tension stemming from unpleasant inner emotional states.

This hypothesis has had limited systematized scientific study, but clinical and empirical data are persuasive of its validity. The prominence of affective disorders in cocaine-abusing patient populations and the emergency reports of successful treatment of cocaine abusers with therapeutically prescribed medication (tricyclic antidepressants [TCIs], and lithium) support the self-medication point of view.

Attention deficit disorders (Gawin & Kleber, 1984) and states of hyperactivity form another related area of exploration which dovetails with the self-medication hypothesis for individuals who select cocaine as their preferred drug, apparently in an effort to "treat" their emotional problems.

Present and future research into the neurochemical mechanisms for cocaine's effect on the brain and behavior will shed light on this intriguing hypothesis. For clinical purposes, awareness of the self-medication hypothesis dictates that thorough diagnostic evaluation is the cornerstone of the initial phase of cocaine abuse treatment.

Accurate diagnosis is desirable, but it is not always easy to achieve. Clinical wisdom warns against the tendency to make definitive diagnoses of conditions other than drug abuse during the acute phase of the process. The combination of the behavioral and physiological effects of cocaine makes it extremely difficult to obtain a representative picture of what the cocaine user looks like while not in the throes of active drug use.

Part of the diagnostic assessment should therefore include attention to the issue of the time at which the cocaine user seeks treatment. An appreciation of what point along the cocaine use-to-abuse continuum an individual is encountered is extremely helpful in making a thoughtful assessment and treatment plan. The regularity of depressive episodes during varying stages of cessation of cocaine use is a common example of a point of potential confusion between a cocaine-induced symptom that may be drug related versus a manifestation of underlying significant affective disorders, perhaps accentuated or amplified during the period of early cessation of cocaine use.

In a similar vein, states of excitement, euphoria, and increased activity must be carefully evaluated and observed over time to help differentiate between a state of cocaine intoxication related to active drug use, which will subside with time, and a hypomanic or manic phase of a major affective disorder, which may be a more long-standing primary diagnostic issue.

The phenomenology associated with the varied stages of cocaine use presents a complex set of diagnostic issues. The widely recognized problems of disinhibition, delusional thinking, transient psychotic behavior, intense suicidal ideation, sleep abnormalities, paranoia, poor judgment, and many others require that the diagnostic evaluation of the cocaine user be done thoughtfully and comprehensively, with an awareness of the potential pitfalls in the process.

The role of diagnosis and evaluation of cocaine abusers in the sequencing of events in the total treatment plan will be addressed later in this chapter.

GENERAL PRINCIPLES OF TREATMENT

Prior to any description of the specific forms of cocaine abuse treatment currently in use, some general principles of evaluation and treatment should be mentioned. Thus far, the need for the clinician to have a firm grounding in the understanding of cocaine and its effects has been emphasized. In so doing, a point is reached where a cocaine-dependent person is clearly in need of treatment, and decisions regarding an optimum individualized plan become the clinician's primary task.

Determination of Treatment Priorities

Several authors have presented general guidelines that are helpful in this endeavor. Millman (1986) states that "appropriate treatment depends not only upon the characterization of the specific drugs and their patterns of use in each patient, but on an understanding of the psychological set and situations attendant to these behavior patterns as well. The nature of the drug-induced psychoactive effects as well as the presence of abstinence phenomena should be evaluated." (p. 123) His conceptualization of substance abuse treatment is a two-stage process, with the early phase aimed at induction into treatment and achieving greater distance from the drug of abuse and a later stage designed to keep the former user in a state of abstinence.

Blume (1984), in discussing treatment considerations for alcoholism, echoes these principles and amplifies them in outlining the components of effective treatment programs for alcoholics. This model may be readily adapted to meet the general requirements of the cocaine-abusing population as well. The first phase of treatment centers around identification of the problem and making an initial intervention with the goal of helping the abuser recognize that a problem exists and that he/she is in need of treatment. Efforts in this stage are directed at countering the denial mechanisms so prominently displayed by substance abuse patients.

Following induction into a treatment process, detoxification becomes the guiding principle of the second phase. Helping the cocaine-dependent person achieve safe and rapid distance from the drug forms the basis for the methods employed during this stage. This closely parallels Gold's (1983) treatment philosophy, which emphasizes getting "the addictive disease under control first." His view requires that drug-seeking and drug-taking behavior must cease and that psychotherapy should not begin until the compulsive drug use is effectively stopped.

Once detoxification is complete, treatment concerns itself with a host of rehabilitative goals. This phase usually constitutes the bulk of the therapeutic process and forms the point in the process during which most psychotherapy takes place. Therapeutic interventions attempt to educate patients and families about cocaine abuse, its risks, and its consequences. Acquisition of insight into the cocaine user's motivation for drug use and efforts to develop alternate means of coping with life issues without resorting to drug use are important initial treatment goals.

A restorative or recuperative aspect of the program includes rehabilitation strategies designed to help repair physical and practical damage accumulated during the course of protracted cocaine use. On the physical level, neglected medical, nutritional, and dental problems receive proper attention. The by-products of excessive, chronic cocaine use, which inevitably complicate the life of the user, also become a central treatment focus during the rehabilitative phase. Practical issues of finances, including plans for current control of money, repayment of debts acquired during periods of serious abuse, and similar concerns typify the kinds of "repair" efforts undertaken during this phase.

Three other important treatment issues receive attention at this point: (1) relapse management, (2) family involvement, and (3) life-style changes. Contingency plans for management of relapses or "slips," during which the patient resumes cocaine use to any degree, must be anticipated. Plans for the management of cocaine use during treatment cover emergency plans, decisions regarding possible hospitalization, and preventive plans. The latter acknowledges the tendency for older, well-established drug-taking behavior to occasionally override newer strategies acquired through therapeutic approaches, resulting in episodic cocaine use or in "runs" or "binges" of cocaine use.

One of the frequently employed safeguards in this process is the use of drug screening of urine samples to test for current cocaine use. Whether routine or random methods of urine testing are utilized, the tests offer an objective method of monitoring progress during critical phases of rehabilitation and recovery.

Family involvement proceeds actively in this phase of treatment. Direct involvement of family members in formal marital or family therapy sessions may become a regular part of treatment. The family as a resource in the rehabilitative process or as an alternative to hospitalization may be utilized by having selected adult cocaine users return to live with the family as an interim measure. Cocaine abusers who have financial and housing problems and those who have families who can help the patient manage his/her money may find that a temporary stay with the family serves some useful function. Short-term relief from financial pressure, the ability to repair damaged family ties, and the provision of a nurturing atmosphere often help during the early phase of trying to stay away from established patterns that led to drug taking.

This type of family involvement must be carefully considered and recommended only when the rewards of the short-term plan outweigh the risks of returning a drug user to a dysfunctional family, which may itself be critical to the genesis and maintenance of the substance abuse problem in the first place.

Third, life-style changes are invariably necessary for cocaine abusers to successfully give up the drug completely. In some instances, radical life-style changes are necessary. Not only must cocaine-abusing patients disconnect from their drug-using interpersonal network, but often the changes required extend into career and family issues as well. It is not uncommon to see cocaine users who are highly motivated to give up the drug make career changes out of fields in which exposure to cocaine is rampant into other aspects of their fields or to change fields entirely. One such patient felt that the rock music world in which she worked made access to cocaine virtually unavoidable. She returned to school to train for business, a second career at which she became successful.

The final phase of treatment addresses the longer-term needs of the former substance abuser. Relapse prevention and the reinforcement of positive gains form the mainstays of this treatment phase. The methods developed during the rehabilitative phase are extended into this phase, and strategies for maintaining and solidifying gains made in treatment are strengthened. Self-help groups are an example of a longer-term experience that helps greatly in this effort.

Provisions for follow-up and plans for contact with formal treatment programs or personnel are explicitly structured during this period to help ensure maximum prospects for drug-free living.

Determination of the sequence of events in treatment is a major consideration for clinicians involved in working with cocaine-dependent patients. The principles outlined thus far reflect general guidelines deemed useful in designing a patient-specific treatment plan. Flexibility in adapting, modifying, emphasizing, or expanding any aspects of the guidelines recommended thus far is regarded as desirable, since no universally accepted treatment method exists. The clinician ultimately must select and combine elements from currently available treatment resources that most aptly fit the unique needs of an individual who no longer desires to be dependent on cocaine.

FORMS OF COCAINE ABUSE TREATMENT

Successful cocaine abuse treatment requires an integrated approach which offers maximum options for positive change to the patient. Collaboration among participants in the treatment team is the guiding principle in effectively combining the best aspects of diverse sources of help in this endeavor. The welfare of the cocaine user suffers when competitive interdisciplinary issues, self-help versus professional mental health, or preferences for specific forms of treatment, individual versus group, psychopharmacological versus psychotherapeutic, and the like, intrude into the process. When, however, all those involved in the treatment plan are in agreement about their roles and a clearly formulated treatment plan is directed by a knowledgeable clinician, the chances for success are maximized considerably.

The general principles of treatment delineated earlier in this chapter serve as an outline for substance abuse treatment. In order to proceed from general principles to a definitive individual treatment plan, one must be familiar with the major forms of intervention in the cocaine abuse field. For classification purposes, treatment may be grouped into the following categories: preventive/educational, inpatient, individual, group, family, and psychopharmacological.

Preventive/Educational Therapy

In principle, prevention provides the ideal first line of defense against any medical or mental health problem. In reality, epidemological data suggest that cocaine use, both recreationally and to excess, has been on the increase. One conclusion drawn from these observations is that traditional methods of prevention may be antiquated or ineffective and that if prevention is to be successful, newer methods are required.

Millman (1986) has reviewed the problem and cites some important findings about the state of preventive approaches to substance abuse. Prominent in this regard is the idea that one reason for disappointing results with preventive approaches to date has been an excessive reliance on the belief that education and scare tactics alone would be sufficient deterrents to drug use. Programs of this sort, often aimed at adolescent audiences, are characterized by large educational components which orient people (teenagers) to the properties of drugs, their physiological and psychological effects, the societal and peer pressure involved, and the deleterious consequences of excessive use.

The use of newer preventive methods based on the concept of substance abuse as a "socially learned, normative, purposive and functional behavior" emphasize the teaching of techniques to help resist the pressures that propel people toward drug use. A corollary to this orientation accepts that limited drug use is a fact of life among contemporary adolescents and aims at teaching methods for containing, limiting, and controlling drug use. Since this point of view considers experimental drug use virtually inevitable among teenagers, it focuses on reduction of negative sequelae of drug taking and/or the presentation of drug-free alternatives for the acquisition of pleasure, self-esteem, peer acceptance, and other issues central to this phase of development in a young person's life.

Innovative preventive and educational approaches play an essential part in the overall cocaine abuse problem. Further study is needed to evaluate the key elements of prevention programs that show promise and efficacy. Work of this sort is a welcome trend and is likely to result in preventive models of intervention that will be influential in reducing the magnitude of the cocaine abuse problem.

Inpatient Treatment

Hospitalization of cocaine abusers is a critical decision in treatment planning. The role of hospitalization differs somewhat from its place in the treatment of alcoholism or heroin addiction insofar as withdrawal from cocaine can be managed on an outpatient basis in many cases. The question logically arises as to when, and under what circumstances, the cocaine user requires hospitalization.

Washton (1985) sees the role of the hospital as being influential initially for the cocaine user who cannot break the pattern of compulsive use. Hospitalization during this phase is designed to interrupt a downward course of drug abuse and to facilitate attainment of a stabilization period for the cocaine user. The function of hospitalization is akin to the model of crisis intervention in other situations that require active punctuation of deteriorating individual, familial, or social patterns to avert further damage.

Authorities in the field tend to agree that although hospitalization plays an important role in cocaine abuse treatment at specific times, it is rarely the place where the entire treatment program takes place. Consensus exists that the ultimate goal of brief or lengthy hospitalization is to return the cocaine user to the world outside the hospital where the pressures to use cocaine must be faced realistically. Successful hospital admission helps pave the way for this process with many individuals.

The indications for hospitalization have been widely discussed in the literature (Millman, 1986; Kleber & Gawin, 1986; Washton, 1985). Millman (1986, pp. 129–130) has consolidated the indications for hospitalization of substance abusers into six primary areas:

1. *"The inability to terminate drug use despite outpatient maneuvers."* Heavy users, including chronic freebasers and intravenous users, have significant difficulty in giving up drug use and can benefit from an

inpatient program. Even highly motivated cocaine users may encounter profound difficulty in remaining abstinent from cocaine. Easy access to the drug, peer or familial pressures that promote drug use, work climate in which drug use is the norm, and a host of other factors may contribute to realistic obstacles in the path of the cocaine user who is sincerely motivated to give up the drug. Hospitalization may be considered for individuals who fall into this category.

2. *"Medical or psychological symptoms that require close observation or treatment, such as psychotic states, severe depressive symptomatology, or extreme debilitation."* During different points in the spectrum of excessive cocaine use, physical and/or psychological crises may occur that are best managed in an inpatient setting. Active suicidal risk in the postcocaine crash period is perhaps the best-known illustration of this phenomenon. Transient psychotic states that require observation and possibly neuroleptic medication form the basis for the decision to hospitalize a patient in many cases. The use of the hospital to prevent harm to the cocaine user himself or to guard against his potential to harm others, as in times of intense paranoid states, is an accepted reason for brief hospitalizations.

3. *"The possibility of life-threatening withdrawal syndrome."* This applies more often to the withdrawal syndromes associated with severe alcoholism and heroin addiction. The after effects of abrupt cessation from cocaine, although not life-threatening, are far from benign and may, on occasion, provide the basis for conducting the detoxification phase in a hospital milieu. Additionally, since cocaine users often abuse alcohol or other drugs, the poly-drug abuse process is more easily managed in the hospital.

4. *"The absence of adequate psychosocial supports that might be mobilized to facilitate cessation of drug use, or a living situation that is powerfully reinforcing for continued drug abuse."* The interpersonal network in which the cocaine abuser is embedded must be carefully evaluated and at times is so pernicious as to require hospitalization as a safe haven from the converging forces that promote cocaine use.

5. *"The inability to enhance motivation or break through denial."* Hospitalization can be effectively utilized to get a patient engaged in effective drug abuse therapy. Inpatient drug education or psychotherapy groups help confront excessive denial by cocaine users as well as providing peer and staff support for positive efforts to remain drug free. The ability to reinforce healthy motivation can be intensified owing to the multiplicity of interactions with other patients and staff, which occur much more frequently on a daily basis as compared with outpatient treatment.

6. *"Repeated outpatient treatment failures."* The hospital is viewed as a "last resort" for the cocaine user who has been refractory to other efforts

short of hospitalization. Length of stay and related decisions are made at a later stage in these cases. The initial priority is to establish a baseline for treatment where the cocaine user will be able to avail himself of badly needed services for which outpatient plans have not sufficed.

Hospitalization, like many other aspects of comprehensive cocaine abuse treatment, calls for flexibility in decision making. Initial hospitalization to accelerate induction into treatment, brief inpatient stays to counter relapses, or long-term hospitalization in programs similar to therapeutic community formats all provide viable options for cocaine-abusing patients at different points in their clinical course.

Individual Psychotherapy

The general goals of the individual psychotherapies designed to treat cocaine-dependent patients cluster around several parameters: (1) the need to acknowledge and accept the injurious effects of cocaine and the need to stop using the drug; (2) the management of personal problems that lead to inability to control drug-taking behavior; (3) increasing awareness of and insight into the role that cocaine has played in the user's life; (4) creating practical channels for expression and resolution of psychological conflicts without resorting to drug use; (5) making lifestyle changes that move the individual away from the drug-abusing subculture; (6) understanding the settings, cues, and interpersonal circumstances that place the individual at risk to use cocaine; and (7) creating a treatment plan that is pragmatic, manageable, and has behavior change as its immediate goal and personality change as its longer-term focus.

The major forms of individual psychotherapy described in the literature to date include supportive, psychodynamic, and behavioral approaches (Gold, 1983). All these efforts emphasize careful evaluation prior to the start of psychotherapy. Evaluation includes assessment of motivation for treatment, a careful drug history, which notes adverse effects in particular, and a thorough neuropsychological assessment of each patient.

Some programs (Washton, 1985) suggest concretizing the issues of commitment to treatment through the use of written treatment contracts. These contracts specify that the patient will stay in treatment for a minimum of six months, consent to urine testing, enter the hospital when deemed necessary, stay abstinent from all psychoactive substances, and permit staff to contact appropriate family, work, or other important people in the cocaine user's life.

The supportive therapies concentrate on helping to educate the co-caine-using patient about the realities of cocaine and its consequences. Advice giving and management of practical issues such as finances and housing are examples of basic elements of supportive approaches. Clari-fication of the goals of treatment and the phases of the process are explained at the outset of therapy.

Blume (1984), in working with alcoholics, uses a cognitive format com-mon to many supportive approaches which explicates the disease model of drug dependency. In addition to the transmission of factual information about cocaine abuse, this method simultaneously addresses psychody-namic issues of excessive guilt and self-blame often found among sub-stance abusers. It helps facilitate self-disclosure in therapy by de-stigmatizing important aspects of drug use that patients often conceal because of shame or embarrassment. In this process, significant feelings emerge, and part of the goal of the supportive therapies is to help co-caine users develop an accurate language for recognition and identifica-tion (acknowledgment) of important feelings. Anxiety, depression, de-spair, guilt, and panic are but a few of the frequently experienced states of discomfort that are habitually numbed by cocaine use.

The line between supportive psychotherapy and psychodynamic ther-apy is impossible to define. Elements of effective psychotherapy are found in both techniques. Psychodynamic psychotherapy has goals that are perhaps more ambitious in aiming to alter personality traits, change self-concept, and effect attitudinal shifts of a permanent sort.

Many of the psychodynamic methods are predicated on an apprecia-tion of the personality issues common to substance abusers. A range of hypotheses have been advanced, based largely on clinical experiences with cocaine users, which attempt to identify the salient psychodynamic functions requiring attention in the psychodynamic therapies. Kleber and Gawin (1984b) have summarized these theories and state that co-caine's appeal to the user may have many possible avenues:

> Narcissistic needs are often served by the glamour associated with cocaine use; the cocaine using subculture may provide a sense of identity; anaclitic needs can be met via cocaine-heightened inti-mate personal interactions. Cocaine may be used to compensate for interpersonal failures; the use and obtaining of cocaine may help to deal with boredom and inadequate leisure time skills; and cocaine may be used to cope with a sense of inner emptiness and to man-age symptoms of psychiatric disturbance. (p. 20)

This impressive array of motives for cocaine use provides the substrate for much of the psychotherapeutic work of insight-oriented psychotherapies. The actual conduct of the treatment process varies as a function of the interaction between the prevailing motivational constellation found in the patient and the theoretical orientation of the psychotherapist.

Behavioral therapies constitute the other frequently employed individual psychotherapeutic technique. The elements of the behavior therapy repertoire that have been used with cocaine abusers are contingency contracting and aspects of conditioning and cognitive relabeling.

Contingency contracting operates through a system of penalties agreed on by patient and therapist. Selection of the specific penalties is made in a manner that will adversely affect the cocaine user by attaching an unpleasant consequence to the use of drugs. Mandatory urine testing for the presence of cocaine metabolites is an integral part of the contingency contracting program. Patients who have cocaine-positive urine test results are subject to the actualization (enactment) of predetermined penalties decided on earlier in treatment. Financial, work-related, or familial venues are the most common areas in which penalties are carried out.

The contingency contracting technique may be useful at any point in therapy, but is frequently undertaken at the very start of treatment to help cocaine users deal with ambivalent feelings about initially relinquishing drug use. The technique relies heavily on the premise that the aversive effects associated with drug use can be powerful determinants in creating new drug-free behaviors.

Conditioning techniques, both operant and classical Pavlovian, have been used to a lesser degree with cocaine abusers. Cognitive relabeling tries to pair the anticipation of the use of cocaine with thoughts of an unappealing, frightening, or dysphoric type. Conditioned abstinence has as its goal elicitation of troublesome cocaine-related states, such as cocaine craving, and extinguishing them through the substitution of specialized behavioral methods, including relaxation and reciprocal inhibition.

The concern with behavioral therapies for cocaine abuse centers around the consistency of the patient's participation in the treatment. The more regular and uninterrupted the therapy, the better the results appear to be, based on the sparse literature on outcome.

Behavioral therapies are finding useful roles as components of multimodal treatment programs in a variety of inpatient and outpatient settings. The ability to easily incorporate behavioral approaches into broader treatment programs enhances their appeal as a promising dimension of comprehensive cocaine abuse treatment.

Group Psychotherapy

Homogeneous groups of cocaine-abusing patients have gained clinical favor in recent years. The two leading examples are self-help groups and psychotherapy groups.

Self-help groups for cocaine-related problems are patterned along the lines of Alcoholics Anonymous. These groups are usually large and provide a network of substance abusers at all stages of the recovery process. Meetings are held daily, and regular attendance is strongly encouraged.

Cocaine Anonymous (CA), Drugs Anonymous, and Narcotics Anonymous are the three best-known self-help cocaine groups. Self-help groups have a supportive, emotionally powerful climate, and although they differ in significant ways from formal psychotherapy groups, they serve a vital therapeutic function for their membership.

Many substance abuse programs currently require participation in a CA group as a condition of acceptance into the program. Cocaine abusers who regularly attend CA meetings report benefit from feeling less isolated, being reminded of the dangers of cocaine, attaining a sense of accomplishment from remaining drug-free, and learning from the life experiences of other group members.

Objection to participation in CA groups requires careful scrutiny to differentiate between avoidance of a beneficial experience and legitimate reasons for being unwilling to attend self-help groups. Consequences that ensue from sacrificing anonymity by attending large group meetings may truly jeopardize the professional standing of cocaine users who function in fields where cocaine use is frowned on. Protestations that the groups are "too preachy or religious" reflect attitudes that often mask ambivalent feelings about full commitment to abstinence.

Psychotherapy groups are being recognized as excellent vehicles for enhancing cocaine abuse treatment. These groups are smaller in size (8–15 members), usually meet less frequently than self-help groups, and are led by mental health professionals, often in collaboration with recovered cocaine abusers.

In addition to high support elements, confrontation is an important aspect of these group experiences. The homogeneous composition of the group (i.e., all members had used cocaine) facilitates self-disclosure, counters the prominent tendency to deny the extent of one's drug use, and helps rapidly establish group norms that promote abstinence. These ongoing groups begin with a detoxification period, but later stages address problems encountered when drugs are no longer a regular part of one's life. At this point in treatment, many of these groups are indistinguishable from non-drug-related psychotherapy groups which deal with the emotional urgencies in the lives of the members.

Family Therapy

Assessment of the family circumstances of the cocaine abuser is essential in the formation of a successful treatment plan. The family of origin as well as the present-day family of the cocaine-dependent patient must be understood thoroughly. Important treatment decisions rest on a realistic appraisal of the assets and liabilities of those family members who are influential in the life of the patient.

Family influences are often extreme in their impact. The clinician is charged with the decision of when and how to directly involve significant family members in the process of treatment of cocaine abuse. Families, like individuals, vary and require understanding on a family-by-family basis. Families have natural resources which could be extremely helpful to the recovering abuser. At the same time, families "enable" or perpetuate dysfunctional patterns resulting in cocaine abuse as the presenting symptom in one of their members.

In a sense, it can be said that the family is always involved in the cocaine problem; the treatment decision focuses on how to involve them in its solution.

There is very little literature on family therapy as a discipline applied to the treatment of cocaine abuse. The family therapy literature to date largely address alcoholism and heroin addiction, and many of the current family interventions for cocaine abuse stem from principles gleaned from the aforementioned populations.

The prevailing approaches in family therapy include psychodynamic, behavioral, and systems-oriented approaches. Of the latter, the structural and strategic family therapy schools are emerging as the two most commonly applied to the problem of substance abuse in the family.

Couples therapy is another family format that is frequently employed. Intimate relationships invariably show the effects of chronic cocaine use. Not infrequently, both partners are involved in cocaine use or in mixed substance abuse. Change in one partner through self-imposed abstinence or by individual participation in a treatment program poses a threat to the homeostasis of the relationship and may trigger sabotaging efforts in the partner.

Relationships in which only one partner is a cocaine abuser involve recognizable issues that are often most easily observed and addressed in a dyadic treatment format. Drug use as an expression of anger at a spouse or as a form of loyalty to a substance-abusing member of the family of origin are two examples of commonly encountered patterns that unfold rapidly in a couples therapy milieu.

The value of family and marital approaches in gaining quick access to clinical data through direct observation of family interaction and dynamics is unparalleled. Early recognition of adaptive and dysfunctional elements of family relationships provides vital information related to diagnosis, evaluation, and the construction of a successful treatment plan. In the process of working with the family, the potential for maximizing and maintaining positive treatment gains can be developed. Similarly, undermining or destructive elements that emanate from dysfunctional family influences can be identified and remedied.

To date, the information on family therapy specifically for cocaine abuse is embryonic, but anecdotal enthusiasm and clinical favor appear with regularity in the recent literature. No doubt the combination of the increasing magnitude of cocaine use and its impact on the family will result in continued efforts to develop innovative, effective, and scientifically reliable (documentable) family therapy techniques, designed to address the problem of cocaine abuse and the family.

Psychopharmacological Treatment

The role of psychotropic medication in the treatment of cocaine abuse is of intense interest in clinical research circles. The appeal of understanding the biological mechanism of action of cocaine through the study of the effects of various medications, as well as the prospect of finding therapeutic agents that might be helpful in counteracting cocaine's undesirable effects, has spurred investigation in the field. This represents the growing edge of psychopharmacological research in cocaine abuse.

The other major way in which therapeutically prescribed medication plays a role in cocaine abuse treatment is as an adjunct to the management of phase-related psychiatric symptoms that develop during the course of cocaine overuse. The arousal and activation caused by states of cocaine intoxication are usually self-limiting; however, selected cocaine users may have intense affective reactions. Acute cocaine intoxication can precipitate hypomania or manic behavior, which ordinarily remits with discontinuation of the drug. At times, however, cocaine users who have underlying bipolar affective disorder will require active treatment to control the problems associated with manic symptomatology facilitated by stimulant abuse.

The phenomena associated with longer-term cocaine abuse may also require employment of psychotropic medication to interrupt a debilitatory psychiatric symptom or problem. This is most often the case in instances of cocaine-related psychotic symptoms. Delusional states triggered by cocaine use are usually paranoid in nature and can be severe enough to require antipsychotic medication for their management. States of agitation, panic, and delirium related to cocaine stimulation also result in clinical syndromes for which brief neuroleptic intervention may be indicated.

In addition to the problems associated with acute and chronic cocaine use, psychiatric problems also occur following the cessation of cocaine use. Depression, dysphoria, and other crash-related symptoms are prominent in this period. Antidepressant medication therapy is employed when the depressive state is unremitting and when active suicidal ideation or intent is part of the constellation of symptoms.

The aforementioned uses of medication are essentially designed to limit disturbing states that occur as a by-product of excessive cocaine use at its various stages. As noted earlier, research into the interaction between cocaine and therapeutic agents has sparked intense investigation. The use of psychotropic medication to prevent, interfere with, or definitively treat aspects of the cocaine dependence problem is receiving intense clinical and laboratory study.

Pilot studies reflect the principal research tracts in the field. These can be categorized either by the nature of the pharmacological agent used or by the correlation considered the target of the medicating treatment. Representative research efforts that reflect this work are illustrated in Table 4.1.

Generally speaking, the categories of therapeutic drugs and the disorders they aim to influence can be understood as follows: (1) Therapeutically prescribed stimulants, most notably methylphenidate and to a lesser extent pemoline, are geared to the subgroup of cocaine users who meet the criteria for attention deficit disorder originating in childhood and present in adult life. (2) Lithium shows promise for cocaine users with bipolar or cyclothymic disorders and in instances where the euphorigenic effects of cocaine are excessive, enduring, and disabling. (3) Tricyclic antidepressants are prescribed for depressive symptoms primarily and, more recently, to promote reduction of cocaine use by reducing the cocaine craving or by interfering with the euphoria produced by cocaine. (4) Trazodone (Rowbotham et al., 1984) is another antidepressant recently utilized to counter the physiological effects of cocaine. (5) Bromocriptine is receiving a great deal of attention for its possible potential as an effective treatment for cocaine abuse. Originally used as a

Table 4.1
The Use of Psychotropic Agents in Cocaine Abuse

Medication	Indication	Research Findings
1. Antidepressants a. TCAs (IMI, DMI) b. Trazodone	1. Preexisting or coexisting major depression 2. Refractory cases of cocaine abuse	Reduction in craving and/or euphoria
2. Lithium	1. Coexisting or preexisting cyclothymia or bipolar illness	Efficacy in cyclothymia or bipolar illness only
3. Methylphenidate (and other stimulants)	1. Coexisting or preexisting ADD	Efficacy in ADD only
4. Bromocriptine	1. Refractory cases of cocaine abuse	Reduction in craving
5. Amino acids (L-tyrosine, L-tryptophan)	Unclear	Unclear
6. MAOIs	Contraindicated	None

ADD = attention deficit disorder.

treatment for Parkinson's disease, bromocriptine exerts dopaminelike effects and is considered promising in reducing cocaine craving. (6) Amino acids, L-tryptophan (a serotonin precursor) and L-tyrosine (a dopamine and norepinephrine precursor), are given in conjunction with tricyclic antidepressants and are felt to be useful in amplifying the antidepressant properties of the primary medication.

Other interesting experimental pharmacological treatments are emerging and will be discussed in greater detail in Chapter 10. It is likely that as new knowledge unfolds, new drugs, alone and in combination, will undoubtedly be tested as vehicles for research and treatment of varied aspects of cocaine abuse problems.

SUMMARY

The broad strokes of general principles of treatment of the cocaine-dependent person have been outlined thus far. The next six chapters focus in greater detail on central components of treatment of cocaine abuse that form regular parts of eclectic treatment models.

REFERENCES

American Psychiatric Association: Diagnostic and Statistical Manual of Mental Disorders, 3rd ed, Washington, DC, 1980.

Blume SB: Psychotherapy in the treatment of alcoholism, in Psychiatry Update, Vol. III, Washington, DC, American Psychiatric Press, 1984, pp 338–346.

Gawin FH, Kleber HD: Cocaine abuse treatment. Arch Gen Psychiatry 41:903–910, 1984.

Gold, MS: National cocaine helpline, 1-800-COCAINE, Fair Oaks Hosp Psychiatry Lett 1(9):1–7, 1983.

Grinspoon L, Bakalar JB: Cocaine: A Drug and Its Social Evolution, revised, New York, Basic Books, 1985.

Khantzian EJ: The self-medication hypothesis of addictive disorders: focus on heroin and cocaine dependence. Am J Psychiatry 142:1259–1264, 1985a.

Khantzian EJ: On the psychological predisposition for opiate and stimulant dependence; Fair Oaks Hosp Psychiatry Lett 3:1–3, 1985b.

Kleber HD: Drug abuse, in Bellak L, ed: A Concise Handbook of Community Mental Health, New York, Grune & Stratton, 1974.

Kleber HD, Gawin FH: Cocaine abuse: a review of current and experimental treatments, in Grabowski J, ed,: Cocaine: Pharmacology, Effects and Treatment of Abuse, NIDA Research Monograph 50, 1984a.

Kleber HD, Gawin FH: The spectrum of cocaine abuse and its treatment. J Clin Psychiatry 45:18–23, 1984b.

Kleber HD, Gawin FH: Drug dependence: cocaine, in Psychiatry Update, Vol. V, Washington, DC, American Psychiatric Press, 1986, pp 160–185.

Millman RB: Drug dependence: general principles of diagnosis and treatment, in: Psychiatry Update, Vol. V, Washington, DC, American Psychiatric Press, 1986, pp 122–136.

Resnick RB, Resnick EB: Cocaine abuse and its treatment. Psychiatr Clin North Am 7:713–728, 1984.

Rowbotham MC, Jones RT, Benowitz NL, et al: Trazadone-oral cocaine interactions. Arch Gen Psychiatry 41:895–899, 1984.

Siegel RK: Cocaine smoking. J Psychoactive Drugs 14:321–337, 1982.

Washton AM: Cocaine abuse treatment, Fair Oaks Hosp Psychiatry Lett 3:951–956, 1985.

Chapter 5

Diagnostic Issues in Cocaine Abuse

Andrew E. Skodol, M.D.

The epidemic-like spread of cocaine abuse has resulted in increasing numbers of individuals seeking psychiatric care for out-of-control cocaine use. As clinics, hospitals, and private practitioners' offices have become inundated by this latest wave of substance abuse, specialty services have been developed for the acute treatment and rehabilitation of the cocaine-abusing patient. In addition to serving as the impetus for the development of new and effective treatment strategies, as discussed throughout this book, these patients pose several interesting diagnostic dilemmas. Since, ultimately, effective treatment selection and accurate prognostic judgment may hinge on diagnostic issues, clinicians should be aware of these problems in differential diagnosis and their current, best solutions.

The two major diagnostic questions with clinical significance are the following: (1) Is there a syndrome of cocaine dependence? (2) What is the relationship of progressive cocaine use to other psychopathology, especially mood disorder? These will be the subjects of this chapter.

COCAINE ABUSE VERSUS COCAINE DEPENDENCE

In the DSM-III classification of substance use disorders (American Psychiatric Association, 1980), there are two general syndromes, substance abuse and substance dependence. Substance abuse is defined as

(1) a pathological pattern of use, (2) resulting in some form of social or occupational impairment, and (3) lasting for at least one month. Substance dependence is limited to cases in which there are indicators of *physiological* dependence on the substance. Evidence of physiological dependence can be either drug tolerance, i.e., increasing amounts of the substance are needed to achieve a desired effect or use of the same amount has a diminished effect, or withdrawal, defined as the development of a substance-specific syndrome on cessation or reduction in the use of the substance. DSM-III includes nine classes of substances that are associated with abuse or dependence. The following five classes have both abuse and dependence syndromes: alcohol, barbiturates or similarly acting sedatives or hypnotics, opioids, amphetamines or similarly acting sympathomimetics, and cannabis. Tobacco has only a dependence syndrome. Finally, three classes have abuse syndromes only; these are phencyclidine and similarly acting arylcyclohexylamines, hallucinogens, and cocaine. Thus, at the time of the publication of DSM-III, in 1980 before the epidemic began, the DSM-III Advisory Committee on Substance Use Disorders concluded that there was no strong evidence that physiological addiction to cocaine, as evidenced by tolerance or withdrawal, occurred (Spitzer et al., 1980). Kuehnle and Spitzer (1981) said that the exclusion of cocaine dependence from DSM-III "may be more of an artifact produced by the high cost of the drug than a lack of potential for dependence from the drug per se. Should cocaine become more available and less expensive in the future, DSM-IV may include the category Cocaine Dependence." The sudden surge in the use and abuse of cocaine observed in the early 1980s belied this economic rationale.

The existence of a syndrome of cocaine dependence has been controversial since Freud first experimented with the drug. Consumption by humans of doses 50 times greater than usual has been offered as evidence of tolerance, and the characteristic dysphoric cocaine "crash" after cessation of use, as evidence of withdrawal. Experimental physiological addiction to cocaine has been difficult to induce in animals (Tatum & Severs, 1929; Post el al., 1976), although some investigators have demonstrated tolerance to cocaine and D-amphetamine, as well as cross-tolerance to both drugs (Woolverton et al., 1978). Recently, several investigators have reported experiments demonstrating acute tolerance to cocaine in humans (Fischman & Schuster, 1982; Van Dyck et al., 1983). Others, however, have postulated a "reverse tolerance" effect of the drug on the central nervous system following repetitive administration (Post & Kopanda, 1976). If physiological dependence on cocaine exists, however, in that tolerance develops or a withdrawal syndrome can occur (DSM-III definitions of substance dependence), this may help to explain how casual cocaine use increases and eventually progresses to heavy use resulting in considerable physical, emotional, and role functioning problems, and even death.

Symptoms of Cocaine Abuse and Dependence in a Clinical Population

In the course of a study to develop a diagnostic screening instrument for use in epidemiological surveys, a colleague* and I assessed a group of individuals with histories of illicit substance use for DSM-III substance use disorders, using protocols based on the NIMH Diagnostic Interview Schedule (Robins et al., 1981).

Individuals were asked if drugs from each of the major DSM-III drug classes had been used to get high, without a prescription, in doses more than prescribed, and every day for two weeks or more. Individuals were also asked if they ever felt dependent on each drug, whether they tried to cut down use, needed larger amounts to achieve an effect (i.e., get high), or experienced withdrawal symptoms (i.e., got sick) due to stopping or cutting down on drug use. Finally, individuals were asked if drug use caused them problems with their health, family or friends, work or school, with the police, or of an emotional or psychological nature. These questions covered the concepts of DSM-III substance abuse, a pathological pattern of use and resultant social and occupational impairment, as well as of substance dependence, i.e., tolerance and withdrawal, regardless of whether DSM-III had a dependence diagnosis for a particular class of drug.

The frequencies of symptoms and/or problems associated with cocaine use were compiled. The report of tolerance (needing larger amounts to achieve effect) and withdrawal for cocaine was also compared to tolerance and withdrawal for four other classes of substances for which physiological dependence is known to exist: barbiturates and similarly acting sedatives and hypnotics, cannabis, and the opioids divided into two groups—heroin and all other opioids.

Sixty-four individuals from a sample of 156 reported symptoms or problems associated with cocaine use, and 40 reported difficulties associated with cocaine use of sufficient severity at some point in their clinical histories to meet DSM-III criteria for a diagnosis of cocaine abuse. Fifty-three cocaine users (83%) reported daily use for two weeks or

*The author would like to thank Bridget F. Grant, Ph.D., for her assistance in the collection and analysis of these data.

more, 15 (23%) tried unsuccessfully to cut down use, 27 (42%) reported larger amounts were needed to achieve the desired effect, 21 (33%) felt they were dependent on cocaine, and eight (13%) reported experiencing withdrawal symptoms on stopping or cutting down use.

Table 5.1 separately compares the proportions of individuals reporting tolerance or withdrawal to cocaine with those reporting tolerance or withdrawal to other drugs known to be associated with physiological dependence. From Table 5.1, it appears that there is no difference in the frequency of reported tolerance for cocaine as compared to that reported for barbiturates and other sedatives or for opioids, excluding heroin. Tolerance is reported less frequently for cocaine than for heroin by individuals who have used both, but is actually reported more frequently for cocaine than for cannabis. As many individuals report withdrawal symptoms from cocaine as from either barbiturates or cannabis; withdrawal is significantly less often reported for cocaine than for all opioids.

The frequency of reported tolerance to cocaine among users of illicit substances is striking and significant for clinical diagnostic practice using DSM-III. If we applied the general DSM-III criteria for dependence, 27 (42%) of 64 cocaine users would warrant a dependence diagnosis, including six who had not met criteria for cocaine abuse.

Since our findings are inconsistent, however, with the most prevailing

Table 5.1

Frequency of Reported Tolerance and Withdrawal Associated with Cocaine Compared to Four Other Classes of Abused Substances in Individuals Who Used Multiple Substances

Combination of Substances Used	N*	P1†	P2‡	X^2	P
Tolerance					
Cocaine-barbiturates	30	.31	.43	.90	NS
Cocaine-marijuana	55	.36	.18	4.05	< .05
Cocaine-heroin	58	.36	.88	24.74	< .001
Cocaine-other opiates	45	.34	.40	.24	NS
Withdrawal					
Cocaine-barbiturates	30	.20	.33	.90	NS
Cocaine-marijuana	55	.13	.04	1.78	NS
Cocaine-heroin	58	.13	.88	39.20	< .001
Cocaine-other opiates	48	.11	.40	8.47	< .005

*Number of clients reporting use of both substances.
†Proportion of cocaine users reporting tolerance or withdrawal to cocaine.
‡Proportion of cocaine users reporting tolerance or withdrawal to the other substance.

opinion (National Commission on Marijuana and Drug Abuse, 1973; Petersen & Stillman, 1977), they raise several important clinical and research questions. Should tolerance, by itself, be considered an indication of physiological substance dependence? Some investigators think that it should not, since, in the case of certain drugs, including alcohol, innate tolerance is more significant than acquired tolerance in predicting behavioral effects of the drug. Therefore, the presence of tolerance does not necessarily imply the prolonged and increasing use usually associated with drug dependence. Innate individual differences in the metabolism of cocaine have also been reported (Brecher, 1972; Caldwell, 1976).

The findings also raise a question of whether drug tolerance can be determined on the basis of subjective report? In our sample, users of cocaine were also users of other illicit drugs, especially heroin and cannabis. A common means of cocaine use among this patient population was "speedballing," i.e., the injection of heroin and cocaine in a single bolus. The effects of cocaine may not, therefore, be differentiated subjectively from the effects of drugs used in combination by the multiple drug user. In favor of real tolerance to cocaine is that tolerance to heroin was reported much more frequently than for cocaine, suggesting that users can make the discrimination.

Inconsistencies in reports of tolerance may also be due to the development of tolerance to some drug effects, but not to others; to differences in drug dosages or routes or patterns of administration; or to interactions between cocaine and other substances that alter the pharmacological properties of cocaine taken alone. Additionally, drugs taken illicitly vary in purity to such a degree that the significance of subjectively reported tolerance is difficult to interpret and to compare with pharmacological studies of drug effects.

I feel that the answers to these questions with respect to cocaine are largely unknown and that further investigations of the phenomena underlying progressive cocaine use, especially in samples of exclusive cocaine users, are indicated. Until progressive use of cocaine is better understood, however, I also believe that the exclusion of a diagnostic category of cocaine dependence from DSM-III was premature.

The following case vignette illustrates a typical progression from casual, recreational use of cocaine to heavy, uncontrolled use, accompanied by many social, physical, and economic problems.

Case vignette 1

P.G., a 39-year-old investment banker, first started to use cocaine 15 years ago. He was introduced to it by a friend at a party shortly after business school graduation. For 10 years Mr. G used the drug at most two or three times per year, always at parties, and always cocaine that was given to him, not bought. About five years ago, he was offered a gram to buy, which he did for $60, and then proceeded to use for the first time outside of a social situation.

Mr. G.'s career had progressed substantially. He was earning approximately $200,000/year. Socially, he did not feel as successful, however, since he had yet to meet someone to marry. In fact, he found that his job interfered significantly with his social life, since on those occasions when he did go out he was exhausted. About three years ago, he discovered that cocaine increased his sex drive and that rubbing cocaine on his penis helped improve his sexual performance.

He started to get high whenever he had a date and especially when he had sexual intercourse. Soon, however, he found that he wanted to get high even on nights when he came home late and was alone, simply to relieve himself of the day's pressures. He found that he preferred the sexual feeling that he experienced while using cocaine to any he had enjoyed with a partner. By this time, the cost of Mr. G.'s cocaine use had grown; he was up to 3–4 g/week, costing $300–400.

Then Mr. G.'s use took an even sharper upward turn. He found that at work he was sluggish in the mornings, and that "taking a hit" before leaving for work made him more alert. Soon, however, he was snorting in his office several times a day, and he couldn't wait to get home at night so that he could stay high. Not only did he use cocaine more often, but he reported that he began to get "used to" the effects of his usual dose. Sleep and appetite became disturbed. Clients began to complain that he seemed disorganized and preoccupied, co-workers observed that he talked too quickly and stuttered, and his boss received complaints. Socially, he stopped dating altogether. His last girlfriend broke off with him because he was late for every date and only wanted to "do coke." He quit his weekly squash game.

Finally, he began to arrive late at work. Deadlines were not met, and clients asked for him to be replaced. When confronted with the decline in his performance and threatened with termination, he admitted the cocaine problem and was referred for evaluation. At this time, his habit was costing $3,000/week.

Proposed Revisions for Substance Use Disorders in DSM-III-R

Other investigators have also had problems with the DSM-III distinction between substance abuse and substance dependence. Critiques have been made (Rounsaville et al., 1986) that social and occupational *consequences* of drug use should not be the criteria for diagnosing a disorder and that tolerance and withdrawal both have limitations as indices of dependence. With respect to the impairment criteria, it has been argued that individuals with pathological compulsive substance use may be missed in diagnostic evaluation because impairment has not yet been detected. Regarding tolerance, large innate individual differences, diverse mechanisms, varying patterns and amounts of tolerance across different drug categories, and reverse tolerance have all been mentioned as detracting from its meaningfulness as a criterion for substance dependence. Withdrawal, also, has been noted in its milder versions to be too nonspecific for a drug dependence diagnosis and in its more severe versions, too insensitive.

The major recommendations for DSM-III-R (Work Group of the American Psychiatric Association, 1985) included removing the abuse/dependence distinction from the classification and broadening the definition of dependence to include a range of clinically significant behaviors, cognitions, and symptoms that indicate a substantial involvement with what will now be called "psychoactive" substances. Specifically, all of the classes of psychoactive substances will have the set of criteria for psychoactive substance dependence that is outlined in Table 5.2. Any three of the nine symptoms would meet the diagnostic threshold for dependence.

This revised concept of psychoactive substance dependence is more consonant with the model of the dependence syndrome recently recommended by a WHO work group for the scheduled Tenth Revision of the International Classification of Diseases (ICD-10) (Edwards et al., 1981). The key feature of this syndrome is impaired control over substance use. The addictive behavior develops and is maintained as a result of rein-

Table 5.2
Proposed Criteria for DSM-III-R Psychoactive Substance Dependence

1. Preoccupation with substance seeking or taking
2. Takes in larger doses/longer than intended
3. Tolerance
4. Withdrawal
5. Used to avoid withdrawal
6. Efforts to cut down or control use
7. Impaired when expected to fulfill obligations
8. Given up activities for substance
9. Continued use despite disorder or problem

forcements that may be both physiological and environmental. Although tolerance and withdrawal continue to be symptoms of dependence according to the DSM-III-R proposal, they are only two of nine symptoms and clearly are not required for the diagnosis. Thus, the physiological aspects of dependence have been deemphasized, with a pattern of compulsive drug taking gaining greater significance. DSM-III-R psychoactive substance dependence corresponds to the ICD-10 proposed category of "hazardous use."

Substance abuse, in DSM-III-R, will be a residual category for an individual who has a maladaptive pattern of use without ever having met criteria for dependence for this particular substance. Evidence of a maladaptive pattern will be continuation of use despite significant impairment in psychological, physical, social, or occupational functioning that is caused or exacerbated by the use of the substance. Some signs of impairment must persist for at least one month or occur repeatedly over a longer period. This category is the counterpart of the category of "harmful use" proposed for ICD-10.

With respect to the controversies over cocaine tolerance and withdrawal, the DSM-III-R proposal begs the issue, since neither tolerance nor withdrawal will be required for a diagnosis of cocaine dependence. Another change proposed for the DSM-III-R psychoactive substance use disorders, however, sheds some light on current views about the physiologically addictive properties of cocaine. The substance-induced organic mental disorders have been regrouped in DSM-III-R with psychoactive substance dependence in the broad class of psychoactive substance use disorders. For several drugs, the number of psychoactive-substance-induced organic mental disorders described has been increased. Cocaine is a notable example. In DSM-III, only cocaine intoxication was described. In DSM-III-R, in addition there are syndromes of cocaine delirium, delusional disorder, flashback disorder, residual disorder, and withdrawal. The criteria for cocaine withdrawal are outlined in Table 5.3.

The criteria describe a depressive syndrome (see also "Cocaine Abuse and Mood Disorder"), rather than one of neuroexcitation or disinhibition. Nevertheless, the syndrome is more likely to occur after prolonged, heavy cocaine use and can be sufficiently dysphoric to interfere with reduction or cessation of use. If a syndrome of withdrawal is now formally recognized, then the consensus seems to be that cocaine is physiologically addictive.

Thus DSM-III-R solves several of the practical problems encountered in assigning a principal diagnosis to persons who abuse cocaine, while being less than totally informative on the question of physical depen-

Table 5.3
Proposed Criteria for DSM-III-R Cocaine Withdrawal

---

1. Prolonged heavy use of cocaine
2. Cessation or reduction leading to depressed mood and two of the following:
   a. fatigue
   b. disturbed sleep
   c. increased dreaming
3. Not due to another physical or mental disorder

---

dence. Greater clarity about the physiology of progressive cocaine use awaits future study. We now turn to problems associated with making other, additional diagnoses in the presence of cocaine dependence.

COCAINE ABUSE AND MOOD DISORDER

The second major differential diagnostic concern in these patients is the relationship of cocaine abuse to other psychopathology, especially mood disorder. The observation that the syndrome of cocaine abuse responds to antidepressant drug treatment raises the question in itself. The frequent highs and lows that characterize the clinical course of cocaine abuse further highlight the issue. Since intoxications are associated with a strong euphoriant effect, are individuals who abuse cocaine treating themselves for a clinically significant depression? Is the depression that characterizes the cocaine "crash" a direct effect of the drug via depletion of a neurotransmitter or a return to baseline dysphoria characteristic of the individual who becomes involved with cocaine? Are those individuals whose cocaine abuse responds to antidepressants suffering from an underlying mood disorder and those who do not respond without such a prior history?

Previous studies (Gawin & Kleber, 1984; Weiss et al., 1983), though few in number, report that as many as 50% of individuals seen for treatment of cocaine abuse have a coexisting affective disorder. Gawin and Kleber (1984) found that 33% of their outpatients had a lifetime diagnosis of major depression or dysthymic disorder by the Diagnostic Interview Schedule, and 17% had a cyclothymic disorder. Weiss and associates (1983) reported almost identical figures for an inpatient sample. The numbers of individuals diagnosed in these studies are very small, however. Moreover, the samples are clinical populations seeking pharmacological treatment with mood-altering drugs and cannot, therefore, be considered representative of the general population of cocaine users or abusers. Finally, the methods of assessment were not rigorous. But these early findings, nevertheless, are consistent with clinical observations that an association exists between cocaine abuse and mood disorder.

Differential Diagnosis of Mood Disturbance

In clinical settings, the use of DSM-III facilitates differential diagnosis of individuals who abuse cocaine in a number of ways. First, the multiaxial diagnostic approach encourages multiple diagnoses on Axis I (Clinical Syndromes) and Axis II (Personality Disorders, for Adults). This means that the clinician is not forced to choose one diagnosis for a given patient, but rather can convey the complexity of the clinical picture by the use of multiple diagnoses, both current and past. Second, DSM-III presents a broad array of diagnoses to describe the mood disturbances that can be seen in association with cocaine abuse. Table 5.4 depicts the diagnostic possibilities in DSM-III for a patient with a mood disturbance.

Although DSM-III does not formally use the primary/secondary distinction in assigning diagnoses, the temporal priority of the syndromes is obviously relevant in attempting to understand the relationship of cocaine use and mood disorder. In the following discussion, I shall first describe problems associated with the diagnosis of the current condition; subsequently I will discuss establishing a past diagnosis.

Diagnosing current mood disturbance

More often than not, the patient presenting to a treatment clinic for cocaine abuse will describe some current dysphoria during the initial interview. The mood disturbance may frequently contribute to the patient's reasons for seeking treatment. A report of depressed mood may not, however, signify a primary mood disorder.

Since many patients will have recently been on a heavy cocaine binge, the first consideration in differential diagnosis is whether the depressed mood described is a manifestation of an organic affective syndrome. Although DSM-III did not include a specific diagnosis for an affective syndrome associated with cocaine, DSM-III-R has the diagnosis of cocaine withdrawal to describe the mood disturbance seen during cocaine crashes (see Table 5.3). This is the equivalent of an organic affective syndrome, except that the organic factor responsible is drug cessation, rather than drug ingestion. DSM-III criteria for amphetamine withdrawal (a drug that has many clinical effects similar to those of cocaine) are exactly

Table 5.4
DSM-III Classification of Disorders
Involving Mood Disturbance as
a Predominant Feature

Organic mental disorders
   Organic affective syndrome
   Substance-induced organic mental disorders
      Intoxication
      Withdrawal
Affective disorders
   Major affective disorders
      Bipolar disorder
         Mixed
         Manic
         Depressed
      Major depression
         Single episode
         Recurrent
   Other specific affective disorders
      Cyclothymic disorder
      Dysthymic disorder
   Atypical affective disorders
      Atypical bipolar disorder
      Atypical depression
Psychotic disorders not elsewhere classified
   Schizoaffective disorder
Adjustment disorder
   Adjustment disorder with depressed mood
V codes
   Uncomplicated bereavement

parallel to those of cocaine withdrawal in DSM-III-R. What was an oversight in DSM-III should not be missed in clinical practice.

The longer the period of abstinence prior to the evaluation, the less likely the persistence of dysphoric mood represents the effects of cocaine withdrawal. Although the course of cocaine withdrawal depression has not been thoroughly studied, experienced clinicians expect this depression to show signs of resolving within one week of being drug-free (Siegel, 1982; Smith, 1984). One recently completed study (Gawin & Kleber, 1986) sheds some light on the symptomatology of the abstinence period following a cocaine binge and its temporal progression. Gawin and Kleber describe a triphasic course for the symptoms occurring in the period after cessation of cocaine use. In the first phase, lasting from several hours up to six days, patients reported typical crash symptomatology consisting of depression, anhedonia, insomnia, irritability, anxiety, confusion, suicidal ideation, paranoia, and gradually diminishing cocaine craving. These syndromes were sometimes severe enough to meet DSM-III criteria for major depression except that they were of short duration and related to organic factors. At the end of the phase, patients were hypersomnolent. In the second phase, termed the withdrawal phase by the authors, mood began euthymic, but as time went by, anhedonia, mild dysphoria, anergia, anxiety, and irritability returned. These symptoms recurred after one to five days of normal mood and could persist for up to 10 weeks, if the person resisted cocaine use. For it was during this period that craving for the euphoriant effects of cocaine reemerged and frequently led to relapse binging. If abstinence could be sustained, then a third phase ensued, with normal mood and episodic cocaine craving, precipitated by environmental cues. Gawin and Kleber believe that it is inappropriate to refer to the cocaine crash as withdrawal, since it is not during this period that the maximum risk to resume cocaine abuse occurs. Rather, they believe that the middle of phase two is associated with the greatest likelihood of relapse. If a neuroendocrine basis for phase two symptoms can be established (Gawin & Kleber, 1985) the process might be better termed neuroadaptation, rather than withdrawal.

When the depression associated with cocaine abstinence does not remit, the clinician should suspect a nonorganic disorder. Since there are many negative effects that cocaine abuse can have on a patient's marital, occupational, financial, and family life, it is possible that persistent depression represents a stressor-induced disorder. If the symptoms are relatively mild or short in duration, this may represent an adjustment disorder with depressed mood. If it is a significant, serious depressive episode, it may be major depression, with the severity of psychosocial stressors recorded on Axis IV of the multiaxial system. Whether or not this is a first episode, or a recurrence of an underlying disorder precipitated by stress, depends on the assessment of the past history, a topic to be discussed below. The following case vignette illustrates the difficulties associated with assessing current depressed mood.

Case vignette 2

C.M. was a 25-year-old single woman, employed as an assistant advertising account executive. Her experience with cocaine began five years earlier, when a friend offered some to her. Two years before coming for her present evaluation, she went on her first cocaine binge, after she and a boyfriend broke up. On that occasion, she used cocaine continuously for 15 hours before being taken to a psychiatric emergency room, in a panic, by a friend.

Since then, she has gone on cocaine binges a dozen times, usually following disappointments with boyfriends or bosses. These have led to absences from work, such that she has twice been fired. The current episode was also precipitated by a breakup. The patient stayed high for two days; she spent her entire paycheck on cocaine, and when she ran out, she crashed and became depressed and suicidal. Filled with intense self-hatred, she scratched both arms numerous times with a razor blade. She had not been to work all week and was told again that she was in danger of losing her job.

The present evaluation occurred five days later. The patient complained of severe depression, loss of appetite, nightmares waking her up, agitation, no interest, no energy, feelings of worthlessness, trouble concentrating, and thoughts that she would be better off dead. She dated the onset as one week ago, the time of the break-up.

In this patient, a full depressive syndrome is present and psychosocial stressors (breakup with boyfriend, threatened loss of job) can be readily identified. The duration of the episode is only one week, however, and coincides with the period of heavy cocaine use and subsequent withdrawal. An organic cause for the dysphoria cannot be ruled out definitively for the present episode, it is probably best characterized as cocaine withdrawal. The pattern of maladaptive reactions to loss and disappointments suggests some other psychopathology, either an Axis II personality disorder or an affective disorder. These would require investigation of the past history at a time when the patient had had a significant drug-free interval.

At the other end of the affective spectrum is the patient who presents to the clinic or emergency service without having abstained from cocaine use at all. Since bipolar disorder has also been found associated with cocaine abuse, the clinician is interested in separating out the acute effects of cocaine intoxication from an underlying bipolar or cyclothymic disorder.

The symptoms of cocaine intoxication include psychomotor agitation, elation, grandiosity, loquacity, and hypervigilance. These may be difficult to distinguish from the symptoms of a manic episode, in a patient who denies recent use of cocaine. Physiological symptoms are also present, however, during cocaine intoxication. The presence of tachycardia, pupillary dilation, elevated blood pressure, perspiration or chills, or nausea and vomiting should alert the clinician to a substance-induced etiology. The diagnosis can be confirmed by urine or blood testing.

Cocaine use may also cause other acute disturbances. As mentioned earlier, syndromes of delirium, delusional disorder, and flashbacks have been described and are listed as diagnoses in DSM-III-R. In diagnosing current disturbances, a suspected organic etiology takes precedence over a corresponding functional disorder.

Establishing a lifetime diagnosis of mood disorder

As mentioned before, research studies have suggested that unipolar, depressive, and bipolar mood disorders are associated with cocaine abuse. It may be easier to understand how a person with a depressive disorder could become involved with a euphoriant drug, compared to a person with an innate tendency toward elevated mood. Clinical experience, however, confirms that both patterns of lifetime mood disorder are encountered frequently. For the person with a depressive disorder, recurrent major depression or dysthymia (DSM-III-R) may be appropriate. For the individual with a bipolar disorder, either bipolar disorder itself or cyclothymia.

The differential diagnosis of recurrent major depression from dysthymia rests on distinguishing a pattern of somewhat more discrete episodes of severe depression from a more chronic pattern of mild to moderate depression. This is not always a straightforward task, since recovery from a major depressive episode is frequently incomplete, leaving the patient with residual symptoms (Keller et al., 1982). In addition, patients with chronic, mild depression may at times develop more severe major episodes superimposed, so-called "double depression" (Keller & Shapiro, 1982). In DSM-III-R, major depression that does not completely remit can be noted to be "in partial remission (or residual state)." For patients who have chronic, milder depression that clearly precedes their developing major episodes, the combined diagnoses of major depression and dysthymia are used. On recovery, these patients would be expected to return to baseline levels of chronic symptoms.

Some investigators have proposed the use of the term atypical depression (Quitkin et al., 1979; Leibowitz et al., 1984) to describe a depressive syndrome in which mood reactivity is maintained and symptoms of increased appetite/weight gain, oversleeping or spending more time in bed, severe fatigue or feelings of leaden paralysis, and rejection sensitivity are prominent. These depressions appear to be associated with a preferential response to MAO inhibitors (Quitkin et al., 1979; Liebowitz et al., 1984). Clinicians working in cocaine treatment centers suspect that atypical depression may be quite common among cocaine abusers. In DSM-III and DSM-III-R, atypical depression, as defined above, is not a separate diagnostic category; patients with atypical features may meet criteria for major depression, dysthymia, or both (Davidson et al., 1982).

In attempting to establish a lifetime depressive disorder diagnosis for a patient with cocaine abuse, it is necessary to focus on the clinical history prior to involvement with cocaine. Because of the commonly encountered dysphoric mood states associated with cocaine withdrawal, the period associated with regular or heavy use is not helpful in establishing the presence of a lifetime disorder. Usually, a patient can focus on the time before involvement with cocaine. Occasionally, however, he or she is so distressed currently that an accurate report of past history is not possible. In such cases, establishing a lifetime diagnosis must be deferred to follow-up interviews, or a third-party informant should be used.

The following case vignette depicts a person with a preexisting depressive disorder who became involved with cocaine as a self-treatment only to find that the "cure" worsened the illness.

Case vignette 3

T.A. is a 42-year-old, self-employed tavern owner who was referred by his internist for psychiatric consultation when he spoke of plots to steal his business, one day during a physical examination.

Mr. A. migrated from Italy to the United States when he was 30 years old. He left because of an overbearing family who he felt would never allow him to become independent. He worked at many jobs and was well liked for his hard work and industriousness. He saved money until three years ago when he bought a tavern from an estate and went into business on his own. He has been reasonably successful, making a comfortable living, which enables him to travel, his primary recreation.

Mr. A. always saw himself as inadequate, especially with women. He thought that he was not physically attractive, sexually experienced, or "smooth" enough in conversation to appeal to women, and therefore, he dated only if it was arranged by friends. Even then, he rarely asked a woman out a second time. He was very disappointed that he was not married.

A regular patron of his bar offered him cocaine two years ago. He found that on cocaine he became talkative, self-confident, and soon developed a reputation as "the life of the party." Since he was actually quite nice-looking, he was able to meet and date women. When he did not use cocaine, however, he fell back into self-doubt and self-deprecation. The cycle of getting high on cocaine and depressed when drug-free became more extreme and more frequent. Mr. A. found himself getting high every day and dreading the down times. He began to snort increasing amounts of cocaine and began to have nasal septal problems. In the course of the physical examination, he told his doctor that he felt that a plot was in effect to take his bar from him.

The psychiatrist found evidence of an organic delusional syndrome during periods of heaviest cocaine use and a lifetime history of dysthymic disorder. There were also two past major depressive episodes when Mr. A. was unable to work for two or three months, although he had never received psychiatric treatment. Family history was negative, to the best of his knowledge, for mood disorder.

The fact that cocaine abuse has become a common ailment of the rich and the successful suggests that not all cocaine abusers are treating themselves for low self-esteem. In fact, some users will describe exactly the opposite pattern of use; they will use cocaine when they are feeling particularly well, "on a roll," as if to extend or "top off" an already "upbeat" period. Such persons are often very driven, high pressured, energetic, and frequently successful. Their temperament suggest a possible disturbance in the bipolar affective spectrum. Some business people and certain athletes may fall into this group.

A lifetime pattern of bipolar disorder, with full-blown manic episodes causing severely negative consequences or leading to hospitalization, is not as hard to discern as more subtle forms of mood disturbance in the bipolar spectrum. Cyclothymia and atypical bipolar disorder (bipolar II) are more difficult to recognize, particularly among the successful.

In cyclothymia, a chronic pattern of alternating periods of mild highs and lows is found with few "in-between" or normal days. When high, the person may sleep less, have lots of energy, feel good about himself or herself, and be very productive, creative, or optimistic. Such periods may be associated with considerable success, unless or until the individual overextends and encounters some difficulties, such as making foolish investments or commitments to projects whose deadlines cannot be met. At such times, the person may suffer a setback, which will then lead to a period of mild depression. In bipolar II disorder, hypomanic periods alternate with more severe episodes of major depression.

In evaluating the patient for a suspected or possible bipolar mood disorder, the period of active cocaine use, with its frequent periods of intoxication and withdrawal, must be discounted, just as in the case of a depressive disorder. Substance-induced mood abnormality would again be expected to color reporting of past history, as well. The following case vignette illustrates the development of cocaine abuse in a patient with a subtle disorder of the bipolar type.

Case vignette 4

S.R. was a 27-year-old salesman who was admitted to the hospital for cocaine binging that had become out of his control. He had spent several days "freebasing" at a friend's apartment, absent from work, having canceled numerous appointments. When his boss threatened to fire him, he agreed to hospitalization.

Mr. R. had a three-year history of cocaine use. When the hospital nursing staff confronted him with their opinion that he must be very depressed, he laughed and said, "Not usually!" The psychiatric history revealed that Mr. R. had had brief periods of mild depression since college when he felt bored, listless, and unable to get out of bed, but that usually he was cheerful, gregarious, energetic, and couldn't get enough out of life. "I've never been able to do things halfway," he told the psychiatrist. "It's all or nothing. If I'm into work, all I want to do is work; I'll make so many sales, my boss can't believe it. If I'm into women, all I want is more women. I've been known to screw three different women in one night!"

Mr. R.'s use of cocaine corresponded to the periods when he was "up" and not when he was "down." In fact, when depressed, he reported no desire, at all, for cocaine. When observed on the ward, Mr. R. was usually animatedly trying to coax some of the more depressed patients into organized ward activities. Family history was positive in that his father had been diagnosed as bipolar, 10 years previously.

The psychiatrist diagnosed cyclothymia and placed Mr. R. on lithium carbonate. Within three weeks he reported a more "even keel" feeling, was observed to be less active, and claimed to have little desire for cocaine.

A positive family history for a mood disorder, as was present in case vignette 4, may be used by the clinician to confirm a suspected mood disorder. As often as not, the family history will be negative, and there-fore, one cannot rely on the family history for making a diagnosis.

Mood disturbance is an important phenomenon for understanding the development of cocaine abuse, for guiding treatment decisions, and potentially for elucidating mechanisms of cocaine's effects on the central nervous system. Future studies should use rigorous diagnostic methods, family history data, and a general population sample, in efforts to further our understanding of the associations.

SUMMARY

In this chapter, I have focused on several challenging problems of differential diagnosis that are encountered when evaluating the patient who abuses cocaine. These have been grouped into two major areas: (1) distinguishing a syndrome of cocaine dependence and (2) differentiating cocaine-induced organic mental disorders from coexisting mood disorders. The problems are illustrated with research data and case vignettes. Strategies and solutions, including those offered by the forthcoming DSM-III-R, are presented.

REFERENCES

American Psychiatric Association: Diagnostic and Statistical Manual of Mental Disorders, 3rd ed, Washington, DC, American Psychiatric Association, 1980.

Brecher EM: Licit and Illicit Drugs, Mount Vernon, NY, Consumers Union, 1972.

Caldwell J: Physiological aspects of cocaine usage, in Mule S, ed: Cocaine: Chemical, Biological, Clinical, Social and Treatment Aspects, Boca Raton, FL, CRC Press, 1976.

Davidson JRT, Miller RD, Turnbull CD, Sullivan JL: Atypical depression. Arch Gen Psychiatry 39:527–534, 1982.

Edwards G, Arif A, Hodgson R: Nomenclature and classification of drug and alcohol related problems. Bull WHO 59:225–242, 1981.

Fischman MW, Schuster CR: Cocaine self-administration in humans. Fed Proc 41:241–246, 1982.

Gawin FH, Kleber HD: Cocaine abuse treatment: open clinical trial with desipramine and lithium carbonate. Arch Gen Psychiatry 41:903–909, 1984.

Gawin FH, Kleber HD: Abstinence symptomatology and psychiatric diagnosis in cocaine abusers: clinical observations. Arch Gen Psychiatry 43:107–113, 1986.

Gawin FH, Kleber HD: Neuroendocrine findings in chronic cocaine abusers: a preliminary report. Br J Psychiatry 147:569–573, 1985.

Keller MB, Shapiro RW: "Double depression": superimpositon of acute depressive episodes on chronic depressive disorders. Am J Psychiatry 139:438–442. 1982.

Keller MB, Shapiro RW, Lavori PW, Wolfe N: Recovery in major depressive disorder: analysis with the life table and regression models. Arch Gen Psychiatry 39:905–910, 1982.

Kuehnle J, Spitzer R: DSM-III classification of substance use disorders, in Lowinson JH, ed: Substance Abuse: Clinical Problems and Perspectives, Baltimore, Williams & Wilkins, 1981, pp 19–23.

Liebowitz MR, Quitkin FM, Stewart JW, et al: Phenelzine vs imipramine in atypical depression: a preliminary report. Arch Gen Psychiatry 41:669–677, 1984.

National Commission on Marijuana and Drug Abuse: Drug Use in America: Problem in Perspective, Washington, DC, US Government Printing Office, 1973.

Petersen RC, Stillman RC: Cocaine: 1977 (NIDA Research Monograph No. 13), Washington, DC, US Government Printing Office, 1977.

Post RM, Kopanda RT: Cocaine, kindling, and psychosis. Am J Psychiatry 133:627–632, 1976.

Post RM, Kopanda RT, Black KE: Progressive effects of cocaine on behavior and central amine metabolism in rhesus monkeys: relationship to kindling and psychosis. Biol Psychiatry 11:403–419, 1976.

Quitkin FM, Rifkin A, Klein DF: Monoamine oxidase inhibitors: a review of antidepressant effectiveness. Arch Gen Psychiatry 36:749–760, 1979.

Robins LN, Helzer JE, Croughan J, Ratcliff KS: National Institute of Mental Health Diagnostic Interview Schedule. Its history, characteristics, and validity. Arch Gen Psychiatry 38:381–389, 1981.

Rounsaville BJ, Spitzer RL, Williams JBW: Proposed changes in DSM-III substance use disorders: description and rationale. Am J Psychiatry 143:463–468, 1986.

Siegel RK: Cocaine smoking. J Psychoactive Drugs 14:321–337, 1982.

Smith DE: Diagnostic, treatment and aftercare approaches to cocaine abuse. J Substance Abuse Treat 1:5–9, 1984.

Spitzer RL, Williams JBW, Skodol AE: DSM-III: the major achievements and an overview. Am J Psychiatry 137:151–164, 1980.

Tatum AL, Severs MH: Experimental cocaine addiction. J Pharmacol Exp Ther 36:401–410, 1929.

Van Dyck C, Ungerer J, Jatlow P, Byck R: Intranasal cocaine: dose relationships of psychological effects and plasma levels. Psychiatry Med 12:1–13, 1983.

Weiss RD, Mirin SM, Michael JL: Psychopathology in chronic cocaine abusers. Presented at the 136th Annual Meeting of the American Psychiatric Association, New York, May 4, 1983.

Woolverton WL, Kandell D, Schuster CR: Tolerance and cross-tolerance to cocaine and D-amphetamine. J. Pharmacol Exp Ther 205:525–535, 1978.

Work Group to Revise DSM-III of the American Psychiatric Association: DSM-III-R in development (10/5/85 draft), Washington DC, American Psychiatric Association, 1985.

Chapter 6

Individual Psychotherapy of Cocaine Abuse

Robert M. Kertzner, M.D.

The dramatic increase in cocaine abuse in this country has challenged psychotherapists to join the ranks of clinicians formulating new and responsive treatments. For those providing individual psychotherapy, the task is one of integrating what is known about the more general topic of substance abuse treatment with the specific properties of cocaine. It is a task requiring a thoughtful blend of different treatment options to fashion a hybrid psychotherapy that works. The individual psychotherapy of cocaine abuse is a treatment with obvious effect despite obscure answers to such basic research questions as for whom, for how long, and for what reasons.

Little in the way of systematic study has established the efficacy of psychotherapy in cocaine abuse, although studies of other substance abusers have indicated the utility of several psychological treatments. Woody and Luborsky (1983) reported the superiority of supportive-expressive and cognitive-behavioral psychotherapies to drug counseling alone in the treatment of opiate addicts. Their data further suggested that different types of psychotherapies had selective effects on outcome measures.

Although research in the area of cocaine abuse psychotherapy is in a nascent state, considerable clinical insight exists, derived from the experience of treating other substance abusers (Millman, 1986) and an increasing familiarity with the natural history of cocaine abuse itself (Kleber & Gawin, 1984b, 1986). Nonetheless, several important issues need to be addressed in the different context of cocaine. How should therapists accustomed to working in a conventional dyadic mode proceed with the cocaine abuser? What conceptualizations, techniques, and strategies are most effective? What is the relationship between individual therapy and other treatment formats?

This chapter will address these issues by reviewing the current knowledge of cocaine abuse pertinent to psychotherapy and then describing the collective wisdom acquired to date in the individual treatment of these abusers. Recognizing that cocaine use ranges in severity from recreational to compulsive, this chapter will concern itself primarily with the latter, defined as: (1) the inability to stop or reduce use, intoxication during the day, and episodes of overdose, and (2) impairment in social or occupational functioning due to cocaine use (DSM-III criteria for cocaine abuse).

Specific guidelines will be offered and case material will be presented to illustrate the above. Since many basic principles apply to other treatment formats as well, discussion of the dyadic setting provides a foundation for a more general understanding of the cocaine abuser in group, family, and inpatient treatments.

THE COCAINE ABUSER

A rapidly expanding literature has described the demographics, psychiatric diagnoses, and psychopathology of individuals abusing cocaine (Khantzian & Khantzian, 1984; Khantzian, 1985; Kleber & Gawin, 1986; Millman, 1986; Resnick & Resnick, 1984; Spotts & Shontz, 1984; Washton & Gold, 1984). Familiarity with this information as well as certain properties of cocaine is useful in formulating the task at hand for treating cocaine abusers.

Figures available for 1982 provided an estimate that 21.6 million Americans had used cocaine at least once, with the number using it in the past month put at 4.2 million (Siegel, 1982). Although it is difficult to generalize about such a large population that runs the gamut from casual to compulsive use, earlier surveys of the cocaine abuser revealed relatively high levels of education, wealth, and employment (Washton & Gold, 1984). Compared to other substance abusers, the cocaine abuser was thought to be less likely involved in multiple substance abuse and to have a lower incidence of antisocial personality. These characteristics suggest a relatively good psychotherapy prognosis, but with the increasing availability and potency of cocaine (Fekel & Podlewski, 1986), the differences between cocaine and other drug abusers are probably diminishing.

As reviewed in Chapter 5 in this book, several studies have examined the prevalence of psychiatric diagnoses in cocaine abusers. Affective disorders are estimated to be present in 50% of cocaine abusers, with the following breakdown: depressive illness, 30%, and manic-depressive illness and cyclothymia, 20% (Kleber & Gawin, 1984a). Others have described attention deficit disorders in cocaine abusers (Kleber & Gawin, 1984b). The prevalence of Axis II disorders was found to be as high as 90% of cocaine abusers in one study, with borderline and narcissistic personality disorders predominant (Weiss & Mirin, 1984).

As diagnostic assessment of cocaine abusers has become more sophisticated, so have psychodynamic explanations of cocaine abuse. In Khantzian and Khantzian's (1984) recent review of psychological predispositions to cocaine abuse, changing psychoanalytic perspectives were presented. Classic drive theory looked to the id for an explanation of drug-taking behavior and invoked pleasure-seeking and, later, regressive and self-destructive motives. The escapism of intoxicated states was another early concept of motivation for drug use and abuse. Subsequent theories shifted focus to the ego-enhancing or adaptive functions of abused drugs; in this sense, drugs are seen as part of an overall coping strategy, although a problematic one.

Wurmser (1974) believed that drug use represented an attempt at self-treatment. Drugs were seen as serving as an artificial or surrogate defense against overwhelming affects, such as rage, shame, and loneliness (calmed by opiates) or feelings of unworthiness, weakness, and resultant depression (relieved by stimulants, including cocaine). The abuser was felt to have a constitutional vulnerability to such affects because of several underlying problems: narcissistic conflicts, faulty ego structures such as the ego ideal, a deficient sense of internal meaning, a desperate search for an object substitute, and hyposymbolization, a specific deficiency of language and abstraction described below. Wurmser felt that these factors comprised a predispositional constellation for compulsive drug use and, together with a specific reason (a narcissistic crisis) and a precipitating reason (drug availability), provided the necessary and sufficient explanation for drug use.

Hyposymbolization, contained in Krystal's (1979) concept of alexithymia, refers to a deficiency or difficulty with experiencing and recognizing feelings and the related inability to adequately verbalize or symbolize them. Individuals with this condition are ill equipped to defuse difficult emotional states. Feelings are vaguely perceived, undifferentiated, somatized, and thus overwhelming; they are experienced as uncomfortable physiological sensations to be relieved by the effects of drugs. Preverbal affects reign supreme without introspection or verbal expression to temper drug use.

Perhaps the most compelling psychodynamic theory of drug abuse is that of the self-medication hypothesis, advanced by Khantzian (1985). As applied to cocaine, this theory submits that cocaine is used to "medicate" the distressful states of depression, self-esteem disturbances, impulsivity, acute and chronic dysphorias, and cyclothymia characteristic of cocaine abusers. These states can be understood in terms of concurrent DSM-III diagnoses or as resulting from the frustration of needs typical of cocaine abusers (and for which the drug is intended). These needs, as described by Kleber and Gawin (1986), are: narcissistic needs for recognition and adulation; anaclitic needs for closeness despite pre-existent difficulties in interpersonal relationships; and needs to provide a sense of identity, a distraction from boredom, and a remedy for an inner experience of emptiness. Rather than experience a sense of personal inadequacy and failure these needs would imply, the abuser uses cocaine to "medicate away" such psychic woes.

In this context, it is interesting to consider Spotts and Shontz's (1984) profile of individuals at risk for heavy cocaine abuse: they are described as achievement oriented, perfectionistic, experiencing intimacy difficulties, and not "team players"—preferring instead opportunities for independent action as a result of counterdependency fears. Cocaine is experienced as a near-perfect drug, providing an illusory feeling of emotional self-sufficiency.

To summarize the above theories, cocaine abuse is now considered primarily homeostatic or prosthetic in function, as opposed to regressive, sybaritic, or masochistic. Although contemporary theories reflect a greater sophistication, it is nevertheless important to consider several caveats about psychopathology and drug abuse. Psychopathology can be a consequence as well as an antecedent of substance abuse; Gawin and Kleber (1986) have recently addressed this issue by documenting cocaine abuse abstinence symptoms as distinct phenomena. Moreover, psychopathology can be a coexistent variable with no etiological significance (Meyer & Hesselbrock, 1984). To some extent, psychopathology can also be considered an adaptation to the experience of being a drug-dependent individual in a society that stigmatizes such behavior (Millman, 1986); consider the treatment many drug abusers receive in busy emergency rooms. Finally, psychopathology becomes less clinically relevant as certain abused substances become more normative in our society (Meyer & Hesselbrock, 1984).

Several features of cocaine itself must be considered in examining the relationship between psychopathology and cocaine abuse. These features also have bearing on clinical issues, as will be discussed. Cocaine has been shown to be highly reinforcing in animal experiments where laboratory rats will self-administer lethal amounts of the drug; this is in contrast to the rats' more tempered use of heroin (Bozarth, 1985). In humans, the reinforcing effect of cocaine is almost equally as profound. A survey of callers to a cocaine hotline revealed that for many, cocaine preempted much in their lives. Callers preferred cocaine to food (71%), sex (50%), friends (64%), family activities (72%), and recreational activities (76%) (Siegel, 1982). The great reinforcing property of cocaine has led to the argument that premorbid disposition may be less relevant and drug availability more important to cocaine use than is true of other drugs (Kleber & Gawin, 1986).

In addition, since cocaine withdrawal is not associated with a classic syndrome of physical discomfort, such as the noxious state of opioid withdrawal, the well-described craving for a euphoric effect seems to be of paramount importance in explaining relapse. As recently described by Gawin and Kleber (1986), the resumption of cocaine use, triggered by craving, seems to occur as the individual is completing the withdrawal phase and about to enter the extinction phase of cocaine abuse. At this juncture, environmental factors play a particularly critical role. Social and physical settings associated with prior cocaine use become powerful conditioned cues for relapse and must be duly considered.

In summary, understanding patients who abuse cocaine requires an awareness of associated psychiatric diagnoses, psychopathology, and the unique characteristics of the drug. Psychological treatment of cocaine abuse can no longer be the psychoanalysis of the "addictive personality." Cocaine abuse is a multidetermined phenomenon, and, accordingly, effective psychotherapy is best conceptualized with several important perspectives in mind.

THE PSYCHOTHERAPY OF COCAINE ABUSE

General Treatment Principles

A flexible and responsive approach is the hallmark of effective psychotherapy with cocaine abusers. Different stategies may be indicated for different patients, and within the treatment course of a single patient, various psychotherapies may be employed either sequentially or concurrently. For reasons discussed in Chapters 7 and 8 of this book, the treatment of cocaine abuse almost invariably includes group and family work. Treatment may shift from inpatient to outpatient settings and may also involve medication, particularly if the patient appears to have a DSM Axis I diagnosis.

Thus, partisans of any one school of thought or those who prefer exclusive therapy rights will not fare well in the provision of psychological treatment to the cocaine abuser. Clinical experience bears this out, as reflected in the observation that therapists too zealous in uncovering psychological causes of drug use—without adequately supporting the patient—risk hastening a relapse (Millman, 1986). Underlying psychological conflicts do not need to be resolved in order for patients to achieve an abstinent state. This will be more fully discussed below.

Treatment itself can be thought of as the gradual transfer of control over behavior from external to internal loci (Siegel, 1982). This is typically a lengthy process which begins with several types of interventions to contain drug use. As abstinence is established, therapy becomes more streamlined and targeted to the specific needs of the patient. Some patients may eventually become suited for insight-oriented psychotherapy, but, as mentioned above, this transition is not thought to be necessary for abstinence (Millman, 1986).

A final treatment principle to consider is that cocaine abuse, like other substance abuse, is a chronic illness with relapses that should be expected and regarded as part of the natural history of the illness (Millman, 1986). Earlier interventions may need to be reinstituted, and the therapist may once again need to be part of a larger treatment team or support network to help the patient return to abstinence.

Clinical Management

Initial assessment

The patient entering treatment for cocaine abuse is assessed along several dimensions: the severity of drug abuse, presence of other psychiatric diagnoses, psychological assets and liabilities, quality of the patient's environment, and previous treatment experience (Kleber & Gawin, 1984a). These parameters are useful in determining the treatment setting (inpatient or outpatient), frequency, format (group, family, individual treatments), and modality (psychopharmacology, psychotherapy). The above factors also suggest what blend of individual psychotherapies is indicated; for instance, nonverbal patients with limited social supports might benefit from a combination of behavioral and supportive strategies with adjunctive medication. More articulate patients with mild to moderate cocaine abuse might respond better to therapy with a cognitive or expressive emphasis.

Stages of treatment

Treatment stages can be thought of as corresponding to the following goals: (1) stopping cocaine use, (2) securing abstinence, and (3) prolonging abstinence. Each will be reviewed with a description of specific treatment decisions required along the way.

Stopping use

Patients need to stop cocaine use completely. Resistances may take the form of a wish to simply reduce the amount of cocaine used or a reluctance to give up other drugs taken, which can impair judgment and precipitate relapse. As denial is the sine qua non of substance abusers early in their treatment, myths and misguided notions must be actively debunked. The therapist should be wary of colluding with the patient who proposes a gradual or incomplete detoxification. This may be expressed in the mistaken belief that the cocaine abuser can control drug use by himself.

At this initial point, a decision must be made as to whether the individual should be hospitalized for treatment. Criteria for hospitalization include: suicidal risk, the extent of psychoses, multiple substance abuse, a malignant environment, past outpatient treatment failures, and the patient's motivation to stop using cocaine (Kleber & Gawin, 1986). There is some debate over how to apply these criteria, reflecting disagreement over the general usefulness of hospitalizing cocaine abusers. Some clinicians argue that hospitalization delays the necessary outpatient confrontation of environmental stressors and conditioned cues for cocaine use (Kleber & Gawin, 1986).

Securing abstinence

If the decision is made to manage the patient on an outpatient basis, family and social supports should be mobilized, as is explained in Chapter 8. A trial of medication may be initiated at this point which, besides the pharmacological effects, may communicate to the patient the imposition of controls. During this stage, the psychotherapist continues to evaluate and monitor the cocaine abuser, determining whether the treatment program is appropriate. Using Gawin and Kleber's (1986) model of post-cocaine-abuse abstinence symptoms, these steps can be accomplished during the initial phase of withdrawal (i.e., the first several days following a binge), characterized by relatively low cocaine craving and some recognition of the consequences of cocaine abuse.

Prolonging abstinence

This stage of treatment anticipates increased craving and possible relapse. A variety of behavioral and cognitive measures can be implemented to restructure the patient's environment, strengthen behavioral controls, and prepare for long-term abstinence.

As described earlier, cocaine craving has critical importance in patient relapse. As the withdrawal phase continues, abusers experience increased craving, which is fueled by mounting dysphoria, selective recall for euphoric drug effects, and the likely presence of environmental cues (Gawin & Kleber, 1986). An effective treatment addresses each of these factors. Medication may play a role in treating dysphoria-induced craving, as reviewed in Chapter 10. Selective recall should be challenged by the therapist: reminders of the crash and its associated irritability, confusion, and dysphoria can help to defuse drug craving, and, over time, such reminders may constitute a type of aversive conditioning.

The role of environmental cues in precipitating relapse frequently requires a change in venue for the cocaine abuser. As much as is possible, patients should steer clear of the cocaine milieu: drug haunts and their habitués, cocaine paraphernalia, and the use of other disinhibiting or cocaine-associated drugs. The myth of cocaine selling without sampling should be confronted.

Several more direct interventions have great utility in maintaining cocaine abstinence. Random urine checks for surreptitious drug use have obvious value in detecting compliance, but they also may strengthen the therapeutic alliance by preventing devaluation of a hoodwinked therapist (Resnick & Resnick, 1984). Without a completely informed therapist, treatment cannot tackle the resistances and denial so characteristic of the beginning stage of treatment.

Urine checks are also an important tool in contingency contracting, a behavioral strategy linking cocaine relapse to meaningful sanctions. For example, a patient participating in such a contract will agree that, in the event of relapse, a previously drafted letter will be sent to his employer informing the latter of the patient's cocaine problem. Kleber and Gawin (1984b) cite the landmark study of Anker and Crowley in which (negative) contingency contracting was found effective in approximately 80%

of those who agreed to participate. Limitations of this strategy are the sizable number of abusers who decline to participate (52% in the above study), the rate of relapse in participants after the contract expires, and the ethical problems inherent in negative sanctions. Others have modified this technique to include positive sanctions for continued abstinence, such as returning patients' money held in escrow.

Cognitive approaches are particularly useful at this stage of treatment. Abusers are provided with an educational model that explains drug abuse as a chemical dependency and chronic illness; this serves to diminish the guilt and self-loathing associated with relapse while focusing attention on issues of compulsive behavior and loss of control (Millman, 1986). Educational models should not, however, absolve the abuser of his responsibility for the task of maintaining abstinence.

To help the patient experience greater control over cocaine use, considerable work can be done to elucidate antecedent feelings that act as conditioned stimuli to induce cocaine craving. Galanter (1983) has described a cognitive labeling treatment for substance abusers in which stimuli or conditioned environmental cues are identified, labeled, and then manipulated. Once recognized, they may be paired with an aversive stimulus (for example, motivational distress), and the conditioned response of craving can be extinguished.

More generally, the identification of antecedent feelings can help the abuser develop a sense of which emotions put him at increased risk for relapse. Some patients derive great benefit from understanding their "itch" to do cocaine in terms of feelings of anxiety or depression, otherwise unrecognized. This facilitates efforts to avoid emotionally difficult situations (when possible) and motivates the patient to create new outlets for poorly tolerated affects. Nonverbal outlets include exercise as a mood regulator and the use of deep relaxation techniques to extinguish craving (Resnick & Resnick, 1984): the abuser induces a relaxation response when he experiences craving or its antecedent feelings, thereby aborting drug use. More generally, as patients progress in treatment, they may develop an increased capacity to experience and tolerate affects, even distressing ones. What was previously acted out can now be articulated or sublimated with far less destructive potential.

Extended recovery

It is not clear at what point a cocaine abuser is beyond risk of relapse, if ever. In this sense, it may be useful to adopt the perspective of alcohol abuse treatment, which considers the abuser recovering, and never recovered.

When abstinence is firmly established, the above techniques may be gradually supplemented by other approaches associated with a more traditional insight-oriented psychotherapy. Interpretative techniques should be introduced cautiously for several reasons. As stated previously, there is no evidence to support the concept that abstinence depends on the resolution of underlying psychological conflict. Moreover, interpretative psychotherapy risks precipitating relapse if excessive anxiety is produced. Therapists must be mindful of many patients' limited verbal abilities and the persistent power of conditioned cues to undermine abstinence.

With these considerations in mind, the therapist can incorporate several directive models of treatment that address underlying psychological faults. Rounsaville et al. (1985) apply the precepts and techniques of interpersonal therapy (IPT) to cocaine abusers. Cocaine abusers, like depressives, are thought to be "symptomatic" because of underlying interpersonal problems: interpersonal role disputes, difficult role transitions, prolonged grieving, and a variety of interpersonal deficits. The task of IPT is to provide interventions that clarify these problems and suggest remedial action. For example, if cocaine abuse seems to be a response to role disputes in a faltering marriage, IPT would direct the couple to articulate their spousal expectations and would suggest techniques for improving subsequent communication.

Kleber and Gawin (1986) write of helping the patient better understand the psychological functions served by cocaine. A self-awareness of underlying needs may lead to an increased sense of control and a decreased need to turn to cocaine euphoria for a sense of omnipotence, described above. Furthermore, once these needs are exposed, alternative and more adaptive solutions can be devised. Patients can develop new activities and relationships that enhance self-esteem and build self-confidence, independent of the cocaine conceits of power and glory.

Millman (1986) cites Blume's review of psychotherapy with alcoholics, which describes treatment goals relevant to this context. They are: (the abuser) reporting spontaneous engagement in new activities, interests, and behaviors; handling unique, potentially conflictual situations in an adult and self-satisfying manner; accepting setbacks without becoming anxious or depressed, or without acting-out; knowing and experiencing feelings as they occur; and, when conflicted, examining and working through the conflict by oneself or in a nondefensive way with the therapist.

Resnick and Resnick (1984) suggest addressing these patients' limited self-soothing mechanisms and limited resources with which to cope with adversity and stress. The therapist facilitates a recognition of these limitations and encourages a higher level of adaptation. Through skillful management of the transference, patients work through previously unresolved feelings, such as despair and rage, which have resulted from early childhood deprivations.

Managing relapses

Relapse can occur at any phase of treatment and should be anticipated. Millman (1986) makes several points regarding therapy with the relapsed abuser. The relapse should be handled firmly to limit the drug-taking episode and psychosocial sequelae. Precipitants should be explored, and, for reasons previously discussed, a chemical dependency model of illness should be reexplained. Although the patient is not "blamed" for the relapse, some degree of patient distress is probably useful to promote vigilance against future relapse. Patients may need to be reminded that drug-craving responses are typically tenacious; abstinence, on the other hand, is tenuous.

Transference

The therapist's response to relapse reflects a larger therapeutic stance which is significantly different than that found in traditional insight-oriented psychotherapy. In working with cocaine abusers, the therapist should be prepared to foster a powerful, positive transference (Millman, 1986). The therapist needs to be direct and directive: patients should be challenged when denial and other resistances are threatening treatment; ground rules must be established, and environmental modifications as described above should be prescribed. Particularly in the early phase of treatment, the therapist is likely to play an active role, with family, significant others, and therapists providing additional treatment.

The therapist should also be involved in planning relapse prevention strategy so that patients will have contingency plans in high-risk situations. The cocaine abuser should know who to call or where to go in such a situation, and patients may need increased contact with the therapist during this time. The awareness of the therapist's availability itself may have a significant deterrent value, even if the patient never needs to call. Such availability communicates to the patient the therapist's interest and dependability; these perceived attributes are greatly stabilizing to patients who may be struggling with feelings of insignificance and impulsivity.

As is true of most psychodynamic treatments, the presence of a concerned, consistent, and nonjudgmental therapist strengthens the treatment alliance and facilitates change. In the context of cocaine abuse, this has a special nuance. The therapist promotes self-respect in the abstinent patient, implicitly and explicitly challenging standards of personal value based on the cocaine subculture. This is accomplished by several techniques such as crediting the patient for stress handled successfully, endorsing new and less self-destructive behaviors, and encouraging activities that reinforce current abilities.

To the extent that many cocaine abusers suffer from alexithymia, patients may initially use the therapist as a template for fashioning appropriate feelings, thoughts, and action. A dependent transference should not be discouraged so that this process of imprinting can occur. As patients develop greater verbal skills and introspective abilities, the relationship between patient and therapist can evolve into a more traditional one.

Countertransference

There are, of course, numerous countertransference pitfalls inherent in this treatment. The therapist should avoid assuming too much responsibility for abstinence for self-evident reasons. On the other hand, therapists should not be too passive, out of therapeutic nihilism, inappropriate neutrality, or general contempt. This is particularly true with regard to relapse; the therapist may respond with a knowing sneer or sense that "he did it to himself" (Millman, 1986). Although relapse is a part of the natural history of substance abuse, therapists unable to heed this reality will find themselves scornful or demoralized by the patient who "fails to get better." In this situation, the more disruptive failure will be the empathic one.

CASE HISTORY

The following case is presented as an example of an ongoing treatment of cocaine abuse. Although there is considerable variation among cocaine abusers in terms of their history, presentation, and clinical course, this patient illustrates many of the treatment principles and interventions discussed in this chapter.

History

S.D. is a 24-year-old, single, employed male who sought treatment 15 months ago for uncontrollable cocaine use. In his own words, he wrote: "My chief complaint is that from enjoying coke and using it socially, now

I feel that it doesn't do the trick any more and causes horrible side effects . . . depression, anxiety, lack of sleep, no eating, and a crazed sex drive. . . . I feel that I have no control of stopping."

S. had been using cocaine since his junior year in college (age 20), when he would occasionally snort a line with friends and experience a pleasurable euphoria. Over the next several years his use slowly progressed to the point where he made regular weekend purchases (1 g). S. graduated from college, began working, and started freebasing several times a year in addition to regular snorting. During this time, he occasionally felt worried that his cocaine use was getting out of hand, and he would consult a psychiatrist for several visits followed by long periods of no contact. He went to an outpatient clinic specializing in substance abuse and began an evaluation there, but interrupted this to vacation with his family.

Several months before seeking treatment with me, S. began a new pattern of weekend freebase binging. Concurrent use of alcohol and Quaaludes increased, and S. experienced these binges as "lost weekends," with less euphoria and more shakiness, sweating, disorientation, and fearfulness (for example, a vague sense that someone was behind him). Binges also led to increased feelings of being sexually "wired" and patronage of prostitutes. After a weekend of spending $3,000, three days of constant cocaine use, and no recollection of these 72 hours, S. became depressed and remorseful and contacted our facility.

Upon presentation, S. attributed his difficulties to a continuing sadness he felt after being rejected by a recent girlfriend. In addition, since many of his college friends were getting married over recent months, S. experienced his social world as contracting. Several of his weekend binges had, in fact, started off as bachelor parties.

S. denied any emotional problems prior to his cocaine use except for a transient feeling of emptiness following a rejection by a high-school girlfriend. Later in treatment he reported sometimes experiencing mildly dysphoric mood, typically in the fall, but without accompanying vegetative symptoms. He gave a history of mild depression on his mother's side of the family and mentioned a paternal relative who was successfully treated for cocaine abuse.

The patient is the oldest of four children in a recently wealthy family. While the patient was growing up, the family's financial status fluctuated widely because of the vicissitudes of S.'s father's business. S. would later describe himself as being a somewhat shy and insecure child, although this perception diminished in high school when the patient played competitive sports and fell in with the "right crowd." S. went to a prestigious college where he was an average student, guided, in part, by his father's injunction "to have fun." Since graduation, S. has become a businessman.

Treatment Course

At first meeting, S. appeared as an extroverted collegian eager to get help. He conveyed some distress over his recent cocaine use, but his mood was essentially euthymic throughout the interview. He appeared comfortable during the meeting, with no evidence of major psychopathology such as paranoid thoughts or suicidal ideation. He reported with disappointment his father's response to his cocaine abuse when the latter was first informed of the problem: his father told S. not to spend money on treatment, but to just stop. Later, S. added that his father had threatened financial sanctions if the patient was not successful in stopping cocaine.

S. ended the initial interview by stating he was about to leave on a two-week vacation.

The patient returned from his trip and treatment was begun. He was told that complete abstinence was the first goal. As part of our clinical program, he was started on daily doses of 500 mg tyrosine, 500 mg L-tryptophan, and increasing amounts of imipramine beginning at 25 mg; the rationale for this medication regimen was to treat any emerging withdrawal symptoms and decrease craving (discussed in Chapter 10). S. was also referred to a support group for cocaine abusers and was begun in once-a-week individual psychotherapy.

Over the next several weeks, S. reported several instances of being tempted to use cocaine and occasionally did (by snorting), but reported no pleasurable high. Therapy focused on supporting his successful avoidance of cocaine, underscoring how physically noxious his recent binges were, and acknowledging the frustrations of a slow period in his business. S. was encouraged to avoid cocaine haunts, and it was suggested he was "allergic" to cocaine. Imipramine was gradually increased to 100 mg.

In the third month of treatment and following a vacation with his family, S. freebased, gambled, and lost a substantial sum of money. He missed work, became demoralized, and had fleeting, nonspecific suicidal ideation. S. told his parents about the relapse; a family meeting was held and a plan devised to increase the patient's financial accountability to his family. Indications for hospitalization were reviewed with the patient and his family; however, it was decided that outpatient treatment could continue with newly imposed external controls. S. was reminded that he could not (literally) afford another slip. The precipitants for this relapse remained unclear despite additional therapy sessions during this period. It was particularly difficult engaging him in a discussion of the recent family trip and its effects on him.

Over the next several months S. remained abstinent. Imipramine was discontinued as the patient was complaining of side effects and seemed to have developed some internal controls. He reported with pleasure the positive comments he was hearing from friends, who found him bright, attentive, and enjoyable company. Sometimes he would comment that "we are doing well," referring to himself and the therapist. He widened his social circle to include straight friends and continued dating, but no longer felt it necessary to use Quaaludes or alcohol to decrease predate anxiety.

In the eighth month of treatment S. reported he felt he was at increased risk of relapse in response to the threatened disruption of his parents' marriage. Although there had been long-standing marital conflict, S. was "stunned" to hear that a parent had filed for divorce. He admitted to the fantasy that if he relapsed, this might forestall such a rupture. He asked if extra sessions would be possible, but never actually requested one.

A month later he again relapsed after a night of drinking. This time a contingency contract was signed stipulating that S.'s father would be called the next time he used cocaine; this would mean greater financial restrictions, which the patient dreaded. Again, no clear precipitant was identified; by this time his parents had resolved not to separate. Nonetheless, S. subsequently did well. Despite a slow business climate, he was able to feel satisfied by resuming sports, enrolling in an evening class, and developing another, more secure business. In therapy sessions he acknowledged being too dependent on his family and began discussing long-standing feelings of inadequacy. He discussed his mounting frustration that his varied and many dates, their fame and glamour notwithstanding, did not fulfill some basic need. These explorations tended to be limited since S. would quickly switch the subject to less conflictual material. This resistance, however, was not confronted.

Over recent months S. has done well. There has been an increase in the wistful recall of past debacles, but S. has countered this with jarring memories of crashes. He identified a woman he was dating as the "right one." S. identified himself as having a "sexual problem"; this was prompted by a relapse in which cocaine use seemed secondary to briefly seeing his college girlfriend. A decision was made not to send the notification letter to his father as the patient had enjoyed eight months of abstinence and had otherwise worked hard to consolidate internal controls.

Issues to be addressed are: understanding the conditioned cues of sexual desire and longings for his past girlfriend, alternative ways to discharge related cravings, and increasing emotional self-sufficiency. If treatment progresses to a point where more exploratory work seems reasonable, therapy should be concerned with: (1) needs for attention and admiration, and (2) underlying feelings of sadness and deprivation, perhaps related to S.'s childhood experience of inadequate nurturing.

In sum, this is a case of generally successful treatment, still ongoing, and with the implied potential of both continued improvement as well as episodic relapse. It began after a series of failed attempts to enter treatment, reflecting an ambivalence characteristic of many abusers who consider giving up cocaine. At its inception, it involved a variety of treatment formats, including group, psychopharmacology, individual, and later family. A variety of therapy techniques were employed, based on cognitive, behavioral, and psychodynamic orientations. The patient gradually assumed more responsibility for his treatment after banking heavily on the direct involvement of the therapist, particularly at the beginning of treatment. Interpretative psychotherapy was limited because of its probable risk and questionable utility, although the patient may eventually be more appropriate for such efforts. Several relapses occurred throughout the treatment, but this was not regarded as a negation of the positive effects achieved.

TOWARD THE FUTURE

Advances in the understanding of substance and cocaine abuse have enabled psychotherapists working with abusers to avoid errors of the past and provide more effective treatments today. Nevertheless, much needs to be done to make treatments more precise and clinicians better informed. The psychotherapist presently working with the cocaine abuser relies heavily on clinical intuition; perhaps this is true of all psychotherapy, but it would be useful to have more clearly defined markers delineating the treatment path.

In terms of the individual psychotherapy of the cocaine abuser, several important questions need to be addressed more fully. Systematic studies are needed to identify subtypes of cocaine abusers and their selective response to different treatment formats and strategies. Studies have already looked at the prevalence of Axis I diagnoses in cocaine abusers (Washton & Gold, 1984), and these findings suggest the utility of psychopharmacological treatments for some patients. Although there is considerable theory about the relationship between cocaine abuse, Axis II diagnoses, and, more generally, psychodynamic attributes (Khantzian, 1985; Wurmser, 1974), virtually no clinical studies exist which look at how these factors influence treatment outcome. For instance, it would be useful to know how defense mechanism styles influence the choice of treatment strategies employed. Studies are needed to determine what patient and treatment characteristics predict long-term abstinence.

Definitive research awaits the resolution of methodological problems such as those reviewed by Kleber and Gawin (1986). They cite several points in need of clarification: what constitutes recovery and which indices should be used to measure it; how to control sample factors such as severity of abuse, self-selection artifact, and heterogeneity of abusers; and an underlying need to better understand the natural history of cocaine abuse. These issues will also need to be resolved before good outcome studies of the individual psychotherapy of cocaine abusers are possible.

With ever-increasing numbers of patients seeking help for cocaine abuse, clinicians must, of course, provide treatment without the clarity the above research implies. In this respect, a flexible, empirical approach provides a sound compass to guide therapy. As cocaine abuse is multidetermined in origin, so should its treatment reflect a variety of approaches. Herein lies the challenge and satisfaction for the psychotherapist providing individual treatment to the cocaine abuser: an active, dynamic synthesis of complex input is required to create a "customized" therapy. The adage that patients let their therapists know how to proceed with treatment is particularly apt here; the clinical course of cocaine abuse is greatly responsive to a variety of factors, treatment among them. This makes for a truly dyadic relationship.

REFERENCES

Bozarth MA: Toxicity associated with long-term intravenous heroin and cocaine self-administration in the rat. JAMA 254:81–83, 1985.

Fekel JF, Podlewski H: Epidemic free-base cocaine abuse. Lancet 1:459–462, 1986.

Galanter M: Psychotherapy for alcohol and drug abuse: an approach based on learning theory. J Psychiatr Treat Eval 5:551–556, 1983.

Gawin FH, Kleber HD: Abstinence symptomatology and psychiatric diagnosis in cocaine abusers. Arch Gen Psychiatry 43(2):107–113, 1986.

Khantzian EJ: Self-medication hypothesis of addictive disorders: focus on heroin and cocaine dependence. J Am Psychiatry 142:1259–1264, 1985.

Khantzian EJ, Khantzian NJ: Cocaine addiction: is there a psychological predisposition? Psychiatr Ann 14(10):753–759, 1984.

Kleber HD, Gawin FH: Cocaine abuse: a review of current and experimental treatments. National Institute of Drug Abuse Research Monograph Series 1984a Monograph 50-111-129.

Kleber HD, Gawin FH: The spectrum of cocaine abuse and its treatment. J Clin Psychiatry 45:18–23, 1984b.

Kleber HD, Gawin FH: Cocaine, in Frances AJ, Hale RE, eds: Psychiatric Update: The American Psychiatric Association Annual Review, Vol. 5, Washington, DC, American Psychiatric Press, Inc., 1986.

Krystal H: Alexithymia and psychotherapy. Am J Psychother 33(1):17–31, 1979.

Meyer RE, Hesselbrock MN: Psychopathology and addictive disorders revisited, in Mirin SM, ed: Psychopathology and Substance Abuse, Washington, DC, American Press, Inc., 1984.

Millman RB: General principles of diagnosis and treatment, drug abuse and drug dependence, in Frances AJ, Hale RE, eds: Psychiatric Update: The American Psychiatric Association Annual Review, Vol. 5, Washington, DC, American Psychiatric Press, Inc., 1986.

Resnick RB, Resnick EB: Cocaine abuse and its treatment. Psychiatr Clin North Am 7(4):713–728, 1984.

Rounsaville BJ, Gawin FH, Kleber HD: Interpersonal psychotherapy adapted for ambulatory cocaine abusers. Am J Drug Alcohol Abuse 11(3–4):171–191, 1985.

Siegel RK: Cocaine smoking. J Psychoactive Drugs 14:271–359, 1982.

Spotts JV, Shontz FC: Drug induced ego states. I. Cocaine: phenomenology and implications. Int J Addictions 19(2):119–151, 1984.

Washton AM, Gold MS: Chronic cocaine abuse: evidence for adverse effects on health and functioning. Psychiatr Ann 14(10):733–743, 1984.

Weiss RD, Mirin SM: Drug, host, and environmental factors in the development of chronic cocaine abuse, in Mirin SM, ed: Substance Abuse and Psychopathology, Washington, DC, American Psychiatric Press, Inc., 1984.

Woody GE, Luborsky L: Psychotherapy for opiate addicts. Arch Gen Psychiatry 40(6):639–645, 1983.

Woody GE, McLellan AT, Luborsky L, et al: Severity of psychiatric symptoms as a predictor of benefits from psychotherapy. Am J Psychiatry 14:1172–1177, 1984.

Wurmser L: Psychoanalytic considerations of the etiology of compulsive drug use. J Am Psychoanal Assoc 22:820–843, 1974.

Chapter 7

Cocaine Abuse: Therapeutic Group Approaches

Henry I. Spitz, M.D.

Group experiences occupy a position of prominence in the substance abuse field. The flexibility that groups afford has led to the development of an array of group formats which is both impressive and potentially confusing.

Therapeutic group experiences are often the central component of integrated treatment programs for cocaine-dependent individuals. The structure, membership, and leadership dimensions of these groups determine the form, scope, and major focus of a given group experience. The thrust of this chapter will be severalfold: (1) to briefly describe the representative group types employed regularly in the treatment of cocaine dependence; (2) to define the rationale for the use of group experiences with patients who abuse cocaine; and (3) to discuss the practical issues involved in operationalizing theoretical concepts into clinically meaningful treatment formats.

This chapter will be clinically oriented in an effort to capture the flavor of the decision-making process of the clinician who organizes and leads groups composed of cocaine-dependent members. Problems or potential pitfalls in successful group work will be emphasized in an effort to shed light on the pivotal issues involved in group experiences with cocaine users.

An understanding of general principles of groups and the specific modifications required when the group is homogeneously composed of cocaine users forms the core of what determines whether or not the outcome of a particular group experience of any design is to be truly "therapeutic" in nature. This chapter addresses the clinical issues that bear directly on this theme.

OVERVIEW OF GROUP APPROACHES TO COCAINE ABUSE

For descriptive purposes, the group formats applied to the problem of cocaine dependence fall into two broad categories: self-help groups and psychotherapy groups. Considerable overlap exists between self-help groups and therapy groups, but it is simpler to arbitrarily divide the situation and treat each group format as a separate entity.

Self-Help Groups

Historically, self-help groups have been categorized as repressive-inspirational support groups. Contemporary models of self-help groups contain some of the traditional elements and incorporate aspects of philosophical, religious, and/or encounter group elements in a large peer group setting. Interpersonal networking and educational and support functions are central elements of many self-help group designs. Almost invariably, self-help groups for substance abusers insist on total abstinence from all psychoactive substances as an organizing concept in their group approach.

Cocaine Anonymous (CA), Narcotics Anonymous, Drugs Anonymous, and similar Alcoholics Anonymous (AA) derived programs typify current examples of this important group work. Allied self-help groups such as Narc-Anon, parents of adolescent groups (Galanter et al., 1984), "Toughlove," ACOA, and similar innovative self-help formats invite the participation of family members and "significant others" involved in the life of the cocaine-dependent person.

The rationale for the use of a self-help group model for cocaine users has positive precedent mainly in the field of alcoholism. The long-standing existence and widely reported usefulness of AA-type programs encouraged scientific speculation and study about the helpful properties of self-help group experiences. Vaillant (1983), Trice and Roman (1970), and many other researchers have attempted to identify, through systematized study, those factors which emerge in the clinical-descriptive literature as essential to the success of self-help groups with alcoholics.

The general purpose of employing self-help groups with cocaine abusers embodies a combination of generic attributes of self-help groups and specific elements clearly originating in the AA model. To explicate the particular components of this premise, it is useful to start with some general observations concerning the nature of the conceptual framework of self-help group experiences.

In the broadest sense, the self-help group movement was created to fill essential voids perceived by its exponents as being unmet by existing social systems. Price (1978) describe self-help groups of this orientation as "voluntary, small group structures for mutual aid and the accomplishment of a special purpose. They are usually formed by peers who have come together for mutual assistance in satisfying a common need, overcoming a common handicap or life-disrupting problem and bringing about desired social . . . or personal change" (pp. 241–242).

Self-help groups may be classified in numerous ways. Levy (1979) conceives of self-help groups as being of four major types: (1) behavioral control or conduct reorganization groups, (2) stress-coping and support groups, (3) survival-oriented groups, and (4) personal growth and self-actualization groups. The cocaine-related self-help groups fall into the first category. These self-help groups consist of members who share a common drug problem which interferes with the successful conduct of their lives. Group membership focuses almost exclusively on the drug problem and avoids addressing non-drug-related life issues in an effort to bring the cocaine problem under control.

Stress-coping and support groups apply to Al-Anon, Narc-Anon, and similar group models in which members support, advise, and share experiences that are deemed helpful to people intimately involved in a relationship with a nongroup member who is substance dependent. Members attempt to assist each other in coping with the stresses engendered by excessive cocaine use.

Katz (1970) has outlined other aspects of self-help groups that define them and differentiate them from other social agencies. Self-help organizations contain or share the properties of small groups. They are problem centered, and any recreational or social outgrowth of the group is considered a "fringe benefit," rather than an essential part of the group experience. Professional leadership is not a part of the self-help model. Groups are peer-led, and members have a sense of parity with each other.

All self-help group members must subscribe to universally accepted group goals which emanate from the membership. In the same sense that goals are group goals, action is also group related. Individuals undertake change on their own but do so in a manner that is consonant with the ideals and prohibitions of the group as a whole. High degrees of altruism and support typify self-help group experiences. Positive value is placed on fellowship, mutuality, and a spirit of cooperation among group members.

Self-help groups function autonomously from the standpoint of minimizing outside influences. Reliance on organizations, professionals, consultants, or other entities is minimized in most self-help groups and actively discouraged in some. The power base in self-help groups comes from the peer vector of the group. Group leadership emerges through the combined efforts of the membership. Designated leaders of particular group sessions may be chosen by the membership for a specific purpose. Members with long-term sobriety or abstinence are often session organizers or nominal leaders of substance abuse self-help groups.

Despite efforts to generalize about similarities of self-help groups, it remains a complex, if not impossible, task. Lieberman (1986), a frequent author on the subject of self-help groups, echoes the caution that "self-help groups represent a variety of activities, processes and conditions." Consequently, the operative mechanisms by which self-help groups exert their beneficial influences must be defined separately for each group. Careful categorization of the varied self-help group types, plus an appreciation of their general properties as just described, helps to increase accuracy of the answer to the most intriguing question in the self-help field: How do these groups work?

Few empirical outcome studies exist in group work as a general discipline. The problems inherent in researching the question of the "curative factors" (Yalom, 1985) in self-help group experiences become even more difficult owing to the diverse nature of these groups, their inaccessibility for regular study by outsiders, and a host of other factors. It is beyond the scope of this chapter to address this research issue in detail; however, Ogborne and Glaser (1985) have written knowledgeably on the subject. At this point, it is possible to delineate the most commonly cited reasons offered to explain the inner workings and beneficial ingredients of the self-help group format.

The larger size of self-help groups, as compared to traditional psychotherapy groups, facilitates development of several critical factors. Group cohesion rapidly emerges, not only because of the homogeneity of group membership, but also because of the broad power base for reinforcement present when many members support and identify with each other in the pursuit of shared ideals. These size and similarity factors promote affiliative ties which are correlated with successful attempts at achieving abstinence with alcoholics (Ogborne & Glaser, 1985).

Galanter (1984) draws a parallel between the properties of self-help groups and those of certain charismatic religious sects, as large groups capable of exerting strong social influence. Commonalities in both groups include consensual belief systems, a climate of optimism, a clear sense of group boundaries, shared attitudinal states, the presence of strong cohesive ties, and emphasis on compliance with the group norms as inextricably linked to the positive affective status of group members. What emerges from this cluster of variables is a picture of a potent force for change and, indeed, at least a clue to the appeal of self-help groups for dealing with symptoms as potentially intractable as alcoholism and cocaine abuse.

Vaillant (1983) addresses the issue of the group dynamics found in self-help settings from a conflict resolution viewpoint. He suggests that "A.A. transforms conflict solution via direct expression of impulses (acting out) into reaction formation (turning instinctual wishes into their opposites); alcohol, instead of being a source of instant gratification, becomes the source of all life's pain" (p. 203). The portrayal of this aspect of AA is an identical prototype of the cocaine abuse self-help models currently in use (CA, NA, DA, etc.). Furthermore, AA and CA groups effectively utilize group pressure and the need for group acceptance in order to maintain abstinence. "Slips" or relapses of group members cease to be an isolated, individual, or secret experience. Guilt, shame, and embarrassment in front of other group members frequently accompany the admission of resumption of alcohol or cocaine usage.

Both AA and CA groups try to instill the substitution of more adaptive attitudes to replace habitual dysfunctional ones. The extreme use of denial and projection of responsibility for chemical dependency onto other people, circumstances, or conditions outside oneself is an example of a target behavior strongly challenged in the substance abuse self-help group. The familiar opening statement of "I am an alcoholic and/or drug addict" epitomizes the concrete representation that defense mechanisms of projection and denial run counter to the group culture and norms.

The codified belief system found in many self-help groups is viewed as essential by many who work in the substance abuse field. Kaufman (1985a) categorically states, "Every successful treatment program for alcoholics I have been associated with has used A.A. principles as an integral part of the program, regardless of its orientation" (p. 93). AA, with its Twelve Steps, is an outstanding example of the construction and implementation of a unified set of beliefs designed to foster substance abstinence and counteravoidance tactics and to promote emotional and physical well-being.

Alibrandi (1982) has condensed the AA Twelve Steps into five major themes: the acknowledgment that alcohol cannot be used under any circumstances; the acceptance of a dependence on a "higher power"; an understanding of one's major personality issues, especially those connected with drinking; attention to interpersonal issues; and establishing patterns of helping others who are alcoholic. Cocaine-oriented self-help groups adopt a similar premise, and despite some minor modifications to tailor the groups to cocaine rather than alcohol, the central group design is the same as it is in AA programs.

Drawing on outcome data collected from another popular self-help constellation, the widows' and widowers' groups, Lieberman (1986) makes some thought-provoking observations. His research suggests that regular attendance at self-help meetings is, by itself, only a partial explanation for the success of the experience for the participants. Equally important, if not more so, is the fact that "the construction of a new social world composed of persons like themselves is the active ingredient of the therapy" (p. 754).

The principles common to all self-help groups are "that all types of helping groups are unified by the simple fact that all are collections of fellow sufferers in high states of personal need, and that all groups require some aspect of the personal and often painful affliction to be shared in public. Regardless of the type of group, participants uniformly indicated that the ability of such groups to provide for normalization (universalization) and support [was] central" (p. 755).

Although self-help groups share many similarities to one another, their particular focus (alcohol, cocaine, widows, medical illness, etc.) determines the manifest differences in actual operation of the group. Emphasis on cognitive, educational, or affective components contributes to the way in which self-help groups show their differences.

Finally, Lieberman (1986) eschews the notion of drawing quick conclusions about properties of psychotherapy groups based on data drawn from the self-help group literature. Psychotherapy groups differ from self-help groups significantly. The similarities and divergences between the self-help group and the psychotherapy group, when both are applied to the treatment of cocaine dependency, are illustrated in Table 7.1.

Psychotherapy Groups

Psychotherapeutic groups illustrate the malleability of the small group to meet an enormous range of cocaine-related problems. There is virtually no individual or family member for whom a productive group format cannot be designed to attend to some important factor in cocaine use.

The capacity for education in the small-group setting is well recog-

Table 7.1
Cocaine Group Formats

	Self-Help Group	Psychotherapy Group
Size	Large (size often unlimited)	Small (8–15 members)
Leadership	1. Peer leader or recovered cocaine user 2. Leadership is earned status over time 3. Implicit hierarchical leadership structure	1. Mental health professional with or without recovered user 2. Self-appointed leadership 3. Formal hierarchical leadership structure
Membership Participation	Voluntary	Voluntary and involuntary
Group Governed	Self-governing	Leader governed
Content	1. Environmental factors, no examination of group interaction 2. Emphasis on similarities among members 3. "Here and now" focus	1. Examination of intragroup behavior and extragroup factors 2. Emphasis on differentiation among members over time 3. "Here and now" plus historical focus
Screening Interview	None	Always
Group Processes	Universalization, empathy, affective sharing, education, public statement of problem (self-disclosure), mutual affirmation, morale building, catharsis, immediate positive feedback, high degrees of persuasiveness	Cohesion, mutual identification confrontation, education, catharsis, use of group pressure re abstinence and retention of group membership
Outside Socialization	1. Encouraged strongly 2. Construction of social network is actively sought	1. Cautious re extragroup contact 2. Intermember networking is optional

Goals	1. Positive goal setting, behaviorally oriented 2. Focus on the group as a whole and the similarities among members	1. Ambitious goals: cocaine problems plus individual personality issues 2. Individual as well as group focus
Leader Activity	1. Educator/role model catalyst for learning 2. Less member-to-leader distance	1. Responsible for therapeutic group experience 2. More member-to-leader distance
Use of Interpretation or Psychodynamic Techniques	No	Yes
Confidentiality	Anonymity preserved	Strongly emphasized
Sponsorship Program	Yes (usually same sex)	No
Deselection	1. Member may leave group at their own choosing 2. Members may avoid self-disclosure or discussion of any subject	1. Predetermined minimal term of commitment to group membership 2. Avoidance of discussion seen as "resistance"
Involvement in Other Groups/Programs	Yes	Yes—eclectic models No—psychodynamic models
Time Factors	Unlimited group participation possible over years	Often time-limited experiences
Frequency of Meetings	Active encouragement of daily participation	Meets less frequently (often once or twice weekly)

nized. Groups have been utilized to help orient and inform cocaine users and their network members about the realities of cocaine and to debunk myths and misconceptions about cocaine usage and its effects. Groups of this sort are often used as initial elements of broader treatment programs in the hope of facilitating program membership and gaining compliance with treatment planning.

Therapeutic groups are also appealing because they lend themselves to incorporation into both inpatient and outpatient programs. A typical in-hospital stay requires minimal to extensive participation in groups for the cocaine-dependent patient. Hospital groups are as varied as assertiveness training, drug counseling, stress management, CA meetings, self-actualization groups, multiple family experiences, discharge and transition groups, and many others.

Outpatient psychotherapy groups also have a variety of forms, including cocaine-related groups with membership populations as broad as couples, families, siblings, adolescents, men's groups, and women's groups. Similarly, different styles of group leadership have been proposed. The combination of group membership and leadership and the locale of the group result in a group format of a very specific nature. Thus, residential therapeutic community meetings, outpatient cocaine multiple-family groups, and inpatient adolescent groups all represent bona fide variations on the theme of the psychotherapeutic group experience.

Discussion of the construction and conduct of the major psychotherapeutic group types forms the bulk of the chapter to follow. The first step in this process lies in the clinician's ability to attain a sense of clarity referable to the understanding of the key dimensions of psychotherapy groups. Once having reached this point, the group leader can make sensible determinations about the choice of "ingredients" and their proportions in the "recipe" for the creation and ongoing management of a group aimed directly at resolution of the problem of excessive cocaine use.

Therapeutic groups are useful experiences, but they are not automatically generated. Not only is there nothing inherently therapeutic about the random assembly of a group of people with similar life issues, there may in fact be high risk attached to such a process. To prevent detrimental consequences resulting from group experiences and, more critically, to optimize the likelihood of success in the group, the group leader has to pay careful attention to several aspects of group structure and function.

Before the actual first session of a new group is held, the group therapist must consider the following general principles concerning therapeutic groups (Spitz, 1977). All effective psychotherapy groups share at least three elements: (1) careful attention to pregroup screening, evaluation, member selection, and patient preparation; (2) sound group composition and organization; and (3) active group leadership based on a firm grounding in group theory and dynamics. When these parameters are effectively managed, the central elements for a positive group experience are enhanced and the risk of adverse psychological consequences is reduced.

It is also useful for the clinician who is forming a group to think about four aspects of groups when interviewing prospective members prior to group entry: leadership style, group composition, time factors, and group membership issues. This clinical orientation is helpful in understanding prior group experiences a patient might have had as well as assisting in the decision-making process concerning future group placement.

The leader's theoretical orientation determines his/her leadership style in group therapy sessions. Psychodynamic, behavioral, transactional, Gestalt, and combinations thereof into technically eclectic styles of group leadership are a few of the varied positions assumed by leaders of groups. The leader's psychological school of thought determines not only his/her ingroup posture, but also the emphasis placed on clinical questions of group composition.

An appreciation of the group composition with regard to homogeneity and heterogeneity is one obvious aspect of group work that directly reflects the orientation of the leader. Most groups are essentially heterogeneous in nature with regard to factors such as age, sex, race, socioeconomic background, history of prior psychotherapeutic experience, religion, and vocation. However, many groups are composed of members who share one trait from which the group derives its descriptive label. Similarity in presenting problem set or other shared factors contribute to characterization of groups described in terms that are more homogeneous than the actual group process in sessions would suggest. The designation "cocaine group" implies a level of similarity among members which belies their actual differences from each other on virtually all other levels, except the drug they all consume.

Whether or not a group functions homogeneously or heterogeneously is largely related to leadership factors. Leaders who emphasize similarities, "groupness," and who intervene at the level of the total group rather than on the individual level promote a degree of homogeneous group function that they regard as essential to the therapeutic work in cocaine-oriented groups. In general, heterogeneous group elements favor the creation of a baseline intragroup tension that prompts interaction. Homogeneous elements form the building blocks for intermember trust and eventual group cohesion.

Time factors play an interesting role in conceptualizing therapeutic group experiences. Time issues yield significant information about the goals and scope of a group. Many groups utilize a brief psychotherapy format employing realistic goals attainable within a fixed time span. Often these groups are task-oriented in nature and stay in existence until the task is successfully accomplished. A current application of this model in the field of cocaine dependence is the detoxification group. Detoxification group experiences have the twofold task of helping the cocaine user gain distance from the drug and its physiological effects and of providing the initial induction experience into a more definitive therapy program for cocaine abuse.

Ongoing or open-ended groups usually have more ambitious goals and begin to approximate the model of insight-oriented group psychotherapy. The principles of psychodynamic or psychoanalytically oriented group psychotherapy are employed to realize the goals of personality change in addition to symptom control.

Finally, group size and whether or not group membership is fixed at the outset, precluding the addition of members, or open to the incorporation of new members throughout its course are important considerations. Broadly speaking, fixed-membership, shorter-term groups are geared to symptom removal and socialization goals, whereas open-ended, longer-term groups aim for the attainment of insight, increased self-awareness, and change in maladaptive behavioral patterns.

With these general principles of group psychotherapy in mind, we can now discuss application of these issues to the cocaine-dependent patient. How the therapist may go about modifying and updating traditional theory and technique to meet the special needs of cocaine users provides the focus for the discussion that follows.

GOALS IN GROUP THERAPY WITH COCAINE DEPENDENCY

Individual Goals

Many concerns face the cocaine-dependent patient and the clinician charged with his/her overall care. A combined effort between the two is geared to provide rapid stabilization and entry into a rehabilitative process. The evolution of a clear set of goals for each cocaine-dependent person helps restore a sense of order in place of the chaos that usually exists in the lives of people who use cocaine excessively.

Detoxification

Certainly, the top priority in the initial phase of treatment of any orientation is detoxification. Cocaine users need to achieve enough distance from the immediate effects of cessation of cocaine use so that they become able to participate in a therapy group in meaningful ways. The process of detoxification usually precedes group entry; however, some cocaine users require rather rapid group placement. In situations where well-motivated cocaine users become isolated as a by-product of having cut their ties to the cocaine subculture, rapid group entry is designed to support and reinforce healthy efforts to remain drug free. A therapeutic and constructive interpersonal network, personified by fellow group members, is substituted for prior counterproductive and addiction-promoting life relationships.

The therapy group functions as an interpersonal anchor during a predictably difficult time. The transition from cocaine use to cocaine abstinence is fraught with pressures for the cocaine user. The temptation to resume drug use is ever-present, as is easy access to the drug when desired. Cocaine users require outside support and guidance in order to successfully negotiate the change from excessive cocaine usage to abstinence from the drug. The peer and staff support elements of the group are extremely helpful in facilitating this process of complete detoxification and establishing an initial abstinence pattern.

Achievement of emotional equilibrium

Once detoxification is accomplished, the cocaine user is far from free of a number of disabling emotional states. Intense experiences of anxiety, often bordering on panic, and degrees of depression, usually intense, characterize the emotional sequelae that emerge when cocaine no longer masks, numbs, or "medicates" these symptoms. The control of intense emotional states is another important early goal in group work with cocaine users.

Under ordinary circumstances, the benefits derived from group participation itself are sufficient to help create a sense of emotional equilibrium in the cocaine users. A group's ability to counter feelings of isolation and alienation plays a prominent part in offsetting feelings of dysphoria related to these psychological issues. Concrete advice giving and other manifestations of interest among group members help contribute to a sense of belonging and being cared for in the group.

Despite the many attributes of group participation, some members still continue to experience extremes of depression and/or anxiety which interfere with their personal or vocational lives, as well as their ability to participate in group therapy. For these group members, the concurrent use of psychotropic medication, in addition to group membership, is indicated. The use of antidepressants or, less commonly, anxiolytic medication, prescribed by the group leader, is viewed as a necessary, but short-term intervention. The goal is clearly not to "substitute one drug for another," but rather to let common sense prevail in determining appropriate treatment priorities. Patients who are incapacitated by these symptoms and who require or desire outpatient treatment fall into the category of group members for whom therapeutically prescribed drugs are appropriate initially.

Integration of the cocaine user into the group is the most important part of this phase of treatment. The more "traction" the member gains which allows him/her to stick with the group, the sooner he/she is able to utilize group properties to gain control over troublesome emotional roadblocks. When initial emotional equilibrium is reached, the cocaine user is in a position to use the group to address important problems that contributed to or were by-products of excessive use of cocaine.

Addressing life issues

Commonalities among group members not only form the basis for group cohesiveness and support, but also facilitate the emergence of shared themes which serve as a focal point for group interaction. In early group sessions, members frequently recount "war stories" or "drugalogues" consisting of experience related to the joys and vicissitudes of life on cocaine. This process is a mixed blessing. In its worst light, the retelling of romanticized versions of cocaine adventures works counter to the establishment of therapeutic group norms, which value drug-free living. If, however, the group leader extracts from these discussions those elements common to the problem set frequently encountered among cocaine users, they provide a constructive basis for organizing the themes of group sessions.

Group themes that reflect unresolved life issues among cocaine users are readily recognizable. Some themes that can be productively used in groups are concerns about work, particularly fears of success and failure; problems with self-assertion; the appropriate expression of anger; issues related to sexuality, including concerns over sexual function and fears related to sexual inadequacy; and competitive feelings and problems concerning the incorporation of pleasure, relaxation, and fun into one's life without resorting to cocaine use.

Through group discussions centered around these themes, members orient themselves to one another and clarify their weaknesses, fears, strengths, and their purpose in being members of a therapy group. These life issues illuminated in early group meetings form a major portion of the content of cocaine abuse groups throughout their ongoing life-span.

Self-monitoring

Part of the purpose of becoming a member of a therapy group designed specifically to deal with cocaine-related problems is to aid in the development of self-monitoring skills for group members. Cocaine-dependent men and women have a very difficult time giving themselves and others an "honest count" vis-à-vis the extent of their drug involvement and their propensity for relapse. Group participation results in the acquisition of skills for self-monitoring that reduce the likelihood of relapse owing to denial defenses of individuals in the group.

Educational and confrontational group factors make a strong contribution to this process. As Brandsma and Pattison (1984) have noted with alcoholics, "There is an interactional relationship between drinking and contextual interpersonal cues. The group provides a congenial setting to observe these relations, to compare them to self-report, to powerfully confront denial and then to use the group as a laboratory for training in new responses and new skills" (p. 19). The case is equally valid for cocaine-dependent patients, and similar principles apply in the group treatment model.

From the very inception of treatment, members are required to make a commitment to remain in group for a minimum of 10 sessions. The rationale for this approach is in the value it has not only in providing a stable group nucleus of members, but also in helping members concretely self-monitor by assessing their level of motivation for change as reflected in the issue of commitment to the treatment program. The initial group contract reflects a treatment philosophy that places high value on honesty, self-disclosure, and engagement, not avoidance, on the individual and interpersonal levels. Encouraging an individual to be sincere and accurate in evaluating his/her level of involvement in the rehabilitative process is one of the central goals of each stage of the group process, from entry through termination.

Groups make a decided effort to help members identify self-defeating attitudes and behaviors that they ordinarily ignore or rationalize. Members are helped to identify stressors or individual risk factors that make them more prone to "slip" back into cocaine use. In one group session, a recovering male member who had just resumed dating women after a long period of isolation reported to the group following his first date. He became aware that his social anxiety, formerly handled by taking cocaine, was intensified by the prospect of going out with a "straight" woman. His impulse to take cocaine prior to the date was present, but he was able to successfully resist. When actually in the woman's presence, he described his inability to avoid having "a glass of wine or two" to allow himself enough anxiety reduction to handle the uncomfortable aspects of the dating situation. Both he and the group were able to constructively identify the sources of his apprehension and the behavioral pattern of handling anxiety with a substance that is itself habit forming, or at least a catalyst for breaking down the solid barriers to use of cocaine, and to plan strategies for handling future experiences of a similar sort.

Development of problem-solving skills

As with the case just cited, the reality testing and feedback provided by many group members contribute to an accelerated capacity for "problem spotting" in individuals.

Once identified, a problem is open for group consideration, advise giving, or other attempts at resolution.

Older members frequently help newer ones with advice or suggestions that were helpful to them at an earlier stage of the rehabilitative process. The new member who has problems controlling the urge or impulse to buy cocaine is taught how to control his sources of money by external mechanisms, such as employer or family rerouting of income, to provide an extra deterrent to cocaine acquisition. Suggestions about how and with whom the cocaine user should disclose his use of the drug are also commonplace. Decisions about the timeliness of when to return to work, resume socializing, and other day-to-day essential plans are openly addressed in the group.

Group norms emphasize engaging with reality issues rather than resorting to drugs to avoid them. In groups this is tangibly expressed by the push to encourage members to pay their accumulated debts, arrange for meetings with the Internal Revenue Service, and plan for any legal problems that might have developed in the course of their cocaine use.

Closely related to the development of new problem-solving skills is the subject of acquiring alternative coping strategies for feelings or problems that were formerly "handled" by excessive drug use. The management of feelings of frustration is a recurrent theme in cocaine abuse groups. Members describe their need for instant satisfaction, their difficulty delaying rewards, their need to be private and to have a secret side to their lives. It is neither possible nor desirable to control and satisfy all these elements in adult life. The member and the group must then decide how best to channel the expression of some of these basic desires to achieve a state of satisfaction rather than frustration.

Certainly attitudinal shifts and some analysis of personality traits are central to this process. In the "here and now" the group can also focus on the present and future and address the question of how to get "high" without drugs. Life-style changes are essential to this process. Group members often get intrigued with the pursuit of innovative and creative solutions to this dilemma. Activities that involve a sense of risk, permit the use of one's hands or some physical expression, and show tangible evidence of reward or success are those which group members describe as most useful to them as substitutes for some of the cravings previously satisfied by cocaine use.

Examples of substitute behaviors abound in groups. One group member who felt the risk elements and ritual involved in preparing cocaine for freebasing were the hardest for him to relinquish developed the hobby of making and flying model airplanes. Construction of the planes was gratifying in ways similar to the "chemistry set" features formerly provided by the freebasing process. Risk was supplied by flying the planes, as was a sense of pride and accomplishment over his success. When he engaged in contests with others, competitive drives emerged which found satisfactory expression in this consuming avocational interest.

Another group member actively involved with a lifelong interest in music described the conscious substitution of buying a piece of musical equipment each time she had an urge to buy cocaine. Over the course of time, she had the equivalent of a professional recording studio at home and had remained drug free during most of the process. This example is testimony to several important issues. First, the recurring impulse to use cocaine occurs at *all* stages of the recovery process. In addition, some members in the group seized on the expense involve in such an undertaking and challenged it as unfeasible for them. Not everyone can do things on a scale as dramatic as the one in the example given, but chronic cocaine use is an expensive process for all users, and the promise of immediate reward as an alternative to cocaine use can be accomplished on much more modest budgets when it would benefit given individuals. In the group, the use of expense alone as a resistance to pursuing viable suggestions for change is frequently confronted by members with the maxim "After you've abused cocaine, everything is cheap by comparison!" Inexpensive alternatives, such as active physical exercise, sports, and planning and structuring weekly schedules, can certainly provide other means by which the elements in cocaine-promoting patterns can be effectively redirected.

Group Goals

The dimensions of therapy groups are broad, and several facets of the group are of particular value when working with cocaine-dependent members. This section will highlight several aspects of therapeutic groups that makes the group setting ideal for working on critical issues that foster excessive drug use.

Peer support

Peer support present in cocaine groups provides the interpersonal cement needed to engage cocaine users in treatment. Once present, the peer and leadership support elements are a powerful influence for change in the drug-free direction. As a consequence, cocaine groups do well to begin with an emphasis on support, encouragement, and affiliative elements.

Vaillant (1983) refers to earlier work by Bales (1962) and emphasizes that "willpower and self-control can be enormously enhanced if they are derived from belonging to a group." This phenomenon is in evidence throughout the course of the cocaine group experience. The desire for acceptance among fellow group members increases as relationships deepen in the group over the course of time. When therapeutic group norms prevail, particularly those of abstinence, group acceptance is directly connected to active compliance with the group's standards.

Support, although desirable, is not unconditional. The esteem of other members is based on a member's ability to make an honest and constructive effort to change. Members do not support behavior such as lying, poor motivation for change, absences, and other negative or sabotaging behavior. As one member stated: "Either you're on the bus to go the full route or get off." Group members commonly have less tolerance for negative behaviors than do the group leaders.

Another vital lesson derived from the peer vector of the group is the model it offers the cocaine user that help can come from varied sources. Peers, as well as authority figures, supply essential benefits historically viewed as coming only from those in positions of authority. Cocaine abusers who have significant unresolved authority issues and those who idealize their therapists in their search for a "perfect parent" can benefit considerably from the development of peer relationships in the group.

Confrontation

High levels of confrontation are present in virtually all group sessions. In contrast to the stereotype of the drug abuse group where affect overshadows all else, an active effort is made to use the group for purposes of providing a cognitive and emotional experience for its members. The group principle of interpersonal honesty, coupled with appreciation of the impact of the confrontation on the recipient, embodies a therapeutic use of reality testing through group interaction.

"Character assassination" is avoided and attack packaged as "authenticity" is interrupted when it is clear that it serves no constructive purpose. Members who minimize the extent of their cocaine problem and those who avoid anxiety-laden areas are the objects of the heaviest confrontation in the group. Group leaders must allow for the expression of affect, including states of intense anger, but have to be on the alert to prevent the scapegoating of unpopular or frustrating group members.

Rachman and Raubolt (1985) describe specific guidelines for the use of confrontation as a therapeutic tool in substance abuse groups. Their concept of the "caring confrontation" blends confrontation with genuine concern. It modifies the extreme posture which reflects a caricature of the encounter group leader's one-dimensionally harsh stance and suggests a confrontational posture which is simultaneously "tough and tender."

Confrontation in the group has to be considered from the standpoint of its timing as well as its form. Confrontational methods are required when a group member's condition is deteriorating or when he/she is not responsive to other interventions that precede confrontation. When no emergency exists, confrontation can be steady and gradual, picking up intensity and frequency if an individual gets worse despite earlier and milder confrontation.

A central goal of both leader and peer confrontation is to keep the group moving in the service of constructing and maintaining a climate that promotes drug-free patterns. Confrontation should not be used as an indirect means of "purging" selected members from cocaine groups.

Peer confrontation has to be supervised by the leader to ensure that members, threatened by attitudes or actions they see in others that remind them of painful aspects of themselves, do not inappropriately attack the person displaying these traits. Some of the most intense group confrontations emanate from this group phenomenon. The leader needs to be clear about the propriety of peer confrontations at critical junctures in the group process. In this way, confrontation as a vehicle for growth through the group can be maximized and its potential untoward affects avoided.

Educational goals

The value of small groups as vehicles for transmitting information and as a form of powerful experiential learning has been accepted since the earliest days of group therapy. Small-group teaching is an essential part of the cocaine group design. Requests for factual information related to cocaine are viewed not as "resistance" to therapy, but rather as a central part of the rationale for seeing patients in the group setting.

Formal educational modules, such as brief lectures to the group on a particular aspect of cocaine, serve both as a way of imparting accurate factual information and as a catalyst for group discussion which follows the presentation. The incorporation of educational elements into comprehensive treatment programs along the model of psychoeducational approaches to schizophrenia is gaining popularity in group circles. Cocaine abuse is a logical field for the expansion of this work to a population in need of being informed about many central aspects of the cocaine problem.

Acquisition of insight and cognitive skills

Cocaine groups try to demystify key elements in the emotional lives of their membership. Education in the group refers not only to factual data, but also to the process of knowledge of oneself acquired through active participation in a group experience. Members are taught how to identify, regulate, and effectively express important emotions without having to resort to cocaine use. Cognitive emphasis helps deal with fears, unrealistic expectations, and the behavior that stems from these irrational beliefs.

Even in groups that are not primarily psychodynamically oriented, acquisition of insight into the motivational, familial, and environmental factors that contribute to cocaine use is apparent to group members. Insight-oriented cocaine groups place high value on self-awareness and structure group experiences in a fashion that promotes attainment of insight for its members. These groups utilize interpretation of ingroup and historical material and may use methods derived from psychoanalytically oriented group psychotherapy, such as discussion of dreams, analysis of transferences manifested between group participants, and understanding of resistant behavior as it emerges in the group process.

Though the routes may vary, most successful groups provide both a sense of cognitive mastery and increased personal insight for members who continue in the program.

Expression of affect

The expression of strong affect is problematic for many chronic users of cocaine. Intense feelings of anger and depression and positive feelings related to the broad category of intimacy are three distinct forms of emotion that require work in group sessions.

Techniques like role playing or behavior rehearsal lend themselves naturally to the group milieu. The cocaine user who is struggling with pent-up anger can be taught how to be assertive and appropriate in the handling of such feelings through the use of these techniques. Similarly, many members benefit from communication skills training, which they can practice with other members in the safe climate of the therapy group.

Members develop an emotional vocabulary for identifying feelings that heretofore may have propelled them directly into cocaine use. The recognition and labeling of painful and pleasurable emotions contributes to creation of a sense of positive commerce with the cocaine user's inner emotional life and an emerging sense of being "in control" of the feelings that precede action.

Universalization and countering hopelessness

Two "curative factors," universalization and countering hopelessness, potentially available to the group therapist are invaluable when working with a group membership that has been dependent on cocaine. Since depression and its manifestations are so prevalent among cocaine users, a sense of hopelessness often resides within an individual and, at times, prevails in the entire group. Group participation helps address these feelings of depression and demoralization in several direct ways.

Most obviously, entry into the group tangibly counters feelings of being cut off interpersonally and supplies new people with whom the cocaine user can engage. Group discussions that illustrate similarities among members help reduce a sense of personal alienation and offset negative feelings of uniqueness or "badness" related to cocaine use. The positive recasting of the image of the cocaine-dependent person from that of a "junkie" to one of a recovering cocaine user helps bolster self-esteem.

Having contact with other group members not only for purposes of identification, but as objects with whom members may get involved, serves to fight excessive depressive introspection and morbid preoccupation with oneself in a manner that only reinforces a sense of demoralization and despair. Members come to accept themselves and others more realistically through the appreciation of imperfections and limitations among all group members.

The sense of identity as part of a functional group emerges as members develop their connections to one another. The group becomes a new and positive subculture which minimizes the feelings of loss associated with the former drug-using group with which the cocaine user identified. This too is helpful in countering feelings of hopelessness expressed as fear that giving up cocaine is equivalent to giving up pleasure, friendship, and other "fringe benefits" of active cocaine use.

In summary, a review of the goals of a group experience for the cocaine user, on both the individual and group level, is a necessary precondition for formulation of a therapeutic group plan. Once clarity has been obtained, the task of the leader forming a new group is to screen, evaluate, and prepare members for the first group session. The components of this process form the basis for the next section.

PREGROUP ISSUES

Prior to the actual first session of the group, much work needs to be done to orchestrate a favorable group experience. This frequently neglected stage of group work, the pregroup phase, is critical in avoiding problems in the ongoing group once it has begun. The essential goals in the pregroup phase are to carefully select, screen, and prepare patients for group entry so that they join with realistic goals and expectations. The pregroup period has three central tasks: evaluation of prospective members, deciding which group suits them best, and providing an orientation to group therapy for each new member.

Evaluation and Group Placement

The total evaluation includes a thorough diagnostic evaluation, drug history, and neuropsychological assessment when indicated. In addition to these elements, a comprehensive evaluation which considers a cocaine user as a potential member of a therapy group has to focus on specific issues that directly affect group participation. High on the list of criteria for group membership is the issue of the cocaine user's level of motivation for treatment.

From a practical standpoint, it is useful to extract a time commitment for the program from prospective members to concretize their motivation. A period of approximately six months is used as an initial part of the group contract. Cocaine users who are unable to agree to this proposal are deemed not ready for the group and are referred to dispositions other than the cocaine group.

Diagnosis forms a pillar of the evaluation process. Formal issues of diagnosis as they relate to cocaine use are discussed in Chapter 5. In the evaluation procedure there are group-related diagnostic issues that require attention at this time. Traditional methods of individual diagnostic assessment yield useful, but often incomplete information regarding aspects of a cocaine user's life that have direct bearing on his ability or difficulty in deriving benefit from a group experience.

The bulk of this issue is the question of the accuracy of an individually derived diagnostic evaluation for group therapy where the primary therapeutic focus is interpersonal. The information gleaned from individual evaluation needs to be extended to include an assessment of interpersonal function, thereby yielding a more comprehensive understanding of personality which will be tapped in the therapy group. Two procedures are helpful in rounding out the diagnostic picture.

During the evaluation interviews, the group leader includes an assessment of group function. This is the group parallel of what the sex therapist does in taking a sexual history with people being evaluated as candidates for sex therapy. A group history can be done chronologically and entails a study of the cocaine user's experiences in "natural" groups in his/her life to date. Sequentially, these include the family of origin, early school history, peer group relations in adolescence, work history, military, religious, or other organized group experience, and a social history with particular emphasis on major emotional relationships.

As a pragmatic point, this may result in outlining the most useful clinical data referable to group suitability and placement. The following examples illustrate this premise: Cocaine users with high levels of authority anxiety will reflect this in work histories characterized by conflicts with superiors; in school situations, through difficulties with teachers and administrators; and, of course, with parents in their primary families. Cocaine-dependent men and women with excessive peer anxiety stemming from disturbed sibling and/or peer group relationships will show a corresponding historical pattern in dysfunctional relationships with their contemporaries. Since the group setting activates both peer and authority relationships, it offers a fruitful medium for the resolution of interpersonal conflicts involving both authority figures and peers.

The group history of a cocaine user may reveal chronic and specific relationship problems. This information is helpful in two ways during the evaluation phase. If a prospective group member's style is interpersonally destructive, as in sociopathy or impulse control disorders, then the therapist is forewarned that inclusion of such a member can be harmful to the group. The information thus becomes a possible exclusion criterion for group membership. If, on the other hand, a pattern of disturbed interpersonal relationships of a more benign type can be identified, the cocaine user can be placed in a group of specific composition, that is, one in which his interpersonal problems can be readily reproduced and, hopefully, resolved.

A second procedure that helps define the appropriateness of group therapy for cocaine users is use of the early phase of the group as an extension of the evaluation process. Early group sessions provide a testing ground in which the group leader can observe individual and interpersonal function simultaneously. In selected situations, a cocaine user's early group behavior will result in a reconsideration of whether or not he can tolerate, or be tolerated in, a particular group. On occasion, the first phase of group reveals a side of a member not seen during the pregroup evaluation. Members whose ingroup role is destructive or those for whom group pressure and confrontation is overwhelming are two types who may need to be "deselected" or removed from groups.

Yalom's (1985) maxim that members in outpatient groups need to be roughly equidistant from psychosis applies in outpatient cocaine groups as well. Diagnosis goes hand in hand with group placement and results in a group membership that is diagnostically varied for factors other than psychotic behavior and cocaine dependence. Matching members to each other is critical to the group design. Less often emphasized, but equally important, is the notion of selecting group leaders who also "fit" the membership. The specifics of leadership variables will be discussed later in the chapter. The issue of proper group placement, however, needs to be viewed as two-dimensional, involving both the membership and leadership lines, in order to construct an effective working group atmosphere and therapeutic alliance.

Pregroup Orientation and Preparation of Members

The group therapy literature of the recent past reflects a burgeoning interest in the issues of preventing dropouts from groups and utilizing methods of pregroup preparation to accomplish this goal. Whether this is done informally or through a structured program (Piper & Marrache, 1981), the group leader is wise to include an organized pregroup preparation component as a final part of the pregroup phase. The pretherapy training literature (Spitz, 1984) suggests that realistic pretreatment expectations for patients, eventual ease of group management for leaders, and positive outcome for the total group are directly enhanced by effective pretraining efforts.

In the author's experience, a pregroup checklist (Table 7.2) facilitates the process of patient preparation for leaders and members. The list is a model for the central issues that need clarification and discussion prior to Session 1 of the group itself. The items on the list may be discussed in greater or lesser detail, depending on how any particular item poses an area of uncertainty or misinformation for prospective members.

It may take one or several sessions to complete an adequate orientation of a member. The time is well spent for the rewards that accrue from understanding the significance of pregroup factors. Early attention to these issues at the first contact with the cocaine user seeking treatment sets the stage for the beginning of a therapy group experience with maximal likelihood of success.

Table 7.2
Pregroup Preparation Checklist

1. General purpose and goals of the group
2. Group composition and size
3. Role and activity level of the leader
4. Observers, audiotaping, or videotaping of sessions
5. Physical arrangement of therapy room
6. Time period of each session; duration of the group (long term versus time limited)
7. Loss and addition of group members
8. Rules about attendance
9. Fees and billing procedures
10. Other coexisting treatment: drugs, hospitalization potential, other therapies (simultaneous individual therapy)
11. Contacts and/or socialization among members outside the group
12. Modifications of the group contract (e.g., individual scheduling problems)
13. Confidentiality
14. Questions and answers about group therapy (try to clarify myths, misconceptions about group and elicit early resistances to group participation)
15. Anything unique about the patient's life situation that might intrude on his/her ability to join, remain in, or participate in the group

STAGES OF GROUP DEVELOPMENT

All therapy groups progress through definable, though intermixed, stages in their development. Information referable to this stage of a group's development is central to the selection and timing of intervention strategies employed at any point in the group experience. Untoward effects including premature dropouts from the group and serious psychiatric sequelae that result from ill-timed and/or inappropriately executed uses of the group milieu can usually be averted by a leader's awareness of the stage of the group life-cycle and what its membership can and cannot accomplish.

In the global sense, group members struggle with the generic themes of affiliation, defining the rules for power and control, achieving intimacy, resolving issues of dependency, establishing a sense of differentiation and autonomy, and ultimately separation as dramatized by ending the group experience. Against this all-purpose backdrop, one can define a set of stages which emerge with regularity when the purpose of a particular group is to deal with the problem of cocaine dependence.

The stages of development in cocaine groups are as follows: (1) crisis management, (2) stabilization phase, (3) induction into group, (4) establishment of group cohesion, (5) working group phase, and (6) transition out of group. This classification scheme defines stages of group development from a clinical perspective and facilitates discussion of stage-specific issues for the cocaine group leader and members.

Since many cocaine users seek treatment following a loss or a crisis, crisis management forms the initial therapy focus. Crisis management entails active attempts to decelerate an escalating pattern of cocaine use which has reached a crescendo in the user's life. During this stage of the group, efforts are designed to make an initial plan for abstinence from all drugs and to mobilize resources for implementation of the plan. Intragroup elements, primarily supportive and educational, are combined with external support elements from family, friends, and other program components in order to interrupt the pattern of cocaine use which is out of control.

Following the establishment of initial abstinence, the cocaine user profits from the group's value as a stabilizing influence which helps maintain abstinence. This stage of the group relies on active leadership direction, the supplying of advice and information by leaders and members, and strong emphasis on persuading new members to stay in the group. The stabilization phase also includes early construction of therapeutic group norms.

Induction into the group overlaps and occurs simultaneously with aspects of the stabilization stage of group development. Members usually have gotten enough initial distance between themselves and cocaine that they are in a position to "look around" in the group and engage with issues of trust, affiliation, and preliminary commitment to the group. Jockeying for positions of power and preferred status typifies the characteristic hierarchical issues that emerge during the group induction stage.

In one group, a member of long-standing, threatened that the entry of a new member who had just recently given up cocaine might jeopardize his established role in the group, dramatized induction stage issues by passing critical judgment on the new member. His comment to the neophyte was "You have a long way to go before you're considered a full-fledged group member. There is a long evolutionary series you have to pass through to get to where I am. Right now you're so early in the process, I think you're probably at the paramecium or pre-Neanderthal level!"

Group cohesion begins to emerge as a by-product of the interpersonal engagement of earlier stages. Increasing degrees of self-disclosure and a sense of emerging trust help bind members to each other in a therapeutic cause. The level of affect in the group increases, and participants reveal important aspects of themselves to fellow group members. A powerful interpersonal network emerges through the group, which directly helps counter feelings of low self-esteem in its membership.

The successful development of group cohesion enables the working-group phase to follow. In cocaine groups with ambitious goals, the working-group phase constitutes the bulk of the group experience. It is during this stage that members "work through" important life issues, feelings, and behaviors that have been problematic. Interpersonal and experiential learning dominate this phase of the group.

Eventually, successful group participation concludes with a transition phase out of the group. Transitional-stage issues include a sense of clear individual and group identity; a facility with effective communication; a review of past accomplishments, problems, and risk factors; an acknowledgment of emotional issues linked to separation; and a concrete plan for remaining abstinent after exit from the group. Postgroup follow-up plans are also an integral part of the termination phase of group membership.

The group leader must identify and monitor stages of group development and especially changes in level of development in groups or individual members. A member who appears ready to "graduate" from the

group may experience an increased desire to use cocaine after a protracted abstinent period. This temporary "regression" or reversion to prior
level of accomplishment may be an emotional manifestation of the anticipated loss of group bonds. Such a reaction in the final stages of a group
is to be expected and usually does not portend anything ominous. The
same tendency to be tempted to use cocaine by a member who has not
yet fully been inducted into the group, and does not share a sense of
solid group cohesion and subscription to the group norms, usually indicates much higher risk for relapse.

Knowledge of the stages of the life-cycle of cocaine groups helps the
clinician and patient to rapidly differentiate between hazardous and
"natural" developmental sequences of behavior observed in group members.

CLINICAL MANAGEMENT ISSUES

Leaders of cocaine treatment groups face many clinical considerations
which shape the fate of the group. Some of the major decisions that
leaders must make form the basis for the following suggestions. For
convenience, these issues have been divided into leadership concerns
and membership concerns.

Leadership Concerns

Single versus team leadership

Solo leadership of cocaine groups can be difficult. The single leader
must perform support and confrontational functions simultaneously.
This is possible, but it is taxing on the leader. This, coupled with the
observation that staff "burnout" is high among those who work inten-
sively with substance abusers, had led us to the evolution of a group
leadership model that uses more than one leader.

Team leadership allows for division or sharing of leadership tasks in
the group. The presence of more than one leader increases the options
for interaction in the group and in so doing may accelerate the pace of
the cocaine group experience.

Coleadership, although advantageous, has potential problems. Leaders need to clarify their roles in the group in order to function collabora-
tively. Leaders must acknowledge their differences and employ them
noncompetitively. Differences in theoretical orientation, professional
disciplines, gender, and other variables when handled constructively are

additive and provide group members with broadened options represented by the attitudes and actions of the group leaders.

A particular form of leadership in the cocaine group revolves around the use of recovered cocaine addicts as special group participants. In contrast to the peer leadership of the self-help group, our leadership model employs one or two permanent staff members from psychiatry or another mental health discipline plus a recovered cocaine user. The recovered cocaine user occupies a position midway between that of a group leader and group member.

The ways in which they are memberlike helps other cocaine users see them as role models for recovery. Credibility of recovered cocaine users among their peers is frequently higher than that of the "straight" professional staff who have not had first-hand experience with "life on cocaine." One of the criteria for selection of recovered addict counselors is a period of at least one year of being totally drug-free. This longer-term sobriety allows for an "elder statesman" role not too dissimilar from the sponsorship models found in AA and CA group programs.

A common occurrence in cocaine abuse groups is the immediate post-session increase, not reduction, in the desire for cocaine following meetings. The intense insession emphasis on cocaine-related topics frequently unsettles the equilibrium of group members who rely on adaptive use of avoidance and denial as coping mechanisms. The recovered addict group leaders are not immune to this process. They frequently report a feeling of discomfort in much the same fashion that members describe. To address this, the professional staff and recovered cocaine counselors meet regularly following each session to "debrief" the counselor as well as to review issues of group process.

Liberal versus strict group norms

Experience with cocaine-dependent individuals has proven how difficult it is for users to self-regulate central aspects of their lives. The structure and discipline required by the construction of fair, but firm group norms assist members in gaining control over excessive cocaine use, one striking symptom of their need for effective controls. The construction of a set of "ground rules" for cocaine groups crystallizes many of the norms that will eventually help members establish a sense of being in control of their own lives.

Total abstinence is a nonnegotiable condition for group membership. Realistically, not all group members are totally drug-free consistently throughout their stay in the group. The group aspires, however, to hold to this value whenever possible. Moreover, countertherapeutic positions, such as limited or recreational cocaine use and the use of alcohol or marijuana instead of cocaine, are actively challenged whenever they appear in group.

A representative set of rules and regulations which we distribute to new group members is listed in Table 7.3.

The general purpose of adopting strong group norms is to help set a therapeutic structure in the group. The leader actively promotes positive group norms through the creation of the group rules and his/her leadership style which models a consistent and nonpunitive stance. Since so many cocaine users come from families in which limit-setting functions or other parental functions were inadequately handled, it is better for them to have a solid group framework within which the therapeutic work is accomplished.

Brief versus long-term group formats

To those who subscribe to a view of cocaine dependence as a chronic condition characterized by exacerbations and remissions, treatment becomes a lifelong proposition. The role played by the cocaine group in

Table 7.3
Cocaine Treatment Program Group Therapy Ground Rules

Purpose
   To support and assist self and other members in abstaining from cocaine.
Rules
1. Absolute commitment to never use cocaine.
2. Absolute honesty about drug use.
3. Regular attendance: you may not continue in the group if you have more than the occasional absence (e.g., once per 2 months).
4. No coming to group under the influence of any drug.
5. "Slips" will be looked on as potential learning experiences. However, you cannot continue in the group if you have a regular pattern of slips (e.g., every week). This is destructive for everyone.
6. Random urine testing for all group members.
7. Group therapists will be in regular contact with individual therapists.
8. No socializing outside of the group.
9. Fee will be on a monthly basis, due at the first session of each month.
10. *Confidentiality:* Anything said in the group must be respected and not used for "gossip" or other purposes outside the group. Serious breaches of confidentiality are grounds for dismissal from the group.

---

managing the drug problem can be viewed from its short- and long-term perspectives.

Brief group experiences are essentially detoxification experiences. It is possible to bring symptoms under control quite quickly and to achieve a state of reasonable stability in a short-term group format. In our view, longer-term groups are better equipped to reinforce the adverse effects of cocaine in ways more acceptable to the user than aversively based behavioral methods found in some short-term groups. Personality, family, and other complex individual and interpersonal issues that contribute to cocaine use must be addressed in order to sustain a pattern of abstinence in the long run. The axiom used by AA reflects an appreciation of this position contained in the expression "You can take the rum out of the fruitcake, but you know what you still have left." This colloquially captures the spirit of the clinical challenge to the group leader of how best to deal with critical issues once detoxification has been accomplished. Ongoing psychotherapy groups serve an excellent function for both learning and maintenance of drug-free patterns, their causes, and how best to master them.

Closed versus open membership groups

The advantages of open membership in cocaine groups seems to far outweigh their limitations. The rationale for adding new members throughout the course of the group rests in part with the ability to maintain a group of sufficient size. Groups consist of 8–12 members some of whom may drop out before successfully completing the group program. The net effect over time is a reduction in the ranks of the membership, which has led us to prefer the option of adding new members when needed.

The addition of new members to an established group presents an opportunity to use several important group factors therapeutically. Temporarily, the established group pattern is broken and the entry of a new member interrupts continuing group themes. Since new members are ordinarily less far advanced in their rehabilitation, they often make established group members anxious by personifying the struggle to stay away from cocaine. Their presence brings many members back into contact with a vivid representation of themselves at an earlier stage of the cocaine continuum.

In this sense, new members can be used as catalysts to test the resolve of older members and to check the degree to which denial is still being used by members who form the nucleus of the original group. Similarly, new members are also welcome additions for established members who benefit from a sense of altruism. Older members show new members "the ropes" and help facilitate their integration into the group. In so doing, they not only provide a useful group function, they also experience the rise in self-esteem that comes from the knowledge that one has been helpful to a fellow group member.

Including new members also models flexibility and encourages members to avoid patterns that are excessively rigid or mechanical. Competitive issues are mobilized by new members, and this, too, provides rich data for group study. Most of the by-products of new membership contribute to the furtherance of growth in the group. The leader's managerial tasks are only to sensibly plan the timing of the inclusion of new members and to inform the group well in advance of their arrival. When this is appropriately carried out, the open-membership cocaine group model broadens the scope of the group experience for its membership.

Family involvement

How to involve the family of the cocaine-dependent group member always forms a part of the overall treatment plan. The family serves as a source of historical data and provides excellent opportunities for amplifying diagnostic issues. Direct observation of the cocaine user and his/her family during the evaluation phase prior to group entry gives the group leader a direct glimpse into the dynamics at play in the primary family group. Along with the value of observing the role of cocaine use in the family system, the group therapist has an unparalleled chance to see the patient's group function in a true-to-life setting with his or her family.

Family involvement may be necessary as a form of intervention to engage a resistant cocaine user in group treatment. Family support and presence, either on their own or as part of a structured network intervention, is effective in propelling cocaine-dependent individuals into necessary therapeutic settings. The cocaine user who has ambivalent to negative feelings about joining a therapy group can get the necessary "push" from thoughtful mobilization of family resources. Recommendations about other family members participating in allied experiences, such as Narc-Anon, can be effected through family interviews.

Psychotropic medication management

We have evolved a combined psychotherapeutic and psychopharmacological approach. Early in the course of treatment, a cocaine-abusing patient may temporarily require therapeutically prescribed medication to assist in managing a disabling depression or in gaining rapid control over extremes of cocaine use. Regardless of the indication for the use of psychotropic medication, the discussion, monitoring, and prescription of the drug become part of the group session itself.

Handling medication issues in the group provides a basis for increasing compliance since all group members understand the rationale for the use of these medications. A strong effort is made to differentiate drugs with abuse potential from medications that are potentially useful to cocaine-dependent individuals in their recovery period.

Medication themes are frequent in group sessions. Members express their reservations about taking drugs of any kind, the physiological and psychological effects of the medication they take, the fears of being excessively reliant on a "chemical crutch," and their desire to get off of medication as soon as possible.

Medication is never presented as a solution to the cocaine problem, and the basic principle is to use a prescription drug for the shortest period necessary for it to accomplish its purpose.

Concurrent individual sessions

Every effort is made to encourage management of a broad range of problems within the group. However, in certain circumstances, sessions outside the group may be necessary. Crisis situations, unusual medication issues, and conditions that involve a nongroup member, as in marital problems, are all instances in which group members may need to be seen individually or with their significant family members. Although the group may be a preferred form of treatment, for many cocaine users it has its limitations, and the group leader must guard against rigidly insisting that everything be handled in the group.

Very often a cocaine user is referred for group therapy by an individual therapist who plans to continue individual psychotherapy sessions. When this is the case, the group leader must get the patient's permission to communicate with the individual therapist. This process aids in coordinating treatment efforts and guards against the splitting defense sometimes utilized by cocaine users who play off one therapist against another in an effort to resist change. When the therapists involved in a cocaine user's care communicate regularly, group and individual therapies work harmoniously and add valuable dimensions to one another.

On occasion, the converse situation exists wherein a cocaine user's group behavior suggests that additional individual work is necessary. The time constraints of cocaine groups, which usually meet only once or twice a week, plus the realistic division of the time of each session among many members, may necessitate referral of selected group members for individual psychotherapy. Observation of the member's participation in the group helps enormously in evaluating the type of psychotherapeutic setting and/or combination of therapies that will be maximally beneficial.

Contact outside the group

Extragroup contact among cocaine users poses a thorny question. In principle, contact among group members outside formal group sessions is either prohibited or, if permitted, serves a purpose directly in concert with the goals of the group. The concept of contact outside the group takes on added significance in groups of cocaine users because of the concern surrounding the risk of members misusing their outside contacts in ways that promote their use of cocaine.

Sanctioning an activity that might possibly lead to the facilitation of cocaine use has to be balanced against the prospective values of extragroup contact. The most important advantage of member contacts outside of sessions comes from the networking function which can originate in the group. Members in groups can effectively use their relationships as deterrents to, not facilitators of, renewed cocaine use.

In light of these considerations, we have formulated a policy that requests that members in new groups refrain from getting together with each other until the group is well launched (at least 10–12 sessions) and the issue of extragroup contact has been openly addressed and resolved in group sessions. The rationale for this position is only partially prompted by the issue of extragroup contact. It serves the dual purpose of confining and directing the early interactions among group members into group sessions where their behavior and feelings are available for group work. The viability of the group becomes the initial priority, and decisions regarding socialization among members are reviewed in conjunction with their effect on the integrity of the therapy group.

Once a sound sense of group cohesiveness is reached, the resources present in a well-functioning group can be made available to the membership. At this point in the group's life, networking elements are incorporated into the group design. The first form this takes in cocaine groups is the exchange of phone numbers among group members. Leaders and members define the procedure for members contacting one another, and agreement among them is established in the group.

Members utilize the telephone network to interrupt their urges to use cocaine. Group members rapidly learn to distinguish between advantageous and improper use of the group support network. Contacts among members between group sessions are reported to the group in the next meeting. When the nature of the contact is at odds with its expressed purpose, or when members feel uncomfortable with the plan, or when an outside "connection" has helped avoid a time of high risk for cocaine use, the subject of members' meeting outside of group sessions becomes a prominent group theme.

The group therapist sees only part of the cocaine user's life. Group leaders who work with substance-abusing patients cannot afford the luxury of being naive about important issues. In selected circumstances, group members will get together outside the group in ways that are contrary to the group's goals. At times, members will collude with each other in a pact of secrecy and withhold this information from the leaders and members of the group. In addition, in a de facto sense, the cocaine group is not the only arena for contact with a population of cocaine users. Many group members attend CA or other drug-related groups, which are exclusively populated by drug-abusing men and women.

Many of these factors translate into the adoption of a clinical stance that places value on access to information in the cocaine user's life as a group priority above prohibiting or sanctioning specific behavior in members. Although group leaders take active stances about issues as important as extragroup contact, they are, at the same time, aware that merely stating a position is not synonymous with its universal adoption by group members. Information related to the nature, extent, and function of extramural relationships among members assists greatly in tracking progress in treatment, identifying roadblocks, and establishing plans for resolution of lingering interpersonal and individual issues demonstrated through the character of the relationships developed among group members both inside and outside of regular sessions.

Management of ''slips''

Mandatory urine testing is essential in the cocaine group format. All members who join the group agree to participate in the urine-screening program as a precondition for group membership. Results of laboratory tests are discussed openly in the group, and an effort is made to understand the significance of positive and negative urine test results in the overall clinical course of group participants.

Relapses into episodic cocaine use are expected in the rehabilitation process. Ehrlich and McGeehan (1985) suggest that there may be predictable "flareup periods" during which abstinent cocaine users will revert to former patterns of drug abuse. Groups that employ urine-testing methods are able to quickly identify members who are struggling to remain free from cocaine use.

Identification of active cocaine use among group members is merely the first step in a therapeutic process. The tangible laboratory report precludes denial of cocaine use by members. Once identified, the group focus turns to formulating a realistic, but constructive strategy for those members who have "slipped."

Peer confrontation is intense, and the group leader has to guard against the group's tendency to scapegoat the member who has slipped. The leader's task is to convert the knowledge of current cocaine use by a member into a form from which all group members may learn something useful. Abstinent members are reminded of the compulsion to use cocaine, their own issues of impulsivity, and the value of total abstinence as a secure plan for distancing themselves from the temptation to take drugs again.

The structure, support, and limit-setting functions of groups assist in reducing the chances of slips in group members. Even though the group philosophy attempts to use slips as learnings experiences, some members are unresponsive to the group effort. There is a ceiling on the frequency of cocaine use with respect to retention of group membership. Cocaine group members who repeatedly slip require a plan other than group therapy alone. In severe instances, inpatient stays may be necessary to interrupt resumption of the pattern of regular cocaine use.

Simultaneous group experiences

The cocaine-dependent person who attends a weekly cocaine group very often requires more involvement with drug-free influences than the group can provide. CA and similar self-help groups are recommended in conjunction with psychotherapy groups.

Membership in more than one group simultaneously has, in our experience, worked synergistically. Recovering cocaine users benefit from the broad base of support present in self-help groups. The additional reenforcement of the value of abstinence lends strength to the principles of the psychotherapy group. Coexisting group membership can create a reverberating circuit between rehabilitation experiences which promotes positive change in cocaine-dependent people.

Psychotherapy group members who report experiences with CA-type groups have found several aspects of the CA group to be helpful. Established CA groups contain members who have achieved long-term (years) of sobriety. In contrast to newly formed psychotherapy groups, the self-help group has peers as role models for living drug-free over an extended period of time. This spurs realistic hope for change and underscores healthy identification processes among former cocaine abusers. Therapy group members also describe being the recipients of a "dose of instant perspective" reflected in the wide cross-section of members who attend self-help groups. Cocaine users get helpful advice and practical information from CA meetings which they regard highly.

Management of problem members

Thus far, the focus of this section has been on problems that regularly relate to having a group with a specific membership of cocaine users. There are, however, many "garden variety" issues which occur in all psychotherapeutic groups that apply to cocaine groups as well. The outstanding example of problematic issues in this category is management of group members whose personality dictates an ingroup presence and posture that is troublesome for the group and the leader.

The author and associates (Spitz et al., 1980) addressed the question and identified a cluster of membership roles and behaviors that pose challenges to the group leader. These findings apply equally to the cocaine group model. The "problem patients" include those who are help-rejecting, complaining, monopolistic, aggressive, or silent in group sessions. Managing the unique problems attached to each role requires more explication than is possible in this discussion. However, the group leader is wise to pay attention to the systems aspects of group as well as focusing on the individual aspects of a member's role. A common example of the confluence of individual and group resistances is a session in which one member monopolizes the group time through lengthy, intellectualized monologues. In addition to exploring this troublesome individual posture which prevents group movement, the leader must also question what it is about the group at this particular time that causes them to not interrupt this member. In cocaine groups, sessions in which one member is "permitted" to go on indefinitely frequently serve the purpose of allowing the silent members to "hide" behind the guise of politeness in not wanting to interrupt the group monopolist. Very often, the cocaine user who has slipped, or one who is concealing some embarrassing information, is glad to allow the group time to be consumed by someone else, thereby avoiding uncomfortable self-disclosure on his own part. Successful group management includes addressing both individual and group roles in order to gain thorough understanding of group dynamics and group process.

Cocaine groups present two other problem patient types in addition to those just noted. The seriously depressed member and the cocaine user who comes to the group while he is "high" on cocaine are examples of two recognizable group phenomena which require astute management. The seriously depressed member requires active evaluation for medication and/or possible hospitalization directly from the group.

The pregroup membership orientation and the setting of clear group limits make it easier to remove members from groups when it is clear that they are under the influence of drugs. Remaining members are also less likely to misperceive this therapist action as arbitrary or excessively punitive once it has been clearly established as a group norm for everyone. In fact, members are more often relieved rather than distressed when active steps are taken to preserve the therapeutic climate of the group.

Monitoring the stereotypic and rigid roles played by members is important. This process helps manage session-to-session character traits that require longer-term psychotherapeutic management, while concurrently providing a basis for handling insession "minicrises" created by extreme demonstrations of role-related membership behavior.

Hospitalization of group members

The cocaine group provides a superb vehicle for monitoring its members' state of recovery or relapse. From time to time, a group member will deteriorate to a point where hospitalization needs to be considered. Intense states of depression with suicidal ideation, evidence of active psychosis, and lack of responsivity to other treatment resulting in a continued and escalating cocaine use are three major circumstances under which inpatient placement needs to be considered.

Groups can be very influential in encouraging a reluctant member to enter the hospital when indicated. Group support expresses concern, caring, and the invitation for the member to rejoin the group upon discharge from the hospital. Group pressure also helps to break through unreasonable reluctance to enter an inpatient setting. Members may be hospitalized directly from the group in settings where inpatient facilities are close by.

Group members who are unable to stop using cocaine and reach the point of requiring hospitalization are often spared the additional stress of being the recipients of the accumulated anger of group members who have been frustrated and defeated in their gestures of help. Groups run some risk of demoralization in circumstances where all efforts to help a cocaine-using member achieve predictable abstinence fall short of the mark. Viewed from this perspective, the hospitalization of a group member "decompresses" a tense period in the group and provides an interim solution for the hospitalized patient and his/her comembers.

Membership Issues

Composition of the group

Variations in group composition may be required in selected subgroups of the cocaine-dependent population. Generally speaking, cocaine groups, as noted earlier, are composed in an effort to strike a balance between homogeneous and heterogeneous elements among members. Groups that are homogeneous for sex may be created if they facilitate entry into treatment for treatment-resistant men and women. Same-sex groups are initial group experiences designed for to engage members who are hesitant to enter treatment in a mixed-sex cocaine group.

Members of cocaine men's groups have repeatedly expressed the concern that "I'd never be able to say certain things in front of women." Because the early treatment priorities include becoming abstinent and reducing anxiety, the presence of anxiety-laden issues related to the opposite sex prompted the creation of men's and women's group formats. Experience with homogeneous groups of men suggests that once members resolve their initial concerns related to entry into treatment, establishing relationships in the group, and having a "test run" of the group experience, they often express a desire to address issues related to women. Concerns about one's own sexual inadequacy, possession of demeaning attitudes toward female cocaine users ("coke whores"), and competitive fears involving "macho" jockeying for position with fellow group members if women were present provided the original areas of trepidation about bringing women into the group.

The members' coexisting desire to have the group more closely represent a "real-life" model, their curiosity about how women see cocaine-related issues, and the prospect of having the opportunity to freely interact with women in the safety of the group eventually have led to a trend toward formation of mixed men and women's groups in the latter stages of therapy for this subgroup.

Another aspect of group membership related to composition is the deliberate attempt to mix older and younger members and those with long-term abstinence with those earlier in the recovery process. This procedure creates an implicit hierarchy in the group and helps members strive for status by being successful at long-term abstinence from cocaine and achieving emotional as well as chronological maturity.

Subgroup formation

A practical problem in all groups is recognition of dysfunctional sub-groupings among group members. Members of cocaine groups may form relationships from which other group members are excluded, resulting in a rash of competitive issues in the group. Subgroups drain off significant information and emotional energy from group experiences, resulting in a threat to group cohesiveness.

The sabotaging influence of subgrouping can be observed in a variety of ways. The most serious consequences of subgrouping in cocaine groups involve instances in which two or more group members get together outside of the group for purposes of using cocaine. The socio-pathic cocaine abuser is a common instigator of disruptive action related to the formation of destructive relationships with group members. Failure to refrain from subgrouping activities that result in cocaine use is considered grounds for dismissal from the group. Other versions of subgrouping, which affect group interaction but do not involve drug use, are dealt with as antitherapeutic issues in the ongoing cocaine group sessions.

Confidentiality

Along with the high value placed on honesty and self-disclosure in cocaine groups, strict confidentiality must be ensured for group members. The issue of confidentiality has added significance in cocaine groups, since cocaine is an illegal substance. Information disclosed in group sessions could be potentially damaging to a group member's life. Therefore, the leader must consider carefully the selection of members for the group who can adhere to the ground rules for privacy.

In many groups, information "fed back" to a given member is useful to him/her in relationship to a nongroup member. In such circumstances, group members are asked to be judicious in discussing information originating in group sessions with outsiders. Under no circumstances is it acceptable to identify the source of the information or to violate the privacy of group members in other ways.

An observation about a member's marital relationship that comes to him/her through the group's perceptions may prove useful to take out of the group and share with the spouse. This is considered an acceptable use of group information. Divulging the identity of a "celebrity," community member, or other group member constitutes lack of proper respect for confidentiality and calls for immediate action on the leaders' part in evaluating whether or not it is possible to retain the involved member in the group.

Attendance, lateness, fees

The "administrative" tasks of the leader require thoughtful planning and consistent implementation. Regular attendance and coming to sessions on time are basic to any cocaine group. The group leader, as role model for members, should subscribe to and demonstrate the principles he/she advocates. Sessions need to begin promptly and end when scheduled to do so. Cocaine users who attend organized, well-run groups begin to incorporate important messages from these experiences. Planning ahead, managing one's time, accepting frustration, delaying reward, and many other elements embodied in the conduct of the group address basic life issues currently under revision in the cocaine user's life.

When fees for cocaine groups are charged, the issue of money also precipitates relevant themes for cocaine users. The policy of paying in advance for sessions tests motivation and tries to encourage attendance at all sessions. Advance fee payment and mandatory urine testing are two examples of how contingency contracting aspects of behavioral approaches can be blended with therapy group plans.

SPECIALIZED GROUP FORMATS

Before concluding this overview of group therapy for the problem of cocaine dependence, it is important to briefly note a few other commonly practiced group forms that address issues of special significance.

Family Groups

Two popular formats that combine group and family therapy to address the problem of cocaine abuse are multiple-family groups and couples groups. Both usually play a role as one dimension of an overall treatment plan that includes other modalities.

Tucker and Maxmen (1975) extracted 11 general functions of multiple-family groups which help explain the current clinical enthusiasm for, and methodology of, these groups for the treatment of cocaine problems. These factors include: deisolation; socialization and support; imparting information; catharsis; problem solving; promoting therapeutic competence; instillation of hope; patient support; interfamily learning; facilitation of group therapy; and data source.

In a selective review of a subject, it is not always possible to reproduce the tenor of group experiences as rich as a multiple-family group for cocaine users and their families. Kaufman (1985b) and Kaufmann and Kaufman (1979) have written clinical descriptive studies that capture the flavor of the multiple-family group experience with alcoholics and drug abusers, a form that serves as the forerunner of many of the approaches adopted with cocaine users. They note the assets of the multiple-family group which allows for "the integration of other family members who have a role in perpetuating the substance-abusing system as well as the power to change the system" (1985, p. 174).

Multiple-family groups rely heavily on educational elements to realize their goals. Families with a chemically dependent member are oriented to a view of cocaine abuse that stresses its relationship to significant family factors. Family, as well as individual, denial defenses are confronted in the multiple-family group sessions. Dysfunctional familial patterns of enmeshment, coercion, scapegoating, and others that promote cocaine use are identified and alternative family adjustments are sought. "Enabling" behaviors in family members are pointed out in an effort to increase awareness among all family members of behaviors that perpetuate cocaine dependency.

Family groups consist of several families and are led by at least two staff members. In very large multiple-family groups, the leadership is team leadership, often employing more than two leaders, each of whom has a clearly designated role in the group. Because of the large size of the group, the leaders have many therapeutic options at their disposal. Initially, families can identify with each other in recognizing the impact of living with a drug-dependent member. Frequently, as is the case in single-parent families, the members of multiple-family groups help "fill in" much needed supports for cocaine abusers and their families.

Cross-family learning is dramatic in these groups. Participants are commonly able to identify, in members of other families in the group, the very things they vigorously deny or avoid in their own family system. As a result, intermember and family-to-family levels of the group become prominent channels for both support and confrontation. This adds therapeutic leverage to the task of trying to change established family patterns in drug-abusing family systems.

The multiple-family group also functions as a resource for its membership. Family members are made aware of and encouraged to join support groups of an Al-Anon type. The emphasis on addiction as a "family affair" helps mobilize important family members who would otherwise resist efforts to be involved in a therapeutic process. The groups aim to counter feelings of despair and demoralization prominent in cocaine-abusing family groups. In addition, an active attempt at teaching appropriate modes for the expression of intense feelings among family members is incorporated into the therapeutic experience.

Groups composed of couples, where one or both partners have a problem of cocaine use, form another category of group experience considered useful as part of multimodal treatment. After work with the family of origin is completed or in life circumstances where the original family is not alive or geographically unable to be involved, the marital dyad is frequently worked with directly. Initially, this work is conducted conjointly for purposes of evaluation and, perhaps, for brief therapy. Many couples also require elements that couples groups provide rather easily.

Elsewhere, the author (Spitz, 1979; Spitz & Spitz, 1980) has described the general principles of couples-group therapy. The cocaine variant of this format includes the same overall concepts and adds its own unique dimensions.

Identifying dysfunctional interactional patterns and similar basic concepts from family and group therapies occurs readily in the cocaine couples group. In relationships where substance abuse is a problem, the presence of other couples helps strengthen identity as an adult pair and demarcates the marital boundary from the edge of the original family. The group lends its support to the consolidation of adaptive behaviors and assists couples in achieving a stable marital homeostasis once cocaine use has ceased.

Theme-oriented couples-group sessions center around cocaine, power and control issues in relationships, the role of the family of origin vis-à-vis the marriage, sexual issues, parenting decisions, money, and other issues all affected by cocaine use. The level of affect is high, and couples learn necessary communication skills in the group. Anger and mistrust, along with submerged feelings of love, emerge routinely in couples groups. The leader strives to balance the cathartic value of the expression of affect with efficacious forms of communicating these feelings to the spouse. It is important to get a sense of closure in session when intense affect has dominated the group in order to oversee the transition process from stormy, chaotic dyadic exchanges to more productive ones.

Structurally, couples groups are usually smaller (three to four couples) and meet weekly for about an hour and a half. We recommend opposite-sex coleadership teams in order to have the group be homogeneous for dyads, and to give the group leaders an opportunity to role-model suggested changes through the use of their own ingroup transactions. Male and female members of cocaine groups often see the same sex therapist as an ally or "kindred spirit," a feeling which, although not necessarily accurate, bridges the initial obstacles to joining the group. Eventually, the distortions or projections that shape members' misperceptions of the leaders, their spouses, and other group members become a central part of the content of group sessions.

Cocaine couples groups are longer-term groups with shifting membership. Their purpose in complementing other treatment efforts initially, and later as a form of enduring maintenance therapy, leads to a group life-span that extends for months or years. The duration of membership is reviewed regularly as a check against fostering excessive dependency on psychotherapy rather than being self-reliant. On balance, the ways in which family and group techniques have been "married" have resulted in forms of treatment that give the clinician, the cocaine user, and the family powerful and readily acceptable experiences which are specific for interpersonal aspects of the cocaine problem.

Adolescent Groups

The increased use of cocaine by adolescents is alarming (Gold et al., 1985). This phenomenon has prompted a renewed search for preventive and therapeutic programs.

Group therapy has traditionally been appealing to teenagers and to therapists who work with them (Sugar, 1975). Recently, some practitioners of adolescent group therapy have turned their attention to the specific problem of substance abuse. Although controlled studies of technique do not as yet exist, the clinical literature reveals strong support for experimentation with groups as a setting for treatment of substance-dependent adolescents. In fact, Rachman and Raubolt (1985) state their view that "group therapy is the treatment of choice for adolescent drug abusers."

Their enthusiasm and the favor shown by others (Raubolt & Bratter, 1974) in the field are based on several factors: (1) Peer group relationships, so central to adolescent development, are mirrored in group experiences. (2) Adolescents often accept peer groups as therapy experiences in preference to being seen alone or with their families. (3) The social elements present in groups blend with age-related social concerns shared by adolescents. (4) Groups provide clinicians with "therapeutic leverage" necessary to promote change, set limits, help test reality, and confront problematic behavior. (5) Groups assist greatly in the consolidation of adolescent ego identity through the evolution of individual and group identifications made through relationships that originate in the group. (6) Groups provide a place where experimentation is encouraged, thereby permitting constructive use of fantasy, the expression of emotion, creativity, and the development of alternatives to self-defeating, drug-taking behavior.

Rachman and Raubolt (1985) have delineated the application of the above principles to the question of adolescent drug abuse and defines several ways in which psychotherapy groups accomplish their goals:

1) Encouraging adolescents to bring their fantasies about drug experimentation before the actual experience;
2) Open, direct and honest confrontation of self-destructive drug abuse by both the therapist and the group;
3) Therapeutic exploration of actual drug experiences to find out the personal meaning to the individual involved.
4) Therapist sharing drug-related beliefs and serving as an ego-identity role model for alternatives of substance abuse;
5) Offering specific recommendations for curbing drug abuse, including total abstinence, reduction in drug abuse, or changes in drugs used, i.e. "hard" to "soft" drugs;
6) Encouraging extra-group activities to supplement the treatment regimen, i.e. joining a drug rehabilitation program; encouraging family therapy sessions; supplemental individual psychotherapy sessions;
7) Developing and maintaining a positive, emotional climate in groups where non-drug taking is considered virtuous. In essence, drug abstinence is reinforced as a positive, sought after life style. (pp. 357–358)

Whether the setting in which the adolescent cocaine group meets is on an inpatient ward of a hospital, in a therapeutic community/residential treatment center, or in outpatient venues, the actual conduct of the group involves therapist activity, authenticity, and careful attention to the selection of adolescents who can tolerate the confrontation necessary in cocaine group experiences. Adolescents who have coexisting major psychiatric illness of which cocaine use is merely one manifestation are usually inappropriate candidates for cocaine groups with high levels of confrontation and pressure.

Groups have also been explored for their preventive, as well as treatment, potential. Educative approaches utilizing small and large groups of adolescents themselves and/or with significant family members are expanding. The influx of "crack," a less expensive and ready-to-use form of freebase cocaine, into the adolescent subculture represents an area where adolescents and their families benefit from the information disseminated in drug prevention groups.

SUMMARY

Cocaine dependence is a complex problem in ways identified earlier in this volume. The flexibility of the group entity holds promise for contributing significantly to the management of troublesome aspects of the comprehensive care of cocaine users.

More formal research is required to elucidate aspects of group work which are most beneficial, as well as those which are potentially injurious, in working with the cocaine-dependent patient populations. As such studies emerge, it appears that group treatment will continue to grow and retain its fundamental position in the treatment of substance abuse.

REFERENCES

Alibrandi, L: The fellowship of Alcoholics Anonymous, in Pattison EM, Kaufman E, eds: Encyclopedic Handbook of Alcoholism, New York, Gardner Press, 1982, pp 979–986.

Bales RF: Attitudes toward drinking in the Irish culture, in Pittman DJ, Snyder CR, eds: Society, Culture and Drinking Patterns, New York, John Wiley & Sons, 1962.

Brandsma JM, Pattison EM: Group treatment methods with alcoholics, in Galanter M, Pattison EM, eds: Advances in the Psychosocial Treatment of Alcoholism, Washington, DC, American Psychiatric Press, 1984.

Ehrlich P, McGeehan M: Cocaine recovery and support groups and the language of recovery. J. Psychoactive Drugs 17:11–17, 1985.

Galanter, M: Professionally directed self-help therapy for alcoholism, in Galanter M, Pattison EM, eds: Advances in the Psychosocial Treatment of Alcoholism, Washington, DC, American Psychiatric Press, 1984.

Galanter M, Cleaton T, Marcus CE, McMillen J: Self help groups for parents of young drug and alcohol abusers, Am J Psychiatry 141:889–891, 1984.

Gold MS, Semlitz L, Dackis CA, Exstein, I: The adolescent cocaine epidemic, Semin Adolescent Med 1:303–309, 1985.

Katz AH, Self help organizations and volunteer participation in social welfare, Social Work 15:51–60, 1970.

Katz AY, Bender EI: The Strength in US: Self Help Groups in the Modern World, New York, Franklin Watts, 1976.

Kaufman E: Substance Abuse and Family Therapy, Orlando, FL, Grune & Stratton, 1985a.

Kaufman E: Multiple family therapy and couples groups, in Substance Abuse and Family Therapy, Orlando, FL, Grune & Stratton, 1985b.

Kaufmann P, Kaufman E: From multiple family therapy to couples therapy, in Kaufman E,

Kaufmann P, eds: Family Therapy of Drug and Alcohol Abuse, New York, Gardner Press, 1979.

Levy LH: Processing and activities in groups, in Lieberman MA, Borman LD, eds: Self Help Groups for Coping with Crises: Origins, Members, Processes and Impact, San Francisco, Jossey-Bass, 1979.

Lieberman MA: Self help groups and psychiatry, in Frances AJ, Hales RE, eds: American Psychiatric Association Annual Review, Vol. 5, Washington, DC, American Psychiatric Press, 1986.

Ogborne AC, Glaser FB: Evaluating alcoholics anonymous, in Bratter TE, Forrest CG, eds: Alcoholism and Substance Abuse: Strategies for Clinical Intervention, New York, The Free Press, 1985.

Piper WE, Marrache M: Selecting suitable patients: pre-training for group therapy as a method of patient selection. Small Group Behav 12:459–475, 1981.

Price AL: Self-help groups: trouble on the frontier. Current Concepts in Psychiatry, Sept/Oct: 6–14, 1978.

Rachman AW, Raubolt RR: The clinical practice of group psychotherapy with adolescent substance abusers, in Bratter TE, Forrest CG, eds: Alcoholism and Substance Abuse: Strategies, for Clinical Intervention, New York, The Free Press, 1985.

Raubolt R, Bratter TE: Games addicts play: implications for group treatment. Corrective Social Psychiatry 20:3–10, 1974.

Spitz HI: Group approaches to treating marital problems. Psychiatr Ann 9:318–330, 1979.

Spitz HI: Contemporary trends in group psychotherapy: a literature survey, Hosp Commun Psychiatry 35:132–142, 1984.

Spitz HI: Indications for and expectations of group psychotherapy, in Flach F, ed: Weekly Psychiatry Update Series, Biomedia, Princeton, NJ, 1977.

Spitz HI, Spitz ST: Co-therapy in the management of marital problems: Psychiatr Ann 10:160–168, 1980.

Spitz HI, Kass FI, Charles E: Common mistakes made in group psychotherapy by beginning therapists. Am J Psychiatry 137:1619–1621, 1980.

Sugar M: The Adolescent in Group and Family Therapy, New York, Brunner/Mazel, 1975.

Trice HM, Roman PM: Sociopsychological predictors of affiliation with Alcoholics Anonymous: a longitudinal study of "treatment success." Social Psychiatry 5:51–59, 1970.

Tucker GJ, Maxmen JS: Multiple family group therapy in a psychiatric hospital. J Psychoanal Groups 27:34, 1975.

Vaillant GE: The Natural History of Alcoholism, Cambridge, MA, Harvard University Press, 1983.

Yalom ID: The Theory and Practice of Group Psychotherapy, 3rd ed, New York, Basic Books, 1985.

Chapter 8

Family Therapy of Cocaine Abuse

Henry I. Spitz, M.D.,
and Susan T. Spitz, M.S.W.

Substance abuse naturally falls within the province of family therapy. Over the years, alcoholism provided an initial focus for these interests. More recently, attention and study has expanded to encompass opiate addiction, barbiturate use, and many other mind- and mood-altering substances. In the evolution of the process, cocaine abuse has only been tangentially addressed.

The purpose of this chapter is severalfold: to review the research and clinical data relative to patterns, phenomenology, and structure in substance-abusing families; to compare and contrast the general observations gleaned from work with alcoholic- and heroin-addicted families with those of the cocaine-abusing population; to delineate the clinical principles involved in family treatment of substance abuse in general and cocaine abuse in particular; and to describe the major ways in which the family is incorporated into an intelligent treatment plan when a family member is abusing cocaine.

GENERAL PRINCIPLES OF FAMILY STRUCTURE

Family influences have long been valued by psychotherapists of all persuasions. Traditionally, the family has been conceptualized as the major shaping force in the individual. Psychotherapies derived from this orientation reflect an individual or intrapsychic focus and a linear orientation as to causality of psychopathology in family members. The intensification of family therapy research and practice over the past two decades has resulted in alternative ways of viewing family behavior and dynamics from an interactional, systemic, and circular framework.

The family systems vantage point regards the family as being in a state of dynamic equilibrium, with the current family form resulting from the interplay of the behavior of *all* its members simultaneously. The focus in the systemic orientation is on the family as a whole and on the elements of family structure that constitute functional or dysfunctional patterns.

Stanton (1985) has consolidated a list of elements in family life that are of particular importance to an understanding of the basis for many family treatment interventions. These principles include: family boundaries, intergenerational coalitions; triads or triangles; family homeostasis; the behavioral context in which symptoms occur; the family scapegoat; family role selection; family life-cycle; and the relationship of the symptom to the family system.

A basic concept in family structure is the notion of familial boundaries, i.e., the dimension of closeness and distance between family members and between the family as a whole and the external world. Patterns of enmeshment and disengagement (Minuchin, 1974) gauge degrees of extreme involvement or detachment between family members and/or among subsystems in the larger family system. A close parallel to this dimension of family structure is the issue of the relationship between the generations in families. Fixed coalitions in which a parent prefers a child and excludes a spouse are common occurrences in dysfunctional families. "Incongruous hierarchies" (Madanes, 1981) occur when intergenerational boundaries are breached, resulting in power imbalances in the family and in a symptom in a family member. As Hoffman (1981) notes:

> The most obvious single characteristic of families with 'disturbed' members is their apparent lawlessness, most strikingly conveyed by the lack of boundaries or appropriate status lines. The family is governed—if that is the word—by a powerful politics of secret coalitions across the generations. (p. 154)

Rigid triangulation, or the formation of inflexible triadic family relationships, is frequently the basis for problematic family function. Two adults and a symptomatic child is a common configuration in dysfunctional families. Specific participants vary, but the principle of three people being involved when there is a significant symptom has received great attention in family circles.

The homeostatic mechanisms that families employ to maintain their steady state form another cornerstone in family systems theory. Losses and separations in the family afford a glimpse into homeostatic processes at work. Actual loss through death of a family member and family re-alignments that occur when an important person leaves the home activate compensatory action in family members aimed at restoring a sense of balance and stability. The pull toward homeostasis can result in beneficial or disruptive family patterns.

In instances where family homeostasis is predicated on scapegoating a family member, an "identified patient" emerges from the process. Despite the fact that all family members participate in this phenomenon, one member reflects or "carries" the family dysfunction in the form of an apparent "individual" problem. Understanding the nature of the symptom, its function within the family system, and the behavioral context in which it occurs is essential in formulating strategies for intervention in symptomatic families.

The psychoanalytic (Bieber, 1980) and the family therapy (Minuchin & Fishman, 1981) literature have recognized the significance of parental attitudes as they regulate role assignments of children in families. Parental selection of children to fulfill unmet needs of adults has been suggested as an essential element of problems as seemingly diverse as eating disorders (Minuchin et al., 1978), homosexuality (Bieber, 1962), alcoholism (Kaufman, 1986), and drug abuse (Stanton, 1977).

Inserting a temporal dimension into the analysis of family life provides data that bear directly on family treatment. Symptoms that emerge at specific points in the life-cycle of the family often reflect developmental issues of unresolved family problems. Examples include families that have difficulty making transitions following births or deaths or when an adolescent leaves the home (Haley, 1980). These events in the family life-cycle may form the basis for a family's inability to progress to the next stage of development.

PHENOMENOLOGY IN SUBSTANCE-ABUSING FAMILIES

The focus on the family has been applied to the problem of substance abuse, resulting in many interesting observations concerning patterns noted in families where drug abuse exists. Kaufman and Kaufmann (1979), working with an urban heroin addict population, delineated characteristic features of families with an addicted member.

(1) The drug addict is the symptom carrier of the family dysfunction. (2) The addict helps to maintain family homeostasis. (3) The

addicted member reinforces the parental need to control and continue parenting, yet he finds such parenting inadequate for his needs. (4) The addict provides a displaced battlefield so that implicit and explicit parental strife can continue to be denied. (5) Parental drug and alcohol abuse is common and is directly transmitted to the addict or results in inadequate parenting. (6) The addict forms cross-generational alliances which separate parents from each other. (7) Generational boundaries are diffuse—there is frequent competition between parents. (pp. 44–45)

Similarly, Stanton and Todd (1982) compared opiate addicts and their families to other dysfunctional, but non-substance-abusing families. Prominent among their findings were the following: a higher degree of chemical dependency, particularly alcoholism, was found among addicts' families, plus a propensity for other addictionlike behaviors, such as gambling and television watching; opiate addicts were more likely to retreat into the drug subculture following family conflict, thereby appearing more independent from the family in a manner that belied their actual degree of connectedness; mothers of addicts got "'stuck' at an earlier stage of childrearing, tending to hold on to their children and treat them as younger than they really are"; pseudoindividuation, pseudocompetence, and pseudoindependence resulted from the symptom of addiction with its accompanying escapes from and returns to the original family; and "greater parent-child acculturation gaps" were noted in families of adolescent drug abusers.

Family studies in the literature often address themes that appear with regularity in the family histories of substance abusers. Coleman et al. (1986) point to the prevalence of death, separation, and loss themes in heroin-addicted populations. This research reports that not only do addicts have a distinct orientation to death, but they are also more suicidal. Their life histories show more family separations and a pattern of separating and reconnecting with the family.

Reilly (1979) echoes the concept of underlying family themes, emphasizing impaired mourning and familial collusion as central dynamic issues in drug-abusing families. He proposes a "profile of a family system which tends to produce drug abusing behavior in its members." Although the sample from which the data were collected was far from universal with respect to important variables such as ethnicity, cultural factors, socioeconomic status, and others, there still remains a group of recognizable phenomena often observed in substance-abusing families. The cluster of family negativism, criticism, and lifelessness sets the stage for stimulating or energizing such families through the use of the substance abuse pathway by an adolescent family member. Parental inconsistency about limit setting and the establishment and maintenance of family norms has traditionally been implicated as a backdrop against which substance abuse emerges in the family. Excessive use of denial on the part not only of parents, but children as well, is another recurrent observation in these families.

Families in which parents vicariously derive some benefit or reward from the child's drug use and covertly "enable," sanction, or encourage it also formed a part of the sample in Reilly's study. Pathogenic parental expectations of success or failure in children were also prominent contributing factors to the patterns observed in these families.

The regulation of affect, most specifically anger and depression, poses a problem for many families. Drug abuse as a symptom of family distress provides a conduit through which intense anger may be channeled. In like manner, the self-medicating aspect of substance abuse suggests that family members resort to drug use to anesthetize or medicate painful affective states seen as unmanageable to them through less extreme measures.

Klagsbrun and Davis (1977) report findings of clinical-descriptive family studies that support this hypothesis. They relate family studies that acknowledge the varied uses of drugs as a solution to family conflicts. Drug use can be regarded as adaptive or functional in protecting the users from painful feelings and in diverting attention away from parental/marital conflict by moving the focus onto the drug-abusing child.

Alexander and Dibb (1977) studied heroin addicts and their families that were more middle class than those usually described in the literature. In their study of interpersonal perceptions among families of addicts, they noted that: all family members, including the addict, held the substance abuser in low esteem; addicts were seen as being "different" from their parents; the major flaws noted in the addict's personality were labeled as passivity and dependency; the parents in the small sample differed from lower-class families particularly in the fact that fathers tended to be present and central rather than peripheral or absent; and mothers were described as more passive than they were in prior studies.

The findings of this study provide further evidence that perception among family members contributes to symptom formation in its members. In this instance, social perception in addict families was seen to perpetuate opiate addiction by chronically undermining the self-esteem of the heroin addict.

Even though the literature is rich with descriptive studies of families where alcoholism and/or drug abuse is the central problem, it seems that family patterns of a more specific sort than those just described are unlikely to emerge. In part, this realization has led to a shift in focus of some family research that aims to study the processes in families considered to be at low to no risk for the development of substance abuse symptoms.

Here again, interest is broad, and many relevant characteristics have been identified. Stanton (1980) has summarized these studies, the highlights of which include a sense of family cohesion; better problem-solving and communication skills; often a firm moral/religious upbringing; less parental/marital incompatibility; and increased assertiveness and self-expression coupled with a sense of goal directedness and purpose in life.

Elsewhere, Stanton (1985) proposes that a therapeutically useful perspective which results from a survey of family studies is to adopt the position that substance abuse involves a "family addiction cycle." This point of view most constructively utilizes both dynamic and systemic family information and permits its incorporation into a treatment model that addresses the major phenomenological issues described thus far. The shift away from the exclusive focus on the individual, coupled with the view of drug abuse as having functional meaning in the family, helps avoid a narrow view of substance abuse linked to poor treatment outcome.

COCAINE ABUSE: FAMILY ISSUES

The study of family issues and cocaine abuse is in an embryonic phase. No body of literature exists from which family patterns, parallel to those for abuse of other substances, might be defined. Certainly, cocaine abuse presents a fertile ground for research into family issues.

At present, one can only speculate about the existence of features unique to cocaine abuse and the family pending the outcome of basic research into these areas. Spotts and Shontz (1980) provide one of the only studies that mentions family patterns of cocaine abusers. Despite the small size and circumscribed nature of the sample, it still provides some interesting data for clinical hypotheses.

Kaufman (1985), in discussing the study, selects the following features of these families:

> Cocaine users described their mothers as warm and their fathers as strong and encouraging and their early family lives as highly positive overall. As adults, they had stronger, more resilient egos than

men in the other drug use groups. They were ambitious, intensely competitive men who worked hard to become successful, took risks and lived by their wits. Their need to be completely self-sufficient was compensation for their intensely denied dependency needs. (pp. 18–19)

These observations raise many controversial points. The stereotype of cocaine as a drug confined to the affluent and successful is open to serious question. As the availability of cocaine has increased and the cost of the drug has dropped, cocaine is reaching the less prosperous. As a consequence, individuals and families appearing for treatment fit the elite stereotype less and less. It is plausible that the initial observations about the type of person attracted to cocaine and the family from which he/she emerged were by-products of a self-selected segment of the population who could afford the drug rather than a true picture of the drug's usership.

The sharp line of distinction between the families of heroin abusers, alcoholics, and cocaine users is changing rapidly. Current experiences shows greater overlap among family patterns of substance abusers in diverse categories than was originally thought. The search for a profile of a "cocaineogenic" family structure appears to be disappearing, not increasing, with the influx of new families into the spectrum of cocaine use and with the widespread use of cocaine and other drugs simultaneously.

The use of denial, prominent in the families of both alcoholics and opiate addicts, appears just as frequently in the cocaine-dependent population. Structural concepts of enmeshment and disengagement, boundary problems, inadequate role definition, and difficulty with separation from the family of origin are prominent in the cocaine patient group as well. Observations concerning the function of substance abuse as a homeostatic family mechanism stand up to scrutiny in the cocaine user's family in a manner that closely parallels those described with the heroin and alcoholic families.

It is important, however, to bear in mind certain phenomenological, behavioral, and clinical observations that occur with regularity in the cocaine subgroup of the substance abuse population. Spotts and Schontz (1980) suspect a pattern of ambition, goal direction, and attainment of academic or career success as a frequently encountered phenomenon in these families. This parallels our clinical experience, which suggests that cocaine abusers in all socioeconomic classes who obtain the drug through their own earnings, rather than by dealing in drugs or other illegal means, have an impressive capacity for work success.

The high cost of cocaine requires the user to be able to sustain major expense over long periods of time. Many cocaine-dependent men and women have managed to finance their drug use through high work performance. When cocaine use escalates to the point where work function is impaired, the user then resembles the prototypical "bottomed-out" user of any substance. At this stage of impairment, cocaine users more closely approximate the "down-and-out" alcoholic or the "street junkie" stage of heroin addiction.

It would be important to study whether the ability to work productively indeed is a consistent finding among cocaine abusers when compared to abusers of other substances. Many cocaine users cite the initial introduction and appeal of cocaine in connection with their work. Cocaine's stimulant properties are regarded as an asset to one's work function, especially when faced with heavy work loads, long hours, and the need to be alert, awake, and productive.

In like manner, it is valuable to analyze familial patterns vis-à-vis success, work function, parental ambition and attainment levels, and other work-related variables to determine whether or not something unique transpires in the families of substance abusers who select cocaine as the drug of choice.

Families of cocaine abusers need to be studied systematically from yet another point of view. The regular observation of the high incidence of affective disorders in cocaine abusers and in members of their original families cannot be overlooked. It appears that a biobehavioral approach that evaluates the family both for its potential biological or genetic contributions and for its learned behavioral influences stands the best chance of accurately interpreting these empirical findings. Depression, manic/depressive disorder, and cyclothymic mood disorders densely populate the families of cocaine abusers. The role of the family in genesis and maintenance of these conditions is a critical area of study.

Family studies have emphasized the age of onset of substance abuse as a distinction between heroin users and abusers of alcohol. Until recently, heroin use was considered an earlier development in the life-cycle and alcoholism a later one. The sharp dividing line between families of heroin addicts and those of alcohol abusers has become blurred with the increase of adolescent alcohol abuse. Cocaine use has followed a similar path.

An offshoot of the infiltration of cocaine into the less affluent population has resulted in widespread use of the drug among teenagers in all social classes and ethnic groups, as well as those from a more heterogeneous group of families than previously expected. The stage of the individual and familial life-cycle at which cocaine abuse becomes a problem is less clearly defined than the heroin and alcoholism studies have historically suggested.

To whatever extent one subscribes to the notion that symptoms are "manufactured" in the family, there is ample room to speculate about family contributions to the adult symptomatology observed in cocaine-dependent people. In addition to mood disorders noted previously, anxiety-related symptoms are characteristic of cocaine-abusing men and women. Two major areas where this is readily apparent are found in intense social anxieties and in apprehension related to sexual function. The use of cocaine as an interpersonal lubricant is a major factor in its appeal. Empirical observations of families of origin, couples where at least one partner is a cocaine abuser, and individuals suggest that the family climate, both historically and currently, plays an integral part in the creation and sustenance of a wide variety of psychological symptoms seen in cocaine users.

This hypothesis coincides with earlier principles originally delineated by Minuchin et al. (1975), Haley (1976), Stanton and Todd (1982), and other family therapists with wide experience in the substance abuse field and forms the basis for the major family treatment efforts with cocaine abuse. The concept of cocaine abuse as a symptom that expresses the final common pathway derived from the interplay of genetic, behavioral, familial, environmental, sociocultural, ethnic, economic, and other variables is the most popular view of the condition from a family therapy standpoint. The emphasis given any of the aforementioned factors by the clinician shapes the form of family intervention chosen and relates directly to the theoretical orientation of the practitioner.

In general terms, the prevailing approaches in the family therapy of substance abuse are systems-derived techniques. Although style of intervention may vary, there is consensus that the "family system is the patient." Cocaine abuse can be viewed as one of many symptoms of family disruption. An appreciation of the symptom, its point of emergence in the life-cycle, and its "function" in the interpersonal context of the family is considered most important to the family therapist charged with treatment of the cocaine abuser. The pharmacological and physiological properties of cocaine, although significant, are largely relegated secondary roles in orchestrating a treatment plan that involves the family.

Owing to the complex set of factors involved when working with families, it is helpful to create a clear, well-formulated, organized framework for therapy which is flexible enough to be modified on a family-by-family basis. Many of the phenomenological observations in the literature have been reported in the hope of drawing conclusions that would ultimately facilitate and simplify treatment of substance abuse problems. The data referable to family process, patterns, and structure guide the formulation of a plan of intervention which must be tailored to meet the specific needs, capabilities, and limitations of each family.

MAJOR SCHOOLS OF FAMILY THERAPY

In the same way that the only commonality shared by cocaine abusers is their attraction to a particular substance, so, too, do the families of cocaine users differ in more ways than they are similar. As a consequence of this heterogeneity, Pattison and Kaufman (1982) emphasize the multivariate nature of substance abuse, citing "multiple patterns of dysfunctional use that occur in various types of personalities, with multiple combinations of adverse consequences, with multiple prognoses, that may require different types of treatment interventions" (p. 13).

The plethora of family therapy formats generally available to the clinician is striking. Paolino and McCrady (1978) have helped to clarify the substantive orientations in the field with respect to their similarities and differences. The family therapies of substance abuse closely parallel their broad classification scheme of psychodynamic, behavioral, and family systems techniques.

In practice, there are considerable areas of overlap among the three major orientations. For descriptive purposes, however, it is simpler to discuss these formats separately with the awareness that as eclectic treatment models continue to emerge, the actual differences among effective family therapies becomes more difficult to discern.

The psychodynamic orientation finds a modern exponent of its application to substance abuse in Kaufman's (1985) "structural-dynamic family therapy." Actually, this approach is more representative of the eclectic model, which builds on a base of psychodynamic elements, blending them with aspects of structural family therapy. The key psychodynamic features of this system of therapy are found in the value placed on understanding past events and their influence on the present and on utilizing primary concepts of intervention through interpretation, overcoming resistance, "working through" (progressing from cognitive to emotional insight), and the judicious use of countertransferance by the therapist. Like many family therapies that originate in psychoanalytic thinking, this approach is more "analytic" in the way in which it synthesizes past and present experience. The actual style of intervention actually combines behavioral and structural family therapies with psychodynamic factors in order to effect lasting change in families.

Behavioral therapies alone or as part of comprehensive treatment programs of substance abuse problems have recently gained clinical favor. Proponents of the behavioral approach advocate its use as a method of symptom control with substance abusers. The initial goal of the behavioral therapies is to achieve a rapid state of abstinence. Following this phase, treatment delineates the stimuli that contribute to perpetuation of the habit of substance abuse and tries to alter, interrupt, or create new behaviors to replace dysfunctional ones.

Cognitive components are a major aspect of the method, which relies heavily on learning theory as its base. Contingency contracting, assertiveness training, behavior rehearsal, cognitive restructuring, and the creation of alternative behaviors other than drug taking are cardinal components of behavioral approaches applied to family therapy models.

The family therapies that derive from systems theory form the bulk of the techniques applied to drug abuse. Stanton and Todd (1982) have detailed a family therapy approach that is rooted in the work of Minuchin (1974, Minuchin et al; 1978) and Haley (1981). This approach typifies a synthesis of principles that have broad-based support in family circles and is exemplified by the work of prominent systems-oriented thinkers such as Bowen (1978), Papp (1983), Hoffman (1981), Boszormenyi-Nagy & Spark (1973), Madanes (1981), the Milan group (Selvini-Palazzoli et al., 1978), Erickson (Haley, 1973), and many others.

Contemporary family therapy is most alive in the areas of structural and strategic forms of intervention. On the basis of current research, this point of view emerges as the most efficacious method for treatment of families where substance abuse is the presenting problem (Gurman & Kniskern, 1981; Stanton, 1980). These techniques are goal-oriented, short-term models that actively involve the family of origin of the substance abuser. The prevailing view in this orientation is that the nature of the symptom matters less than the family's structural organization at the present time. As Stanton and Todd (1982) succinctly state,

> Therapy is concerned with the repetitive interactional patterns that maintain the drug-taking. The thrust of treatment is to alter these sequences. Although it is interesting to speculate about the etiology of drug abuse, it is our experience that historical data are generally of very little utility in actually bringing about change. (p. 133)

As a direct result of this treatment philosophy, family therapy of substance abuse focuses on the present, observes concrete behaviors and sequences of interactions in the family, and aims to construct a family system that achieves and sustains a pattern of abstinence from drugs. Particular emphasis is placed on behavioral sequences that precede and follow episodes of drug taking by family members.

The combined structural/strategic model employed by Stanton (1981) is a hybrid of elements from both schools applied in the following sequence: "Initially deal with a family through a structural approach—joining, accommodating, testing boundaries, and restructuring." Second, "switch to a predominantly strategic approach when 'structural' techniques either are not succeeding or are unlikely to succeed." And finally, "following success with strategic methods, and given that a case is to continue in therapy, it may be advisable to revert once again to a structural approach" (p. 431).

The shared properties of structural and strategic therapies are evident and result in a family treatment model that is brief, pragmatically oriented, emphasizes family process more than content, and requires that the therapist be active in formulating diagnoses, setting treatment contracts, hypothesizing about relevant family patterns, timing interventions properly, and assigning out-of-session tasks that tap relevant family dynamics which hinder change in a positive direction.

PRINCIPLES OF FAMILY TREATMENT

Initial Phase Issues

Formulation of treatment goals

The overriding goals of family treatment are twofold: to make a comprehensive evaluation of a family system and to formulate a treatment plan that includes all family members. Family evaluation is broad-based and considers many dimensions of family function. Family therapy of cocaine abuse aims at creating a plan of abstinence that the family can maintain consistently.

During both the evaluation and treatment phases, the therapist should observe a few general guidelines. Communication with the family should be clear and direct in an effort not only to serve as a role model for these qualities, but also to help achieve family compliance in the treatment plan. The clearer the clinician's formulation of a plan for evaluation and treatment, the greater the likelihood for success in both these areas.

An appraisal of the family, with the resultant sense of what constitutes attainable goals for them in family therapy, is vital to the process. Not only must realistic goals be set, but the sequencing of work on these goals should be thoughtfully considered and presented to the family in positive and nonconfusing terms. The family needs to be engaged in construction of treatment goals and priorities. Therapists who are sensitive to the family's sense of what is emotionally urgent to them stand a better chance of joining the family constructively.

Other qualities on the part of the therapist help facilitate engagement in treatment and foster family cooperation in ongoing sessions. The ability to be active in providing structure for the therapeutic experience is essential. The therapist should have an integrated point of view concerning treatment in general, but it should not be rigid or inflexible. The knowledge of the family over time serves as a roadmap for inclusion or deletion of elements available to the clinician working with cocaine abusers and their families.

A general therapeutic climate of support, clarity, firmness, fairness, and availability on the therapist's part sets the stage for a positive working alliance with the family. When these essential ingredients are present, the realistic pretherapy expectations for success are heightened in both clinician and family members.

Family evaluation phase

The initial stage of family therapy for cocaine abuse begins with an evaluation of the family. Although observation is the cornerstone of this process, it is an observational stance borne out of active interaction and exchange with members of the family. Starting with the initial interview, the therapist is both participant in and witness to the characteristic patterns present in the family.

A wealth of data emerges from this process and has to be quickly synthesized by the therapist into a clinically relevant and realistic treatment format. It is essential, therefore, to have an organized evaluation plan that concentrates on aspects of family structure and function relating to the problem of cocaine abuse. A useful evaluation phase model assesses the family along the following parameters: (1) family structure, (2) diagnostic issues, (3) family strengths, and (4) drug issues per se.

1) Family structure. The general principles of family structure outlined in the beginning of this chapter form the basis for this dimension of family evaluation. Boundary issues, role assignments, coalitions, enmeshment, triangulations, and communication patterns are some of the central components of family structure that relate to treatment planning. Concretizing aspects of family structure may be extremely helpful and can be accomplished by construction of formal genograms or informal family "maps." Genograms (McGoldrick & Gerson, 1985) provide information across at least three generations of the family and add historical perspective to the evaluation of the family in the present. Family maps outline family systems and identify important alliances, splits, or boundary blurring in families, which often fluctuate during the course of therapy.

Whether through a process of gathering direct observational data about families and/or combining it with specific techniques such as genograms to elucidate family structure, the effective family evaluation results in a three-dimensional family picture ready for framing into a treatment approach.

The shift from observation of family structure into a plan for therapy is analogous to Kaufman's family typology (1985) with alcoholism. Using the dimension of family reactivity to the substance abuse symptom, a classification of family structures emerges that offers some recommendations for therapeutic approaches to the problems in each family system. Experience with cocaine-dependent individuals and their families lends itself to the adaptation of Kaufman's (1985) classification scheme to a cocaine-abusing population as well.

The categories described include: functional, enmeshed, disintegrated, and absent families. The first group has a homeostasis that reaches a point of equilibrium through the avoidance of open family conflict. For these patients, short-term family therapy with an educational, cognitive, and behavioral slant is recommended. An emphasis on family roles and rules, coupled with an avoidance of uncovering or insight-oriented techniques, rounds out the treatment philosophy. Established family defenses of denial and emotional isolation are respected rather than challenged once the substance abuse has ceased.

Enmeshed families form the major group for whom family therapy is the treatment of choice. These families are highly reactive, levels of affect are more dramatic than with functional families, and the tendency for relapse is high. Consequently, family therapy strives for rapid control over substance use but expects that the intrafamilial structure and dynamics are such that repetitive, dysfunctional patterns are likely to re-emerge during the course of treatment.

Flexibility in forming an integrated treatment strategy is a sine qua non with enmeshed families. Elements of cognitive and behavioral methods are helpful first-stage efforts geared to attaining drug abstinence, but definitive treatment requires attention to systemic issues in the family through structural and possibly strategic family therapy approaches. Kaufman (1985) recommends inclusion of an external support group of the Alcoholics Anonymous (AA) type to aid in the disengagement and enmeshing phase of therapy.

Disintegrated families show the scars of deteriorated family function over time. These apparently disconnected families and marriages have often been assisted in their downfall by the interpersonal side effects of cocaine. It is hard to evaluate the degree of involvement in families that act as though there are no remaining family ties. Family approaches with this group begin with rehabilitative efforts directed to the individual substance abuser, followed by exploration and appraisal of family structure. Reconstitution of the family is not a goal of the first phase of treatment. Once family evaluation is complete, treatment decisions center on family therapy to attempt reconnection among disengaged members or other agendas such as brief family therapy designed to consolidate effective separation among family members.

Absent families show no overt connection of the substance abuser with the original family and an absence of nonfamily relationships of a major emotional sort. Supportive and social therapies utilizing nonkin networks (AA, church, etc.) have both rehabilitative and affiliative goals simultaneously. This approach may ultimately provide the basis for establishing new marital and family relationships in the future.

2) Diagnostic issues. The diagnostic evaluation for family therapy of cocaine abuse relies on data from family process and structure and does not use diagnosis in the traditional DSM-III sense of individual psychopathology. Familial interactional patterns and interpersonal transactions offer the most useful information for purposes of treatment planning. The focus on the identified problem in the family has replaced the concept of the identified patient as the focal point in treatment.

Family therapists are more concerned with ideas related to "what is the nature of the problem" as opposed to "who has the problem." Many examples of this viewpoint exist in clinical practice. The phenomenon of "scapegoating" provides a case in point. In families where conflict is "detoured" (Todd et al., 1982) through a symptomatic family member who becomes the family scapegoat, the family therapist has a specific set of diagnostic concerns. Therapists are concerned about the significance of detouring as a reflection of family function. Is the detouring "protective," as originally thought with some psychosomatic families, or is it "attacking," as in families of heroin addicts? Family therapists do not concern themselves with issues such as the existence of a masochistic personality disorder in the scapegoated family member.

Other significant factors in the diagnostic appraisal of cocaine-abusing family members relate to sociocultural issues, life-cycle considerations, and thematic content that regularly appears in these family histories. Socioeconomic status and ethnicity are two important variables that influence the patterning of cocaine-abusing families. McGoldrick and colleagues (1982) have detailed both the diagnostic import of these factors and the treatment implications with families from different racial, religious, and cultural backgrounds.

Life-cycle issues also have a prominent place in family evaluation. The family with an adolescent cocaine abuser often requires a therapy which differs from that of the family whose equilibrium is disrupted by the death of an important family member. Similarly, certain family themes such as death and loss are given strong weight in the assessment of families where substance abuse is the presenting problem.

In principle, diagnostic assessment of families with a cocaine-dependent member is multifactorial, placing largest emphasis on systemic issues and decentralizing aspects of individual phenomonology. Family-based treatments follow this diagnostic paradigm and intervene at the level of the family system with a teleological view of cocaine abuse as a symptom of family dysfunction.

3) Family strengths. The potential risk of a diagnostic focus geared exclusively to the evaluation of dysfunction in families is the tendency to undervalue or ignore the family's assets. Elucidation and recognition of the strengths of a family can be a difficult task. In cocaine-abusing families, the chronicity of the drug use usually leads to strain or rupture of important family ties. Parents often tire of "bailing out" their offspring from the legal, social, and financial consequences of long-term cocaine use. Similarly, adult children resent being "lectured" about their behavior in a way they feel belies their chronological age and demeans them. The common result is a family sorely in need of therapy and dramatically distant from any sense of the positive attributes of their family system.

The therapist must elicit evidence of constructive forces in the family. These "natural resources" form the basis for positive gains in subsequent family therapy. Many cocaine-addicted families have their first contact with organized therapy at a point where the user has "hit bottom" or has "gone public" with a confession of drug use to one or more significant family members. Anger, demoralization, frustration, and emotional depletion characterize the entry posture of these families when first encountered. Obviously, this is a difficult climate in which to try to get family members to discuss or demonstrate what they admire and respect about each other, how they collaborate, and what shared areas of interests and goals they possess.

A potential problem for the clinician exists when this demoralized family configuration is taken literally as a statement of a lack of familial assets or strengths. The therapist may have to take a historical focus to gain entry into an earlier stage of family life during which strengths were less camouflaged by cocaine use and its by-products.

An active search for true family strengths allows the therapist to take a positive, enthusiastic approach in treatment that is realistically rooted in a family's shared resource pool. Identification and labeling of strengths of the family helps counter their feelings of despair and hopelessness and gives them a firm basis for the expectation that change is possible through family treatment.

4) Drug issues. Evaluation of the family is best done in an atmosphere where common sense and sound clinical judgment prevail. Despite a preference for a systems orientation, astute clinicians realize that there are properties of the drug of abuse itself that require evaluation in order to obtain a thorough portrait of the family.

Two prominent features of this aspect of the evaluation include provisions for taking a thorough drug history and the incorporation of drug-screening methods into the treatment plan. In order to make a workable therapeutic model, the therapist needs to know specific information about the pattern of cocaine use in the drug-dependent member. The route of cocaine administration ("snorting" versus "freebasing" versus intravenous use), duration of use, the positive and particularly the negative physical effects on the user, prior treatment efforts, major mood changes, the means by which cocaine use was financed—all form part of this initial appraisal. Whether cocaine was used by itself or in combination with other substances, most notably marijuana, alcohol, or heroin, is another core issue.

Much, if not all, of this information can be obtained during the initial interview with the family. There, again, the therapist's skill is required to facilitate the process of taking a drug history with the family present. Feelings of guilt, embarrassment, and anger influence the type of drug-related information disclosed by the cocaine user in front of his/her family. This, coupled with the tendency for massive denial noted in cocaine-dependent individuals, skews the data obtained in family interviews. The therapist must be tactful but persistent in pursuing information related to drug use. An accurate approximation is required prior to embarking on any family therapy plan.

Monitoring drug use or abstinence through urine-testing techniques can be helpful in objectifying issues related to active cocaine use during the course of treatment. Urine screening for cocaine metabolites is done on a regular or random basis. An individual's agreement to participate in this aspect of a treatment program helps demystify the question of the extent of cocaine use per se and also simultaneously serves as a rough measure of motivation for treatment, demonstrated by willingness to acknowledge patterns of current drug intake.

The end point of a thorough evaluation and screening of a family where cocaine abuse is the chief complaint should be a clear understanding of what makes sense as a treatment plan. In the next section, specific techniques of implementing and actualizing these ideas about treatment will be discussed.

Initial treatment contract

The desired end of the first family interview is formulation and presentation of an initial contract for treatment. Creation of the contract encompasses several important areas. An initial plan for gaining control over the use of cocaine is the cornerstone of a universal initial contract for cocaine-dependent individuals. In attempting to achieve an abstinence plan, the therapist must be sure to include the whole family in the process in order to circumvent the pitfall of inadvertently supporting the family's view that the cocaine user alone is in need of treatment.

This ties in directly with another initial contract goal: redefining the problem. Contracting emphasizes the family system nature of the drug abuse problem and avoids the family's tendency to single out members to blame for their current state. Redefinition of the problem puts it into therapeutically workable form. It permits the family to help determine their treatment course by inviting their participation in goal-setting discussions. The initial contract works well if it acknowledges the family's priorities and incorporates them into any plan for therapy. Goals have to be agreed on by family members, and if disputes about goals exists, these become part of the focus in the early phase of therapy.

Just as initial goals are negotiated through family discussion, the ongoing treatment contract is also viewed as flexible and open to modification as family therapy progresses. The use of outside support groups is an example of a decision that must be made when initial family therapy sessions indicate a need for additional resources outside the original family.

The initial treatment contract should include a brief orientation segment which helps the family understand the basic philosophy of family therapy and the "ground rules" for the therapy sessions. The former emphasizes the need for all family members to contribute to the treatment process, to make themselves available, and to participate in a productive manner. The latter concerns itself with the logistics of treatment. Matters of format, including length and frequency of sessions, fees, location of meetings, and other procedural factors, are presented to the family at this time.

A well-conducted initial treatment contracting session results in a family that is properly prepared to understand and participate in family therapy. They view the therapy as practical and problem-focused, occurring in a relatively short-term format which requires active family involvement for the realization of mutually agreed upon, positive, and achievable goals.

Sequencing of events in family therapy

Determining appropriate treatment priorities is privotal in family work with cocaine abusers. Sequencing of treatment events can enhance or destroy a family therapy plan. Clinical experience suggests some rules of thumb that are applicable to the family therapy of cocaine abuse and are acceptable to families in treatment.

As previously noted, a plan for abstinence is a basic requirement at the outset. Second, the initial treatment focus integrates some variation on the theme of the family's presenting problem in the "here and now." This is accomplished by starting treatment with the family of origin in the first phase of the therapy. Attention is paid to the identified problem, which is worked on until its resolution is complete. Plans to work on marital issues or family problems other than cocaine abuse are deferred until the presenting problem is well under control. This sequence advises therapy for the family first, with the emphasis on drug-related issues. Once abstinence is achieved and maintained over some time, other family issues that emerge during therapy may be considered when expanding the therapeutic vista into non-drug-related areas.

In enmeshed families with a married cocaine-abusing child, the therapy is doomed if the sequence does not start with the family of origin before tackling the marital problems that inevitably ensue in families where the cocaine user is incompletely separated from his/her parents.

Treatment of this sort stresses treating the family first and viewing the father and mother primarily as parents and secondarily as spouses. Family therapy addresses the substance abuser's marital problems *after* the original family has worked on "releasing" him from the primary family attachments. This orientation to the family parallels an atomic model in which all of the sites for bonding on the molecule are already taken by the original family, leaving no spaces for connection or attachment to new relationships owing to strong preexisting family ties.

In families where the cocaine abuser lives at home, the sequence of treatment priorities proceeds from abstinence, to construction of an independent work or schooling plan, and perhaps to the eventual quest for an autonomous living situation out of the familial home.

Treatment priorities and sequencing of events must be constantly reevaluated by the therapist throughout the course of the therapeutic process in order to keep the family engaged and to provide a meaningful treatment focus.

Family recruitment

A common concern for the family therapist centers around the decision regarding which family members to include in therapy sessions. Although systems-oriented family therapies pay attention to the larger family system over three generations, it is not always the case, nor is it desirable, to include all family members in all family sessions. To do so routinely would be more mechanical and stereotypical than systems theorists ever intended. Flexibility in treatment design is necessary when considering the choice of significant family participants at various stages of family therapy.

Stanton and Todd (1982) advocate the principle of "vary[ing] the composition of the session in accordance with structural goals, rather than routinely including all family members" (p. 382). In order to make this determination, the clinician has to get an early view of as many family members as possible. This provides a glimpse into the range of choice available to family and therapist in the resolution of family problems.

In surveying the family landscape, the clinician looks at the extended family and the influential subsystems within it. Siblings, a commonly underaddressed segment of the family of the cocaine abuser, can be extremely influential in supporting or sabotaging family therapy plans. Care must be taken to consider whether or not the presence of a sibling is necessary in connection with the treatment goals. Siblings who are also enmeshed with the family and who may themselves be drug users differ from those who are supportive of the cocaine user and can shore up initial treatment gains in other family members. The treatment objectives guide the selection of family members whose participation is necessary at a given point in time. Clinical examples, such as when to include very young children, when to split off the parents to discuss issues related to their marriage, and when to have a session with siblings only, are recognizable decisions that embody inclusion and exclusion criteria.

Once a decision is reached regarding the specifics of family participation, the therapist has to help the family comply with his/her recommendations. The subject of family recruitment has been prominent in the family therapy literature. It is a clinical issue in all family therapy, especially in therapy of cocaine-abusing patients and their families.

Stanton and Todd (1981), Van Deusen et al. (1980), and Wermuth and Scheidt (1981) have all made cogent proposals for recruiting the family for therapy. In summarizing this extensive body of work, one can extract noteworthy principles concerning recruitment in families with a drug-dependent member. Therapists are cautioned not to rely solely on the drug-dependent patient to bring his/her family in, but rather to get permission from the patient to contact family members immediately. Speed in contacting the family is essential, and the sooner the contact with the family, the more likely is their chance of participating in treatment. Direct therapist-to-family-member contact fosters involvement in therapy and averts undermining efforts by the substance abuser.

The presentation of therapy to the family is of critical significance in their ultimate recruitment. The stance of delivering nonblaming, nonjudgmental messages to the family, coupled with a suggestion that the initial treatment focus will be on helping the drug abuser, is desirable. This approach aims to enlist the family's aid in the drug abuse problem, regarding them as interested helpers, not pathological influences, in the life of their drug-dependent child. In adopting this tack, the clinician therapeutically double-binds the family so that their refusal to participate on this basis can only be equated with a desire on their part to keep the drug abuser in a symptomatic state.

The personal qualities of the therapists are tapped continuously during the recuitment phase of family therapy. The constellation of authority, enthusiasm, perseverance, flexibility, activity, and a willingness to expend great effort is the cluster of therapist attributes deemed most influential on the basis of current research.

Finally, the context in which any therapeutic effort is conducted influences the success or failure of the venture. In organizations that value family work and support the efforts necessary to recruit families, the consequences are invariably in a therapeutic direction.

Middle-Phase Issues

Gaining entry into the family system

When efforts to involve the family in therapy are successful, the therapist must contend with their struggle around stability versus change. The interplay between these forces creates the sense of tension present in family therapy sessions. The therapist has to choreograph the route through these opposing influences and fashion a treatment milieu that maximizes the options for productive movement.

It is beyond the scope of this chapter to completely explicate the complex process of family therapy with the cocaine abuser and his/her family. Instead, we shall present a representative cross-section of techniques employed in some typical issues that arise in the course of treatment.

A common early treatment strategy involves the therapist's efforts to affiliate with the family. This provides entry into the family system and forms the basis for the leverage needed later in treatment. The therapist respects family defenses and initially avoids excessive confrontation. Without "joining" maneuvers, the therapist is unable to influence the family to attempt insession changes that are later carried out in their lives at home. In Kaufman's (1985) terms, "the therapist enters the family as a supporter of family rules but makes the rules work in the direction of therapeutic goals for the family" (p. 140).

The therapist must be "in charge" of the sessions to direct the flow of communication in a useful direction. Destructive family exchanges must be limited, and viable alternative forms of communication must be provided. This process takes many different forms. Reframing changes the labels put on objectionable behavior and converts it into a more acceptable and hence workable form. For example, blame, complaining, and criticism are relabeled as manifestations of concern and apprehension by family members. The therapist's insistence that families confine their discussion to the present avoids the repetitious and unproductive recitations of past injustices. Family members who talk in the "past punitive" tense are blocked from perpetuating dysfunctional patterns which only serve to alienate others.

The therapist uses his own alliances with different family members to effect change by achieving a sense of shifting balance in the family system. Lending support to a peripheral or weak father helps bolster him and reinstate his position in the family. In a similar vein, the therapist rapidly attempts to work with the parents to get them to align with each other in helping their cocaine-abusing offspring. In so doing, efforts to restore weak generational boundaries are reinforced and the seeds of healthier family structure are sown.

Management of resistance

Management of resistance forms a major portion of the overall family therapy program with cocaine abusers. Anderson (1983) has written in depth on the subject and defines resistance in family therapy as "all behaviors, feelings, patterns oı styles that operate to prevent change" (pp. 151–152). Resistances vary in the forms they take and the times at which they occur in the course of family therapy. Astute identification of resistant forces and making effective plans for their management consti-tute the bulk of the therapeutic work in family treatment.

The most fundamental resistance encountered in families with a co-caine-abusing member is outright refusal by the user to enter a treatment program. Under these conditions, the group leader's task is to mobilize the concerned people involved with the drug-dependent person to exert their influence in motivating the drug abuser to avail himself of treat-ment services. A guided family intervention is one effective technique for addressing this form of resistant behavior.

Significant figures from the extended family, work, friendship, and neighborhood sectors of the cocaine user's life are linked together to form a network. The group is instructed and rehearsed in positive, non-angry ways of expressing their concern for the deteriorating trend in the abuser's life. Through a process of support and group pressure, the cocaine user's defenses can be overcome, resulting in a commitment to immediate treatment. The form of treatment is agreed upon before the meeting with the cocaine user, as are the conditions under which treat-ment is monitored. When possible, the patient's employer is part of the network, and continued employment is predicated on active participa-tion in the therapy program over a predetermined time period. Guided interventions have met with considerable success in the field of alcohol-ism and work equally well with a cocaine-abusing population. When drug abuse extends into the workplace, the availability of important co-workers and superiors, in addition to family members, is critical to the success of the network intervention.

Earlier in the chapter, the extreme use of denial was reported as a prominent component of the lives of cocaine abusers and their families. It is no surprise, therefore, that excessive denial emerges as a central resistance in family therapy with this group. Families of cocaine abusers often suffer from feelings of shame and social embarrassment and the need to be viewed as a "healthy family" in the eyes of the outside world. These, plus other powerful, dysphoric feelings, increase the likelihood of reinforcing defense mechanisms of denial. The practical translation of this denial is the need for an assortment of techniques which break through denial mechanisms that contribute to continued cocaine use.

Excessive intellectualizing, rationalizing, and merely incessant chatter are forms of denial that prevent a true picture of the family from emerging. Other elements of denial include actively editing what is said in sessions or deliberately concealing information in order to minimize the extent to which cocaine use is a significant problem. The net effect of these denial patterns is persistence of a dysfunctional family structure which fosters cocaine use.

The family therapist can employ one or more strategies to help counter extremes of family denial. Educational efforts designed to increase realistic understanding of the cocaine problem and to destigmatize cocaine abuse in the eyes of the family may be useful initially. In families where denial seems intractable, more active maneuvers are required. Intensification of family patterns by insession amplification covers an array of structural and strategic family interventions which "push" family interaction to dramatic and, consequently, undeniable levels.

Experiential and actualization techniques, such as family sculpting, the use of metaphors and paradox, and the assignment of tasks, are central to the process of overcoming denial resistances in families. All these approaches are selected on the basis of their capacity to create states of intensity, heightened affect, and experiential learning in family members who avoid such states. The therapist intervenes constructively to punctuate the sequence and alter the form of family interaction in an attempt to dislodge rigid family defenses and set the stage for restructuring more adaptive family patterns.

Excessive blaming, often to the point of scapegoating family members, and attempts to undermine the position of the therapist through questioning his/her competence or by efforts to "triangulate" him are two other avenues of resistance requiring vigilant monitoring throughout the course of therapy.

Since depressive symptoms abound in cocaine-abusing families, the family therapist is faced with extreme versions of garden-variety family resistances. Defeating the therapist or the therapeutic effort through the posture of excessive hopelessness, pessimism, despair, and often open hostility are all commonplace examples of amplified resistances found in cocaine-abusing family groups.

Management of crisis situations

Crises in the family therapy of cocaine abuse are of two types: spontaneous and planned. Spontaneous crisis situations are to be expected during the course of family therapy with cocaine abusers. Most often the crisis situation centers around the user's "slips" or "binges" of repeated cocaine use. It is essential for the therapist to understand the context in which the crisis occurs, as well as the nature of the crisis and its meaning for the family when it happens.

A crisis usually emerges at a point where change has developed in the family system via the treatment process. Crises, in this view, can be regarded as behaviors that endeavor to restore the prior state of family homeostasis. The therapist's goal is to identify the meaning of the crisis and to harness it as a force for learning and change in the family. In order to accomplish this goal, it is critical to try to keep the crisis confined to the family so it can be worked on in therapy sessions.

Crisis situations are familiar to the families of cocaine abusers, and for many families they are a recognizable life-style. The therapist has to use the crisis situation to activate the family and to engage them in the work of crisis resolution. This orientation suggests that several interventions be avoided or delayed if possible during the crisis phase. Hospitalization of the cocaine user, increasing the dose of medication used for cocaine abuse, and banishment of the user from the family home are examples of "last-resort" efforts during family crisis which dilute the impact of the crisis in the family.

From the standpoint of technique, it is important to avoid the use of certain paradoxical interventions during crises that involve escalated cocaine use. Symptom prescription and similar paradoxical interventions which encourage the amplification of the troublesome symptom (cocaine use), either to dramatize its ineffectiveness or absurdity or to demonstrate the family or individual's control over its occurrence, are potentially dangerous during these crisis periods. In contrast to alcohol abuse, where paradox has been used creatively (Bergman, 1985), cocaine is illegal and acutely damaging on a physiological basis; therefore, suggesting its increased use as a family therapy strategy is difficult to justify.

Relapses into repeated cocaine use are not the only crises that regularly occur in treatment. Other behaviors that require attention are threats by family members to discontinue therapy; suicidal threats, gestures, or actual attempts; job-threatening crises; and some form of trouble with the law.

Planned or therapist-induced crisis situations deserve brief mention here. In extremely resistant families, it may become necessary to intervene in order to "shake up" the inflexible, static, treatment-resistant family. As Mowatt et al. (1982) have stated,

> The therapeutically-induced crisis might be seen as the "royal road" to functional reorganization and change in the family. In

these families, the lack of crisis—or the aborting of therapy prior to the occurrence of a crisis—usually means that no change will occur. (p. 202)

When a therapeutically induced crisis is indicated, it is achieved by judicious, but very active interventions designed by the therapist. Techniques of unbalancing family alignments, assigning tasks that intensify emotion in family members, reframing, and other interventions aimed at stimulating the responsivity of the family system are employed at these times. The use of paradoxical interventions, other than prescribing increasing cocaine use, is most often included in this phase of family therapy.

Confidentiality issues

Guidelines for handling information inside the family and between the family and other systems require sensitive study (Rinella & Goldstein, 1980). Traditional concepts of confidentiality derived from individual psychotherapy fall short of what is desired when working with families. When the problem for which the family seeks assistance involves the use of an illegally obtained drug, the issues of privacy, confidentiality, and the disclosing or withholding of relevant information take on even greater significance.

From a therapeutic standpoint, a climate of openness is ideal, but difficult to reach with cocaine abusers and their families. Information must be evaluated from the standpoint of both its content and the role its revelation or obscuration plays in the family dynamics. One useful rule of thumb with cocaine abusers is to support the notion of privacy among family members except when the reluctance to share information functions as an outgoing resistance to therapeutic progress.

This stance respects and supports appropriate boundary issues in the family, encourages healthy individuation with its attendant rights of privacy, yet is not naive in assuming that secrets in families are to be honored and unchallenged categorically. The therapist has to avoid entering into collusive alliances of secrecy with family members. Pressures to fall into this trap are enormous with cocaine abusers and their families.

The therapist is constantly tempted to learn new information, as yet unknown to other family members, on an individual basis from some person in the family. One-to-one attempts to engage the therapist take the form of out-of-session phone calls, letters, or the creation of "pseudo emergencies" that require exclusive, individual attention to one family member by the therapist. These events must be rerouted into sessions with the full family present in order to direct the information into the setting most likely to use it constructively. In so doing, the therapist simultaneously makes a position statement by his/her actions that he is not available to assist in perpetuating dysfunctional family patterns by rewarding individual attempts at contact outside the family sessions.

In cocaine-oriented families, the use and misuse of "secrets" in the family elucidates important issues of family structure. The frightened adolescent who confides information about his cocaine use to his mother, the person to whom he feels the closest in the family, yields data about alliances and family affiliations which may be merely descriptive. If, upon hearing the son's disclosure, the mother suggests or encourages keeping this information from the father and/or other family members, a more dysfunctional collusive pattern is suspected. Utilization of private information in a form that excludes others in the family invariably signals the type of family patterning that fosters cocaine abuse.

Cocaine-dependent individuals and their families frequently share in the collective myth concerning "secrets" related to drug use. Often what is called a secret is merely the lack of open, verbal acknowledgment of behavior or information that is known to all family members on some level. The therapist has to search for respectful, yet aggressive means of determining how and when to help "expose" concealed information. He/she must also assist the family in appreciating the mechanics of their participation in conspiracies of silence which only delay or preclude resolution of the cocaine problem.

Later-Phase Issues

Management of termination

When the family reaches a point of success that is maintained for a consistent period of time, the issue of ending therapy sessions naturally arises. The termination phase of family therapy with cocaine abusers and their families has three components: Reviewing the therapy experience, reinforcing gains made over time, and planning for return to therapy when indicated.

Conducting a review of the family therapy experience accomplishes several things. The family can concretely see how their participation in specific ways has resulted in the resolution they experience at the end of therapy. Identification of risk areas in the family and development of the family's ability to diagnose their own symptoms can be learned during the latter phase of treatment and incorporated into a plan for prevention of similar problems in the future. In the process of reviewing the therapy experience, the therapist tries to simultaneously effect disengagement from the family by acknowledging their independent ability to handle many of the circumstances for which they originally sought help.

An active effort is made to positively reinforce realistic gains made by individual family members and by the family as a whole. Maintenance of abstinence patterns and substitution of adaptive family interaction are emphasized in this phase of the termination process. False reassurance by the therapist and last-session "testimonials" by the family must be avoided and differentiated from an objective inventory of family assets that have helped contribute to their success.

Plans for returning to future sessions are discussed explicitly prior to formal termination. When the cocaine abuse is under control, other family issues may be the basis for a new stage in family work. Commonly, elements in the parental marriage become more prominent when no longer masked by the cocaine abuse issue. In selected families, the family therapy concludes its first phase and the parental marriage may require attention in a separate venue that does not include family members other than the spouses themselves. In families where successful resolution of cocaine problems occurs, conflict may be detoured onto another sibling. These families may continue to meet, but the treatment focus ceases to be exclusively cocaine oriented.

Plans for aftercare follow-up

It is important to end the family therapy on a positive note to enhance the probability that family members will return for scheduled follow-up sessions or in the event they experience temporary relapses. Aftercare planning includes provision for monitoring progress and providing the family with a "battery charge" at regulated intervals following the formal conclusion of family therapy.

In the termination phase, it is wise to build in a face-saving procedure for the family to reenter therapy should there be a future need to do so. Although it is desirable to place the responsibility for change on the shoulders of the family, the therapist must realize that relapses often occur even after successful treatment. A contingency plan for management of setbacks has to be explicitly presented to the family for their agreement.

The orientation to termination as the end of a successful phase of family work permits both therapist and family to comfortably resume work at a future date if circumstances in the family so dictate. Attitudes that returning to therapy equals failure and that the family must be "cured forever" at the end of formal sessions work against the view of the family as an ever-changing group with different needs at key points in its life-cycle. Family therapy in general, and particularly family work with a symptom as unpredictable and volatile as cocaine use, has to be flexible enough to adapt to the family's needs at different points in time.

SUMMARY

Family therapy provides an exciting dimension to the treatment of cocaine abuse. Systems-derived techniques with a structural family therapy focus are emerging as the most promising formats to date. The family has been involved in other ways that acknowledge its power and necessity with respect to resolution of cocaine abuse problems.

Preventive and educational programs are currently being tested in the family setting in hopes of utilizing the family as a first line of defense against the vulnerability of its members to cocaine dependency.

Couples approaches are employed with regularity in a variety of formats. Work with couples usually follows completion of family therapy with the original family. In instances where the family of origin is unavailable because of geographical limitations or in cases where they are deceased, marital therapy constitutes the initial approach to cocaine abuse treatment.

The two predominant forms of couples therapy are the conjoint method and group therapy where the group is composed exclusively of dyadic relationships. This important body of family work is discussed in Chapter 7. That chapter also includes a discussion of multiple-family group therapy and other group formats, such as couples groups, which involve family members. These technical variations represent the growing interface between group and family therapies for the treatment of cocaine abuse in the family.

REFERENCES

Alexander BK, Dibb GS: Interpersonal perception in addict families. Fam Process 16:17–28, 1977.

Anderson CM, Stewart S: Mastering Resistance: A Practical Guide to Family Therapy, New York, Guilford Press, 1983.

Bergman JS: Fishing for Barracuda: Pragmatics of Brief Systemic Therapy, New York, WW Norton, 1985.

Bieber, I: Cognitive Psychoanalysis, New York, Jason Aronson, 1980.

Bieber, I: Homosexuality: A Psychoanalytic Study of Male Homosexuals, New York, Basic Books, 1962.

Boszormenyi-Nagy I, and Spark GM: Invisible Loyalties, New York, Harper & Row, 1973.

Bowen M: Family Therapy in Clinical Practice, New York, Jason Aronson, 1978.
Coleman SB, Kaplan JD, Downing RW: Life cycle and loss: the spiritual vacuum of heroin addiction. Fam Process 25:5–23, 1986.
Gurman AS, Kniskern DP: Handbook of Family Therapy, New York, Brunner/Mazel, 1981.
Haley J: Uncommon Therapy: The Psychiatric Techniques of Milton H. Erickson, M.D., New York, WW Norton, 1973.
Haley J: Problem Solving Therapy, San Francisco, Jossey-Bass, 1976.
Haley J: Leaving Home: The Therapy of Disturbed Young People, New York, McGraw-Hill, 1980.
Haley J: Reflections on Therapy, Chevy Chase, MD, The Family Therapy Institute of Washington, DC, 1981.
Hoffman L: Foundations of Family Therapy, New York, Basic Books, 1981.
Kaufman E: Substance Abuse and Family Therapy, Orlando, FL, Grune & Stratton, 1985.
Kaufman E: The family of the alcoholic patient. Psychosomatics 27:347–359, 1986.
Kaufman E, Kaufmann PN: Family Therapy of Drug and Alcohol Abuse, New York, Gardner Press, 1979.
Klagsbrun M, Davis DI: Substance abuse and family interaction. Fam Process 16:149–173, 1977.
Madanes C: Strategic Family Therapy, San Francisco, Jossey-Bass, 1981.
McGoldrick M, Gerson R: Genograms in Family Assessment, New York, WW Norton, 1985.
McGoldrick M, Pearce JK, Giordano J, eds: Ethnicity and Family Therapy, New York, Guilford Press, 1982.
Minuchin S: Families and Family Therapy, Cambridge MA, Harvard University Press, 1974.
Minuchin S, Fishman HC: Family Therapy Techniques, Cambridge, MA, Harvard University Press, 1981.
Minuchin S, Baker L, Rosman BL, Liebman R, Milman L, Todd TC: A conceptual model of psychosomatic illness in children. Arch Gen Psychiatry 32:1031–1038, 1975.
Minuchin S, Rosman BL, Baker L: Psychosomatic Families: Anorexia Nervosa in Context, Cambridge, MA, Harvard University Press, 1978.
Mowatt DT, Heard DB, Steier F, Stanton MD, Todd TC: Crisis resolution and the addiction cycle, in Stanton MD, Todd TC, eds: The Family Therapy of Drug Abuse and Addiction, New York, Guilford Press, 1982.
Paolino TJ, McCrady BS: Marriage and Marital Therapy: Psychoanalytic, Behavioral and Systems Theory Perspectives, New York, Brunner/Mazel, 1978.
Papp P: The Process of Change, New York, Guilford Press, 1983.
Pattison EM, Kaufman E: Alcoholism syndrome, definition and models, in Pattison EM, Kaufman E, eds: Encyclopedic Handbook of Alcoholism, New York, Gardner Press, 1982.
Reilly DM: Drug-abusing families: intrafamilial dynamics and brief triphasic treatment, in Kaufman E, Kaufmann PN, eds: Family Therapy of Drug and Alcohol Abuse, New York, Gardner Press, 1979.
Rinella VJ, Goldstein MR: Family therapy with substance abusers: legal considerations regarding confidentiality. J Marital Fam Ther 6:319–326, 1980.
Selvini-Palazzoli M, Boscolo L, Cecchin G, Prata G: Paradox and Counterparadox, New York, Jason Aronson, 1978.
Spotts JV, Shontz FC: Cocaine Users: A Representative Case Approach, New York, The Free Press, 1980.
Stanton MD: The addict as savior: heroin, death and the family, Fam Proc 16:191–197, 1977.
Stanton MD: Drug abuse and the family, in Andolfi M, Zwerling I, eds: Dimensions of Family Therapy, New York, Guilford Press, 1980.
Stanton MD: An integrated structural strategic approach to family therapy, J Marital Fam Ther 7:427–439, 1981.

Stanton MD: The family and drug abuse: concepts and rationale, in Bratter TE, Forrest EG, eds: Alcoholism and Substance Abuse: Strategies for Clinical Intervention, New York, The Free Press, 1985.

Stanton MD, Todd TC: Engaging resistant families in treatment, Fam Proc 20:261–293, 1981.

Stanton MD, Todd TC: The Family Therapy of Drug Abuse and Addiction, New York, Guilford Press, 1982.

Todd TC, Berger H, Lande G: Supervisors' views on the special requirements of family therapy with drug abusers, in Stanton MD, Todd TC, eds: The Family Therapy of Drug Abuse and Addiction, New York, Guilford Press, 1982.

Van Deusen JM, Stanton MD, Scott SM, Todd TC: Engaging resistant families in treatment: I. Getting the drug addict to recruit his family members, Int J Addictions 15:1069–1089, 1980.

Wermuth L, Scheidt S: Enlisting family support in drug treatment, Fam Proc 20:261–293, 1981.

Chapter 9

Hospital Treatment of Cocaine Abuse

Michael Sheehy, M.D.

The lack of scientific knowledge about hospital treatment of cocaine abuse invites uncertainty on the one hand and dogmatism on the other. Few health care providers would disagree that persons who are suicidal or extremely disorganized because of psychiatric illness, regardless of its cause, belong in a hospital. But after this, agreement ends. Partisan views about length of stay, the role of the hospital, and goals of treatment fall prey to personal experience, ideology, sensitivity to costs, and unproven notions about outcome. These influences are exaggerated when the focus of treatment, in this case cocaine abuse, is a relatively recent and growing problem.

This chapter will view the hospital as a social institution in which treatments are delivered. Nearly all therapeutic approaches to cocaine abuse derive from older treatments for other drug dependencies, especially alcoholism. Hospital treatments are designed to relieve initial personal and symptomatic distress, improve physical health, start the repair of family and social injuries, and develop new skills and knowledge with which to resist relapse. Because of these several aims, the hospital is more than its medical treatments. It is a school, and insofar as it fosters a belief system, it is a church.

The discussion of hospital treatment of cocaine abuse will include answers to common questions about hospital treatment which have been asked by persons who make referrals, work in treatment programs, have a friend in apparent need of treatment, or need treatment themselves. Because a minority of readers may want to start inpatient treatment programs of their own, an attempt will be made to provide some guidance concerning the creation of hospital-based cocaine abuse services.

The information in this chapter is based on the clinical practice of the Silver Hill Foundation, a private, not-for-profit hospital in New Canaan, Connecticut, which has maintained a drug dependency service for many years.

SPECIAL FEATURES OF THE HOSPITAL

Two special features characterize inpatient, as opposed to outpatient, treatment settings. Foremost among these is the denial of a patient's access to drugs of abuse. The hospital also provides intense, organized, and informal contact with other persons who have acknowledged a serious problem with cocaine or other drugs. These range from other patients still struggling with acknowledgment of their problem to experienced professionals and nonprofessionals who offer medical knowledge, social comfort, and in some cases the hope that stems from years of recovery.

WHO IS IN THE HOSPITAL?

In 1984, the charts of 30 randomly selected patients who sought treatment for cocaine dependence at the Silver Hill Foundation were reviewed. To be included, each patient's chart had to demonstrate clear evidence that the DSM-III criteria for cocaine abuse could be attributed to cocaine and not to other drugs that were used concurrently. Twenty charts were rejected on this basis because it was not possible to disentangle some of the effects of cocaine from those of alcohol, barbiturates, and opioids. This problem was as difficult in reviewing the pattern of pathological use as it was in the determination of social and occupational impairment. Charts of the 30 patients who were included in the sample were also reviewed to determine the presence of other psychiatric disorders. Additional diagnoses were made only if there was clear evidence of this psychiatric disorder in the hospital two weeks after admission for the treatment of cocaine abuse. The Silver Hill sample was compared to the nonpatient, randomly selected 500-telephone-call sample of Washton and Gold (1984) (Table 9.1).

The Washton and Gold sample used a structured 20-to-30 minute sur-

Table 9.1
Comparison of the Washton and Gold and the Silver Hill Samples

	Washton and Gold	Silver Hill Sample
Source	800, cocaine callers $n = 500$, random	Inpatients, 28-day program $n = 30$, random
Method	Telephone survey: 20–30 minutes	Intake and discharge summaries plus progress notes
% Male	67	73
Mean Age (years)	30	31
Mean Years of Use	4.9	4.6
Route %	N = 61 S = 21 i.v. = 18	N = 47 S = 30 i.v. = 30
$ Spent (1 G at $100)	637.00	1,370.00

N = nasal insufflation; S = smoking (may have nasal use too); i.v. = intravenous (may use other routes as well).

vey; the Silver Hill sample was based on lengthy intake and discharge summaries as well as progress notes. Both samples were similar in sex distribution, mean age, and mean years of use. Striking differences were noted when the route of cocaine administration was examined. The percentage of inpatients who had smoked cocaine was greater than in the nonpatient sample, and the percent of intravenous users was almost twice as great among inpatients. Most strikingly, the dollars spent on cocaine by the inpatient sample averaged $1,370 per week, in contrast to the $637 per week reported by Washton and Gold's noninpatient sample.

Viewed naturalistically, both groups were comprised largely of males about 30 years old with nearly five years of cocaine use, but the hospital seemed to fulfill its expected social role of treating individuals who were "sicker" by virtue of a more direct route of administration and a larger quantity of drug.

Differences in methodology used by the Washton and Gold sample and the Silver Hill sample did not permit an item-by-item review of symptoms and consequences of drug use. Despite this, all hospitalized patients had experienced adverse social consequences on the job, within their family, or with friends, and 57% experienced psychiatric symptoms, including extreme irritability, marked hypersomnia as part of a crash, bouts of depression, socially disruptive, grandiose and paranoid ideas, and hallucinations. Thirty-seven percent of the inpatient sample had medical problems such as overdose, hepatitis, car crash with injuries, abscesses, and seizures. Among the inpatient sample, other drug disorders were prevalent. (See Table 9.2.)

Seventy-three percent of patients with cocaine abuse met criteria for another drug disorder as well. In contrast to the expectations of many clinicians working on the service, the prevalence of sedative/hypnotic (especially benzodiazepines) disorders was relatively low.

Findings from the inpatient sample on the prevalence of non-drug-related psychiatric disorders must be regarded with caution. The professional literature on drug dependency has been plagued for many years by wide disagreements, especially on the topic of associated affective disorders. Many studies of outpatient alcoholics show that 30–50% of individuals meet the DSM-III criteria for an affective disorder (Cadoret & Winokur, 1972; Guze et al., 1971; Rounsaville et al., 1986; Weissman et al., 1980; Woodruff et al., 1973), while rates are much closer to what prevails in the general population when a long-sober group is studied (Behar et al., 1984).

The inpatient sample charts were reviewed for the presence of a psychiatric disorder in the hospital after two weeks of treatment. Not only may this be an insufficient amount of drug-free time for patients abusing cocaine alone to be rediagnosed, it may be even more problematic for the majority abusing other drugs such as alcohol and opioids. Despite these caveats, 33% of the population met DSM-III criteria for an affective disorder (almost always a depressive disorder) after two weeks of hospitaliza-

Table 9.2
Other Substance Use Disorders
in the Silver Hill Sample

Any other substance use disorder(s)	73%
Alcohol disorder	40%
Cannabis disorder	23%
Opioid disorder	16%
Amphetamine disorder	6%
Sedative hypnotic disorder	6%

tion. Personality disorders, by contrast, were infrequent (10%) in this population of largely upper-middle-class inpatients.

Whether due to the severity of social problems incurred during the course of cocaine abuse, the relative absence of personality disorders, or the attractiveness of the treatment program and environment, only 6% of the inpatient sample signed out of the hospital against medical advice before completing the 28-day-stay program.

THE GOALS OF INPATIENT TREATMENT

Detoxification

The detoxification* at Silver Hill of nearly 700 patients with a cocaine disorder over the past five years has rarely required the use of psychiatric drugs. Although reports in the literature suggest a role for the use of tricyclic antidepressants such as desipramine (Gawin & Kleber, 1984), stimulants such as methylphenidate (Khantzian, 1983), or the dopamine agonist bromocriptine (Dackis & Gold, 1985), these drugs were not essential to the detoxification process based on clinical experience. Although many patients enter the hospital having just completed a final cocaine run, oversleeping, lethargy, cloudy thinking, and, less commonly, overeating spontaneously disappear within a few days. The acute development of suicidal urges during the crash period *in hospital* has been exceedingly rare on our service and has also quickly subsided. This author believes that the temporary use of tricyclics, stimulants, or bromocriptine medications in the hospital setting has potential medical dangers in excess of their clinical utility for detoxification. This is not to deny the role that such medications may play in outpatient detoxification programs or in continued treatment following discharge of persons with a history of frequent relapses.

In contrast, a minority of patients are delusional, agitated, and experiencing hallucinations at the time of admission. Because of the personal distress and disruptive behavior that result from such a state, antipsychotic drugs such as haloperidol or chlorpromazine can be used in standard doses (5–20 mg of haloperidol, 200–800 mg of chlorpromazine daily) with good results in a brief time span. Continued use has not been

---

*The term detoxification is used to describe the clinical management of signs and symptoms during the first few days after cessation of heavy cocaine use.

necessary in the absence of a separate psychiatric disorder, e.g., bipolar disorder, manic type.

During the detoxification period, which usually lasts for only a few days, the hospital provides an unstimulating environment with limited involvement in psychosocial therapies. Encouragement by a physician, a counselor, and especially nurses, along with a physical examination and monitoring of vital signs every two hours while awake for the first three days, is all that is necessary. Based on admission history, urine toxicology, and vital signs, individual patients may require detoxification from other drugs, particularly alcohol, opioids, or sedative/hypnotics. Detoxification from these drugs complicates the care considerably and may require as much as three weeks of medical treatment. To simplify these detoxifications, the Silver Hill Foundation has developed a standard, detailed detoxification manual for all patients which has proven very helpful in eliminating the practice idiosyncrasies of multiple physicians. Whenever possible, this hospital uses clonidine to detoxify patients from opioids, chlordiazepoxide for alcohol dependence, and phenobarbital for sedative/hypnotics or sedative/hypnotics plus alcohol dependence. The rare patient who suffers a seizure is typically treated with intramuscular phenobarbital, given an immediate neurological workup, and placed on therapeutic levels of diphenylhydantoin until the electrocephalogram normalizes.

Medical Complications

Medical complications due to prolonged use of cocaine are common (see Table 9.3). Most are not serious, but a few require emergency treatment. Some complication can be expected in at least a third of hospitalized patients.

Nasal use alone frequently produces a rhinitis marked by sneezing, runny nose, and local pain. When chronic, it is sometimes associated with mucosal erosions. Treatment with steroid-containing nasal sprays can be helpful, but sympathomimetics should be avoided. In the case of a nasal septum perforation, surgery may be required. Some patients develop sinusitis from the nasal use of cocaine which is occasionally complicated by infection. In such an instance, antibiotics as well as a steroid inhaler are useful.

Smoking cocaine or intravenous injection produce more serious problems, though fortunately most are uncommon. Ventricular fibrillation can occur owing to the sympathomimetic effect of the drug. This usually takes place during the course of a cocaine run and is almost never seen in

Table 9.3
Medical Complications Associated with Cocaine Abuse

From nasal use	Rhinitis
	Mucosal erosion
	Nasal septum perforation
	Sinusitis
From smoking or intravenous injection, uncommon from nasal use	Bronchitis
	Ventricular fibrillation and arrest
	Respiratory arrest
	Cerebral hemorrhage
	Hyperpyreia
	Seizures
From intravenous injection	Abscesses
	Hepatitis B
	AIDS
General complications from all routes of administration	Weight loss
	Malnutrition

hospitalized patients. Such an emergency requires immediate cardiac conversion. Extrasystoles are more common during a cocaine run but usually subside spontaneously. Respiratory arrest can also occur, but is typically a reflection of an overdose and not likely to be seen outside of an emergency room setting. Cerebral hemorrhage, from increased blood pressure, and hyperpyrexia also occur but are rare. Smoking commonly causes or aggravates bronchitis, but this usually subsides quickly except in heavy cigarette smokers.

In contrast to these emergencies, a history of seizures is common among patients hospitalized for treatment of cocaine dependence. Rarely do these occur in the hospital when access to the drug is prevented.

Intravenous injection of cocaine produces a particular group of problems including abscesses, which can be noticed by direct inspection of the skin, venous thrombosis, which can make phlebotomy difficult, hepatitis B, and AIDS. It is imperative to test all intravenous drug users for hepatitis B at the time of admission. Screening for antibodies to the AIDS virus remains controversial, though the nature of the test and its current interpretation should be explained to patients in order to give them an opportunity to receive screening if they wish. Patients with a fully developed case of AIDS will demonstrate the usual history of unexplained fevers, cough, adenopathy, weight loss in the absence of anorexia, and other characteristic features of the syndrome.

All patients treated in a hospital for cocaine use should have a brief nutritional screening. Many have lost weight and suffer malnutrition. Since cocaine users commonly abuse alcohol as well, weight loss may have been prevented despite the presence of significant malnutrition.

Rehabilitation

The goals of rehabilitation in a cocaine treatment program include:

- Systematic undermining of excuses for cocaine and other drug use
- Imparting current knowledge about cocaine and its consequences
- Learning coping skills to deal with cocaine craving and drug-using friends
- Renewal of former leisure time interests
- Active participation in the fellowships (AA, CA, NA)
- Conflict resolution in the family ·
- Development of new social links with recovering persons
- Treatment of any other complicating psychiatric disorders discovered during hospitalization

Patients in the hospital are introduced to rehabilitation gradually. As soon as physiological and mental functioning appears to have stabilized, patients begin participation in individual and group psychotherapy as well as fellowship meetings and recreational and occupational therapy. Individual meetings are scheduled with drug counselors on a regular basis. (See Table 9.4 on pp. 242–243.)

THE TREATMENT PROGRAM

The hospital environment provides several advantages from the clinician's viewpoint. Patients have almost no choice with regard to attendance unless they leave the hospital; unlike outpatients, they show up regularly for all scheduled sessions. Dropouts are rare, and there are no intoxicated participants. In the hospital, many different treatments operate at the same time. This provides a broad support and an alternative "viewpoint" if a particular treatment does not seem to work for a patient. Finally, the brief duration of the hospital period (14–28 days is usual) compresses treatment efforts; particular treatments occur much more frequently than is the case on a standard outpatient basis.

The inpatient program also poses points of frustration for the staff. The clinician has almost no opportunity to exercise choice on who should participate in a given treatment. Patients who are at different stages of recovery participate together, based largely on when they entered the hospital. Of necessity, treatments are time limited, and there is little opportunity to "work through" problems. Few real, current life events occur which can be brought into a particular treatment aside from resentment of one patient toward another or toward staff, or a hospital romance. There are almost no temptations and triggers to drug use except for memories and the comments of other patients. Because of time, little consolidation of new learning can take place, and this may be complicated by the "honeymoon" phase induced in many patients by abstinence after protracted intoxication. During this honeymoon, the world seems wonderful, fresh, and inviting, a perception not likely to be confirmed by postdischarge experience.

The comments that follow about each treatment modality will take these assets and liabilities into account. All treatments collectively try to combine strong feelings, new ideas, and behavior change.

Individual Psychotherapy

This is both a treatment and a service since patients expect it. It is very difficult to offer patients different frequencies of individual psychotherapy in a hospital setting without generating resentment, jealousy, feelings of neglect, or specialness. Whatever frequency of individual psychotherapy occurs, it should be hospital chosen if at all possible rather than clinician chosen, unless medical emergencies, dementia, or other pressing psychiatric reasons dictate to the contrary. In individual psychotherapy, every patient has the opportunity to feel somewhat special and to develop an ally. Because hospitalization is short, individual psychotherapy should focus largely on current issues, instead of childhood ones. The principal goals of this treatment in hospital are to undermine a patient's denial of drug dependency and break down the mystique often associated with cocaine use. Individual treatment allows tailor-made strategies for resolving social, family, financial, and work problems which can be rehearsed in other hospital treatments and on passes when permitted. Individual treatment permits a careful review of peer relationships and planning for the development of new ones. Unfortunately, individual psychotherapy in hospital entails reporting events experi-

Table 9.4
Silver Hill Substance Abuse Program

	Monday	Tuesday	Wednesday	Thursday	Friday	Saturday
7:45 A.M.	Breakfast	Breakfast	Breakfast	Breakfast	Breakfast	8:30 Breakfast
	9:15 Group therapy	9:15 Group therapy	9:15 Group therapy	9:15 Group therapy	9:15 Group therapy	10:00 TR opens
			10:30 Fitness class	11:15 House activity	10:30 Fitness class	12:30 Lunch
	11:15 Recovery skills	11:15 AA step meeting		11:15 Transition/ alumni group		5:00 Tapes
						6:00 Dinner
12:15 P.M.	Lunch	Lunch	Lunch	Lunch	Lunch	SUNDAY
			1:00 House activity			8:30 Breakfast
						10:00 TR opens
						10:30 Rap session

Time						
1:00						Dinner
1:30			Assertive training			
2:00	Leisure counseling					
2:30		Men's group / Women's group				
3:00				Film	Lecture or film	
3:15			Stress management			
3:30	House community meeting					
4:00	Relaxation class				Relaxation	
5:00				Community meeting main house		
5:45 P.M.	Dinner	Dinner	Dinner	Dinner	Dinner	Supper
7:00			AA discussion group			
7:30	NA meeting off grounds					
8:00					CA meeting off grounds or	CA meeting or
8:30	AA meeting off grounds	AA, Alateen meeting		AA meeting off grounds	AA and Alanon meeting	AA meeting off grounds

Patients are *required* to attend all activities if physically able.
Exceptions: Assertiveness training program (by doctor's order); transition group (by assignment).

enced in other treatment modalities, particularly group psychotherapy and fellowship meetings. In general, patients should be discouraged from doing this since the "facts" are rarely accessible to the individual therapy clinician.

Some patients with a psychological bent of mind take to individual psychotherapy and wish to extend their hospitalization in order to resolve broad life conflicts from childhood or marriage which cannot be resolved within a reasonable time in hospital. It is important to discourage patients from this expectation while opening the door to such work on an aftercare basis.

By tradition, the hospital's most senior clinicians tend to conduct individual psychotherapy despite the absence of solid evidence that this works better. There is little doubt, however, that the seniority and additional credentials of the individual therapist promote use of this treatment by patients as a "court of last resort" in dealing with hospital as well as extrahospital topics.

Group Psychotherapy

Tradition and economy of scale result in many group psychotherapy sessions in most hospital programs. Whenever possible, these should be scheduled in the morning at a fixed hour to allow for intellectual mastery, reflection, and consolidation later in the day when less cognitively demanding activities such as stress management or relaxation exercises are highlighted. Most group leaders prefer groups with 8–12 members.

Because the composition of groups is continually changing, it is difficult to design these with a large-scale architecture in mind. In contrast, a stand-alone model, in which each group session is impelled toward a start, a middle ground, and a denouement, rarely works effectively in a consistent manner. Some consistency does exist regarding patient issues as well as the ingroup postures assumed by patients. The "help-rejecting complainer," the "intellectualizing monopolistic member," and the "silent, withdrawn role" are a few typical stances adopted by members of cocaine groups.

Because patients usually seek treatment for a cocaine dependence problem in a crisis, they have rarely selected any particular treatment modality and may come to group therapy hesitantly or with unrealistic expectations of rampant aggression, "letting it all hang out," and gut-wrenching encounter. The most effective groups seem to tread a middle ground between sweat-inducing silence and leader-generated charisma. This promotes attention to the *patient's* problems instead of to the leader and helps each patient to develop new insight into his problem.

The focus of group psychotherapy in an inpatient program should be on interpersonal learning and on a review of the triggers to drug use. Extensive discussions of drug use as self-reward, stress relief, and for conflict avoidance can occur productively while non-drug-dependent social behavior improves. In contrast to outpatient groups, relatively few drastic life crises occur to patients in the hospital. They rarely get divorced or terminate their jobs while in the hospital. They also do not have the opportunity to bring the experience of familiar environments, old friends, and the sight of drugs to group, except briefly, based on a pass.

In a time-limited hospital setting, the fortress mentality that develops in some outpatient groups is weak, and newcomers tend to be readily welcomed. But departures from the group occasioned by hospital discharge, while frequent, can be emotionally intense because of the frequency of group meetings (often five days per week) and the strong bonding that the hospital environment can generate. There is also the fearful anticipation associated with departure, separation, and the sense of a new and frightening mission. Group leaders must work hard to prevent these dramatic issues from becoming the exclusive focus of the therapy as opposed to the more mundane learning about how to live drug-free.

Although group treatments in hospital are not complicated by intoxicated attendees and the anxiety over dropout members, patients who discharge themselves against medical advice have a significant emotional impact. Attempts to deal in group with the occasional "drug bust" on campus are also difficult and may ally several or all of the members of a group against the leadership and the hospital administration.

Leadership of groups can be performed by a single individual or by a pair. Team leadership is more expensive, but it is generally helpful for the leaders and gives the patient alternative role models with whom to identify. Groups may be led by experienced clinicians from the disciplines of psychiatry, psychology, social work, nursing, or drug counseling. A combination of disciplines often seems helpful for its breadth of perspective. This is particularly true when a drug counselor leads a group with another mental health professional.

Family Therapy

Unlike participants in a typical outpatient therapy setting, the families of patients hospitalized for a cocaine dependence problem may not be readily available because they live at some distance. Accordingly, some, but not all, patients can participate in family therapy. Whenever possible, family therapy should be included as a part of treatment since it offers an opportunity to educate family members about the patient's drug problem, identify drug problems in other members of the family, encourage attendance at allied fellowships such as Alanon and discuss likely role stresses following discharge. Families who attend these sessions are often unsettled as they bring their resentments toward the patient into a setting where the patient may for the first time hear them clearly. Most families have remarkably unsophisticated views about the causes of drug abuse and need all the assistance they can obtain in gaining a sense of perspective, developing realistic expectations, and resolving strong and hard-to-handle emotions. Financial problems, extramarital affairs, and abdication of child-rearing responsibilities are common themes in this modality of treatment.

Multiple-family groups in which spouses and, in some cases, children can get together without the patient to air common experiences and learn from one another are also valuable. These promote a sense of participation, shared frustration, and shared optimism.

Family therapy groups conducted by the combination of the patient's primary clinician and a drug counselor are often effective since the leadership combines knowledge of the disease and knowledge of the street.

AA, CA, and NA

Attendance at these sessions, which should occur daily if possible, is critical to a hospital treatment program. These meetings bridge the gap between in- and outpatient settings. Individual patients can find sponsors, see other people coping with slips, and identify with models of long-term sobriety. Many patients are initially resistant to these meetings because of their religious flavor and the tendency of some members to view hospital treatment as suspect in its motives. We have found that this resistence decays with time for most patients as they listen to personal biographies with elements similar to their own and develop a sense of camaraderie with a larger group. Because many patients with a cocaine dependence problem have developed a disorderly, self-centered, and exploitative life-style from their drug use, the altruistic and spiritual values of the fellowships are an effective antidote and the organizing grain of sand around which old, or in some instances new, values can coalesce.

In our experience, AA groups remain the most effective meetings because of the long sobriety of some members and their infectious impact on other patients. CA groups are relatively new and often have a younger membership, one that seems to many patients less seasoned and humble in the good sense. Some patients complain that CA meetings tend to perpetuate the feeling of "specialness" about cocaine as a drug, though this is by no means universal. By contrast, some dedicated CA members complain of a gilt-edged self-concept on the part of AA.

Developing fellowship meetings within a hospital setting poses special problems of its own since attendees cannot be screened thoroughly by hospital staff and actively drug-dependent individuals are welcome so long as they appear reasonably motivated and are not disruptive. The clinical and legal implications of assigning patients to attend inhospital fellowship meetings that are open to outsiders should be considered carefully by hospital staff and administration.

Drug Counseling

In contrast to most other treatment modalities inhospital, drug counseling is usually more informal and varied in its frequency. Drug counselors, who are usually recovering alcoholics or drug-dependent persons, can disclose their own experience, pain, and satisfaction of recovering. We have found this modality to be most effective at undermining drug argot and confronting the temptations of the street.

Recovery Skills

These sessions are typically led by drug counselors for 10 or 12 patients at a time. Learning how to say no to cocaine, learning how to handle oneself in the company of associates where pressure to use cocaine is active, and developing specific plans to avoid locations where drugs were purchased or used are core themes of this group treatment. Patients and counselors share tactics and discuss their effectiveness. The content of these sessions commonly overlaps what is done in leisure counseling and reinforces the ethics of fellowship meetings. The limited goals of recovery skills sessions lend themselves ideally to the brief period of hospitalization.

Assertiveness Training

It is not exactly mysterious that the early, more romantic phases of cocaine use encourage garrulousness, comfortable self-assertion, and a subjective feeling of social ease, not characteristic of everyday life or the later states of cocaine dependence. Many patients who once felt that cocaine was a magic ticket to social stardom confess that in the later stages of their addiction, they sat in silent terror on the toilet waiting for the cocaine rush. Relearning or learning for the first time healthy self-assertion does not necessarily come easily, though compared to patients suffering a major depression, cocaine-dependent individuals seem quick studies. Assertiveness training lends itself to fairly large groups comprised of up to 20 individuals and by tradition draws a number of clinicians fond of activity and high-energy therapeutics. The therapeutic strategies used in assertiveness training consist of role playing, confrontation, and group feedback. These sessions can focus on overassertion as well as underassertion in an attempt to discover a reasonable medium. Assertiveness training sessions are usually much more leader-centered and education-oriented than other group therapy undertakings, and their long-range effectiveness is compromised by the limited opportunity for many sessions during hospitalization.

Stress Management

In stress management sessions, usually led by members of a therapeutic recreation department, patients are encouraged to identify their personal, stressful experiences. Typically, these are life changes such as divorce, moving, promotion, demotion, changes in financial status, and the like. Patients rate them in terms of severity. Many patients with drug-dependent problems quickly identify chemicals as their best friends in coping with these stressful events. After individual profiles of stressful life events are developed, individuals are taught relaxation techniques such as muscle relaxation and deep breathing. Regular physical exercise is encouraged as an alternative to drug use. Some time in stress management is spent on developing a list of anticipated postdischarge stresses, which can also be coupled with the relaxation exercises in an attempt to practice new, nondamaging coping strategies. Stress management groups are almost universal components of inpatient treatment programs because of the abundance of time, at least in the short range. They are relatively rare in outpatient settings. Stress management is usually combined with time management exercises which deal with the fact that stopping drug use frees up many hours in a week which can suddenly seem empty and anxiety-provoking. Individual reviews of free time and the development of a menu of activities that fit the individual's preferences can be discussed in these sessions.

Transition and Alumnae Groups

Hospital programs for the treatment of cocaine abuse that are successful tend to generate a strong feeling of gratitude on the part of "graduates." Many of these individuals serve as fellowship sponsors and informal links to patients in the hospital and help them bridge the transition to real recovery. An organized meeting of inpatients with successful graduates is an effective link to the outside and should occur on a weekly basis, if possible. These groups are typically led in a low-key style by drug counselors, but other clinicians may serve just as well. The lack of drama and the spiritual focus in these meetings is highly effective for many patients and generates real-life friendships that persist following discharge. Because of graduates' familiarity with the particular hospital program, they can speak knowledgeably to patients undergoing treatment about "good" and "bad" parts of the program as well as the problems and satisfactions of life postdischarge.

Other Hospital Groups

Fitness groups are almost never a component of outpatient treatment programs but comprise a staple of inpatient treatment. Besides improving general physical condition, these programs help to put in practice what has been learned in leisure counseling and relaxation exercises and offer relief from the condensed and sometimes emotion-laden therapies which occur earlier in the day. Similarly, gender groups have become popular as a response to feminism, gayism, and the traditional predominance of males in drug treatment programs. These groups are led by a same-sex leader sensitive to role behavior and its interface with drug use.

ADMINISTRATIVE POLICIES

Visitors, passes, urine screens, and drug use while in hospital are the principal problem areas that require administrative, as opposed to strictly therapeutic, management. For each, we have found the development of a clear, public, reasonable if not "right," and almost never violated set of standards to be helpful.

Visitors

We do not allow any visitors for one week following admission to the treatment program. For patients who require active detoxification from other drugs of abuse, visitors are not permitted until after this procedure is completed, even if it requires more than seven days. Subsequently, visitors are screened by the nursing staff and permitted to visit patients during nonprogram hours in small numbers. Visitors are informed politely that they may be searched.

Passes

Patients are reviewed for pass eligibility, typically after they have completed two weeks in the program. The determination of eligibility is made by the entire service team after the patient completes a form stipulating the nature and purpose of the pass. Final authorization is given by the patient's doctor. Passes are usually granted for discharge-related activities or as a "test." We have found the latter quite productive toward the end of a stay for a patient who denies experiencing any craving in the drug-free hospital environment. The home environment is more likely to trigger a desire to resume drug use, demand the use of coping skill, and provide useful material for discussion in both individual and group psychotherapy following return. Overnight passes are almost never authorized.

Urine Screens and Drug Use in Hospital

Urine screens are obtained on a random basis during the program and invariably following return from a pass. This is despite the absence of evidence that urine screens improve outcome. Urine screens are universally viewed by staff as keeping the program "honest." Whenever possible, passes are not given to patients whose urine remains "dirty" during hospitalization. This is not always possible since benzodiazepines and cannabis especially may contaminate the urine throughout most or all of a 28-day-stay program without any active drug use. Patients whose urine is found to be "dirty," either during the program or on completion of a pass, have their privilege level dropped. Patients discovered to have given drugs to other patients in the program are discharged administratively or transferred to another service if their psychiatric condition (e.g., active suicidal ideas) forbids discharge.

STAFFING LEVELS

Full-time equivalent (FTE) staff work equals 40 hours/week, for 10 acute-care (detoxification) beds and 12 subacute-care beds housed separately (see Table 9.5).

QUESTIONS AND ANSWERS

Patients, families, and staff often inquire about important aspects of inpatient cocaine abuse treatment programs. Following are commonly

Table 9.5
Staffing Levels

Class of Personnel	FTEs
M.D.	3.5
Counselor	4.0
R.N., L.P.N., aide	24*
T.R. (recreational therapist)	1.5
O.T. (occupational therapist)	0.5

*This figure is high because two geographically separate units comprise the 22-bed service.

encountered questions and responses related to the treatment of cocaine abuse in the hospital.

Question—What are the pros and cons of a single-drug, e.g., cocaine, as opposed to a mixed-drug treatment program treating patients with different dependencies?

Answer—A mixed-drug service undermines the sense of specialness which goes along with the use of a particular drug, especially cocaine. Participation in a mixed-dependency service is also more conducive to participation in the fellowships and reflects the commonality of triggers to psychoactive drug abuse.

Question—What are the indications for hospital versus outpatient treatment?

Answer—All 30 patients reviewed in our sample had participated in prior treatment efforts that were unsuccessful. Thus, it appears that the hospital gathers persons unresponsive to simpler and less expensive treatment interventions. All staff agreed that patients suffering psychosis or severe personal, financial, and social disorganization as a result of drug abuse require hospitalization regardless of prior treatment experience.

Question—What is the best length of stay?

Answer—Drug counselors favored a longer length of stay than our 28-day program permits. Our program, like most others, is determined more by insurance reimbursement practices than scientific logic. The architecture of the rehabilitation program is designed

along the lines of a school curriculum with its elements of introduction, new learning, and review. Other lengths of stay could be
used. We have found it less successful to highly individualize the
length of stay in the program because of the curriculumlike design.
Patients requiring a longer stay for psychiatric reasons other than
substance abuse are transferred to another service at the completion of the 28-day program. This has been rare.

Question—What are the essential elements of discharge planning?

Answer—Every effort is made to involve the patient's family and social
network in discussions that are both educational and therapeutic
prior to discharge. Additionally, each patient is referred to a particular sponsor in his or her hometown in order to make a connection
with a fellowship meeting. Approximately half the patients admitted to our service are not referred for medical/psychiatric follow-up
after discharge.

Question—How do you handle the conflicts between AA, NA, CA, and
medical treatments?

Answer—In a closed-staff hospital this is less of a problem than in an
open-staff hospital where treating physicians are less familiar with
the fellowships, their philosophy, and procedures. Radical disagreements can occur over the use of medications, particularly after
completion of detoxification. Differences also occur about the role
of psychotherapy and whether or not drug use alone can explain
deviant social behavior. (Fellowships say, "Yes"; many psychiatrists
say, "No.") In a closed-staff hospital fellowship participation, including attention to its "spiritual" nature, creates less conflicts. The
AA steps are viewed as the cornerstone in developing a new set of
values with which to replace practices and standards that have
accrued around chronic drug abuse. These "spiritual" values constitute the positive ingredients with which a patient can develop a
new, drug-free identity. We have found that resolution of disagreements between members of our treatment staff on these values is
extremely important to the success of the program.

THE OUTCOME

Because widespread cocaine abuse is a relatively new phenomenon in
this country, no sound follow-up studies have been performed and
published. This is in contrast to the alcoholism literature, where large-
scale studies such as those performed by the Rand Corporation (Polich et

al., 1981) or Vaillant and Milofsky (1982) shed considerable light on the long-term outcome of a drug dependency. Despite the drastic limitations of the method, the 30 patients who comprised the Silver Hill sample were surveyed using a short questionnaire between four months and two years after they completed discharge. The questionnaire and the answers of 10 respondents are shown in Table 9.6.

It is arguably true that patients who were doing well after discharge were more likely to respond to this questionnaire than those who were not. Of this responding group, improved social life, role performance, and attendance at AA or NA appeared most powerfully associated with a positive outcome. Half the respondent group continued in psychiatric treatment.

SUMMARY

The inpatient treatment of cocaine dependency is decidedly similar to the treatment of other drug dependencies. Although the "detoxification" procedure is typically simpler than is the case for alcoholism and much less complicated than for opioids or barbiturates, the standard elements of a rehabilitation program appear effective. Cocaine's declining mystique is nowhere more evident than in its treatment and in the recovery that can begin.

Table 9.6
Silver Hill Sample Surveyed After Discharge

Age 20–54 average = 33.7	
Sex 6M 4F	
Cocaine use since discharge	yes 2 no 8
Cocaine use in past month	yes 2 no 8
Amount spent on cocaine weekly *now*	one "lost count"
Do you have a current problem with alcohol?	yes 2 no 7 one?
Is your social life more stable than before your admission to SHF?	yes 9 no 1
Is your work productivity, or homemaking, or schoolwork better than before your admission to SHF?	yes 9 no 1
Are you in psychiatric treatment?	yes 5 no 5
Do you attend AA or NA at least once a week?	yes 8 no 2
Are you taking antidepressants (Lithium, Tofranil, Nardil)?	yes 1 no 9

REFERENCES

Behar D, Winokur G, Berg CJ: Depression in the abstinent alcoholic. Am J Psychiatry 141:1105–1107, 1984.

Cadoret R, Winokur G: Depression in alcoholism. Ann NY Acad Sci 233:34–39, 1972.

Dackis CA, Gold MS: Bromocriptine as a treatment of cocaine abuse. Lancet 1:1151–1152, 1985.

Gawin FH, Kleber ND: Cocaine abuse treatment: open pilot trial with desipramine and lithium carbonate. Arch Gen Psychiatry 41:903–909, 1984.

Guze SB, Woodruff RA, Clayton PJ: Secondary affective disorder: a study of 95 cases. Psychol Med 1:426–428, 1971.

Khantzian EJ: An extreme case of cocaine dependence and marked improvement with methylphenidate treatment. Am J Psychiatry 140:784–785, 1983.

Polich JM, Armor DJ, Braiker HB: The course of alcoholism, New York, John Wiley & Sons, 1981.

Rounsaville BJ, Spitzer RL, Williams JBW: Proposed changes in DSM III substance use disorders: description and rationale. Am J Psychiatry 143:463–468, 1986.

Vaillant GE, Milofsky ES: Natural history of male alcoholism. IV. Paths to recovery. Arch Gen Psychiatry 39:127–133, 1982.

Washton AM, Gold MS: Chronic cocaine abuse: evidence for adverse effects on health and functioning. Psychiatr Ann 14(10):733–743, 1984.

Weissman MM, Myers JK, Harding PS: Prevalence and psychiatric heterogeneity of alcoholism in a United States urban community. J Stud Alcohol 41:672–681, 1980.

Woodruff RA Jr, Guze SB, Clayton PJ, et al: Alcoholism and depression. Arch Gen Psychiatry 28:97–100, 1973.

Chapter 10

Pharmacological Management of Cocaine Abuse

Jeffrey S. Rosecan, M.D.,
and Edward V. Nunes, M.D.

The use of medications in the treatment of substance abusers is controversial, and most alcohol and drug treatment programs proscribe rather than prescribe them. There are several reasons for this. First, the clinician does not want to give alcoholics and drug abusers the message that their problems can be "solved by a pill." This attitude often led them to seek alcohol or drugs in the first place. Wurmser has proposed that drugs are used by addicts to protect against painful feelings (rage, shame, and loneliness) that they were psychologically unable to cope with because of defects in their ego defenses (Wurmser, 1974). Khantzian has taken this observation one step further and has proposed that drug abusers "self-medicate" not only painful emotional states, but also psychiatric disorders (Khantzian, 1985). Using this rationale, cocaine abusers may be medicating themselves for mood disorders (depression, manic-depression, cyclothymia) or behavioral disorders (attention deficit disorder). Preliminary diagnostic studies of cocaine abusers, reviewed by Skodol in Chapter 5, support this view.

Another reason that most alcohol and drug rehabilitation programs discourage the use of medication is tradition. Alcoholics Anonymous (AA), the largest and most influential provider of substance abuse treatment in the United States, has been dogmatically opposed to the use of any mood-altering substance, including psychotropic medication, since its founding in 1935. Narcotics Anonymous (NA), Drugs Anonymous

(DA), and Cocaine Anonymous (CA) are similar self-help organizations based on the 12-step model of AA, and all share its antimedication views.

Many substance abuse programs, however, have combined the AA model with other modalities, including medication treatments. We feel that there have been major advances in the treatment of substance abusers in the past generation with the development of effective pharmacotherapies. To the extent that addictions have a physiological basis, appropriate pharmacological interventions are rational. Furthermore, the tremendous addictive potential of cocaine, as demonstrated in laboratory animals and humans, suggests that pharmacological interventions might be applied. Preliminary research on the psychopharmacological treatment of cocaine abuse will be presented in this chapter.

HISTORICAL BACKGROUND

Freud used cocaine himself beginning in 1884 as a curiosity, as a research interest in experimental pharmacology, and probably as a self-medication for his own depressions (see Chapter 1). He also used it therapeutically in the treatment of morphine addiction after reading reports of successful treatments by physicians in the United States (see Byck, 1974). Freud administered cocaine to his friend and colleague Von Fleischl, who had become addicted to morphine, and who, to Freud's horror, proceeded to develop the first case of iatrogenic cocaine psychosis ("a delirium tremens with white snakes creeping over his skin"). Freud subsequently moderated his views on the effectiveness of cocaine as a treatment for morphinism.

Dr. William Halsted, the renowned surgeon who discovered nerve block (local) anesthesia with cocaine, unfortunately became addicted to it in the process. Ironically, Halsted "cured" his cocaine habit by becoming addicted to morphine, a dependence he continued for the rest of his long and distinguished surgical career.

These two historical examples point out a clear danger in the treatment of drug dependence with another drug; the substitution of one dependency for another. This is a rationale for the antimedication tradition of AA and other self-help organizations.

CURRENT MEDICATION TREATMENTS OF SUBSTANCE ABUSERS

Several pharmacological approaches to the treatment of substance abusers are already accepted in clinical practice. In these examples, medications appear to be helpful only if used as an adjunct to a comprehensive treatment program.

Disulfiram (Antabuse), although technically not a psychoactive medication, has been used by many alcoholism treatment programs and individual practitioners worldwide, although not without controversy. The principle behind disulfiram treatment is that patients taking the medication have an unpleasant and often aversive reaction to alcohol. Disulfiram works by inhibiting alcohol dehydrogenase, an important enzyme in the metabolism of alcohol, causing the buildup of acetaldehyde in the body. This produces the flushing, nausea, and vomiting that are characteristic of the alcohol-disulfiram reaction. Although disulfiram is not the panacea that was initially hoped for when it was introduced in Denmark in 1948, it remains an important adjunct in the treatment of alcoholism when used in conjunction with AA or individual or group psychotherapy. Many clinicians find that disulfiram taken on a daily basis complements AA's credo of "one day at a time," with the spiritual values and group support of the latter augmenting the external control of the former.

Methadone maintenance has been a major advance in the treatment of opioid (mainly heroin) dependence since it was introduced into clinical practice in 1964. Methadone, a long-acting (once-a-day dosage) opiate, reduces the heroin craving and euphoria when given in adequate doses. Methadone maintenance programs have been helpful for addicts in several ways. For one thing, the need for illicit opiates is negated, and the criminal behavior associated with their procurement is often reduced. The methadone maintenance patient is capable of socially productive behavior. Although he is still addicted to an opiate, the addiction is medically and socially controlled.

A major recent advance in the treatment of opiate addiction involves the use of nonopiate medications. Clonidine (Catapres), an α-adrenergic receptor agonist, has been used successfully to suppress the opiate withdrawal syndrome. This is often followed by maintenance treatment with naltrexone (Trexan), a long-acting opiate antagonist (Charney et al., 1982). The advantage of this medication combination is that an opiate-free withdrawal and maintenance is possible for motivated addicts. Naltrexone, like disulfiram, is often used in conjunction with a self-help group or individual or group psychotherapy.

Cigarette smoking produces a physical dependence on nicotine, which often makes stopping unpleasant and hence difficult. Nicotine chewing gum (Nicorettes) has recently been introduced to help smokers stop smoking by alleviating the nicotine withdrawal. Again, nicotine gum seems to be most effective when combined with a comprehensive smoking cessation program incorporating behavioral or other psychotherapeutic strategies.

The medications described appear to be useful (to a greater or lesser extent) in the treatment of alcoholism, opiate addiction, and cigarette smoking. Are there medications that are useful in the treatment of cocaine abuse? As noted in Chapter 1, cocaine has only recently been reconceptualized as a physiological as well as a psychological dependence. In addition, it has only been in the past decade that cocaine abuse has reemerged (after a relatively quiescent period of 70 years) as a major public health problem in the United States. For these reasons, the use of medication in the treatment of cocaine abuse is in its infancy, although the medications to be discussed have been used for various medical and psychiatric illnesses for decades.

PRINCIPLES OF MEDICATION TREATMENT OF COCAINE ABUSE

There are several guiding principles for the pharmacological management of cocaine abusers. First, medications should always be used as an adjunct to a comprehensive cocaine abuse treatment program. We have found that they can be effective when combined with individual psychotherapy (see Chapter 6), group psychotherapy and self-help groups (see Chapter 7), family and marital therapy (see Chapter 8), and inpatient treatment (see Chapter 9). Second, the treatment must be tailored to the individual patient. Preexisting or coexisting psychiatric disorders that may require psychotropic medication should be identified by careful diagnostic interview (see Chapter 5). Patient and family member attitudes toward medication should be assessed to ensure that magical expectations regarding medication and idealization of the medication giver are minimized. Patients and their families often think of medication as a "cure." This is usually a combination of misinformation and denial. It is important for the clinician to emphasize that cocaine abuse can be a lifelong problem requiring a commitment to total abstinence from cocaine, and that a "cure" in the traditional medical sense is not possible.

INDICATIONS FOR MEDICATION

Medication is indicated in the treatment of preexisting or coexisting psychiatric illness. As discussed in Chapter 5, chronic cocaine abusers appear to have a greater prevalence of affective disorders (depression, manic-depression, and cyclothymia) than other substance abusers. However, it is often difficult to make an accurate diagnosis of affective illness in the patient who is actively using cocaine or withdrawing from it. To further complicate this issue, it is our clinical impression that chronic cocaine use can intensify preexisting affective illness, especially depression, and appears to be depressogenic for some patients. The neuro-chemical changes produced by chronic cocaine use, reviewed in Chapter 3, appear similar to the changes found in depression. Further studies are clearly needed to clarify the clinical and biochemical interrelationships between cocaine abuse and affective illness.

Table 10.1 summarizes the use of psychotropic medication in the treatment of preexisting or coexisting psychiatric illness. Lithium is indicated in the treatment of cyclothymia or manic-depressive illness. Tricyclic antidepressants (or trazedone) are indicated for major depression. Methylphenidate (or a similar stimulant) is indicated for attention deficit disorder, and neuroleptic (antipsychotic) medication is indicated in the treatment of paranoid (or other) psychosis that doesn't resolve within 24 hours after cessation of cocaine use.

Medication may also be indicated for the refractory patient, when previous inpatient and outpatient programs have been unsuccessful. It is

Table 10.1
The Use of Psychotropic Medication in Preexisting
or Coexisting Psychiatric Illness

Medication	Indication	Research Findings
1. Antidepressants a. TCAs (IMI, DMI) b. Trazedone	1. Preexisting or coexisting major depression 2. Refractory cases of cocaine abuse	Reduction in craving and/or euphoria
2. Lithium	1. Coexisting or preexisting cyclothymia or bipolar illness	Efficacy in cyclothymia or bipolar illness only
3. Methylphenidate (and other stimulants)	1. Coexisting or preexisting ADD	Efficacy in ADD only
4. Bromocriptine	1. Refractory cases of cocaine abuse	Reduction in craving
5. Amino acids (L-tyrosine, L-tryptophan)	Unclear	Unclear
6. MAOIs	Contraindicated	None

ADD = attention deficit disorder.

our experience that these patients often experience intense and pro-longed craving for cocaine. This craving, which may well have neuro-chemical correlates (i.e., neurotransmitter depletion and receptor super-sensitivity), often results in a relapse to cocaine use, which in turn can further intensify the craving. In this way, many cocaine abusers find themselves caught in a vicious cycle of increasing craving and increasing cocaine use. Preliminary evidence, to be reviewed in this chapter, indi-cates that medication may help some cocaine abusers break this cycle by reducing this craving and/or blocking the cocaine euphoria.

MEDICATIONS USED IN THE TREATMENT OF COCAINE ABUSE

In this section, we will first review the theoretical rationale for the use of each medication and then the experimental evidence for effectiveness in the treatment of cocaine abuse. Finally, we will propose a clinical decision tree to help the clinician decide which medication might be indicated.

Tricyclic Antidepressants (TCAs)

TCAs have been used empirically by clinicians for years in the treat-ment of cocaine abuse since depression is so prominent in many of these patients. This in itself is an important rationale for the use of TCAs in this setting, since self-medication of underlying depression may fuel cocaine addiction.

Another theoretical rationale for the use of TCAs is that in laboratory animals and in preliminary human studies, they appear to reverse some of the neurochemical effects of chronic cocaine administration. The pre-synaptic and postsynaptic actions of TCAs can be looked at separately (see Table 10.2).

Presynaptically, both cocaine and TCAs block the reuptake of the neurotransmitters dopamine (DA), norepinephrine (NE), and serotonin (5-HT), possibly at the same presynaptic sites. Cocaine does this within minutes, TCAs within hours. It is possible that TCAs antagonize cocaine by displacing it presynaptically or by blocking a putative cocaine recep-tor. Although it is theoretically possible that TCAs may potentiate the actions of cocaine presynaptically, we are not aware of case reports of adverse sequelae to the TCA-cocaine combination.

Postsynaptically, chronic cocaine administration produces a supersen-sitivity ("upregulation" or proliferation) of the DA, NE, and 5-HT recep-

Table 10.2
Presynaptic and Postsynaptic Actions of TCAs

	Presynaptic Actions	Postsynaptic Actions
TCAs	Reuptake blockade	Downregulation
Cocaine	Reuptake blockade	Upregulation

tors, which may result as a compensation for the neurotransmitter depletion also resulting from chronic cocaine administration. As noted previously, neurotransmitter depletion and receptor supersensitivity may be the neurochemical basis for cocaine craving. TCAs produce receptor subsensitivity ("downregulation" or reduction in number) and may reverse the cocaine-induced receptor supersensitivity. This effect occurs over several weeks along the same time course as the antidepressant action of TCAs (Charney et al., 1981).

To date, there have been several uncontrolled and two controlled studies of TCAs in cocaine abusers. All of these studies have been on outpatients. Tennant and Rawson (1983) reported that desipramine (DMI) helped 14 cocaine abusers become abstinent. However, 11 of these patients were on medication for less than a week, and follow-up was limited. Rosecan (1983) reported that imipramine (IMI), in combination with the amino acids L-tryptophan and L-tyrosine, helped 12 of the 14 cocaine abusers become abstinent over 10 weeks. Seven of the 12 noted, in addition, a reduction in cocaine craving and an attenuation of the cocaine euphoria. Rosecan and Klein (1986) also found a blocking of cocaine euphoria after a double-blind challenge with cocaine in four patients on IMI, L-tryptophan, and L-tyrosine. In addition, the expected elevations in pulse and blood pressure were blocked in three of four patients. Gawin and Kleber (1984) found prolonged abstinence (greater than 12 weeks) and diminished craving for cocaine in a six-patient trial with DMI. In the latter study, DMI was effective in depressed as well as nondepressed patients. Gawin, Byck, and Kleber (1985a) have recently completed a placebo-controlled, double-blind study of DMI in nondepressed cocaine abusers. They found that DMI was significantly more effective than placebo in promoting abstinence and reducing cocaine craving. In both the Rosecan and Gawin studies, the reduction in craving and/or blocking of euphoria occurred over two to four weeks, which is the usual time course for the antidepressant effect of TCAs. In addition, the TCAs in these studies were administered in antidepressant doses (i.e., 150–300 mg). A double-blind study of DMI by Tennant and Tarver (1984) failed to show a superiority of DMI over placebo in promoting abstinence or reducing cocaine craving. However, in this study both the average duration of treatment and the average dose of DMI were probably subtherapeutic. Perhaps the attenuation of cocaine euphoria reported by Rosecan and Klein with IMI is a reflection of IMI's serotonergic actions which DMI does not share.

Based on these preliminary data, it appears that TCAs may be effective adjuncts in the outpatient treatment of cocaine abusers, whether or not they are depressed. It is our clinical impression that cocaine-abusing patients who have significant cocaine craving are those who are most helped by TCAs. Although the use of TCAs in the treatment of cocaine abuse without depression is not FDA-approved, it is probably justified in carefully screened treatment-resistant cases. As noted, there have been no reports of adverse effects of the cocaine-TCA combination in any of these studies, and in one study, the tricyclic antidepressant amitryptyline protected laboratory animals from sudden cardiac death from cocaine (Antelman et al, 1981). Clearly, further research is needed in this area to determine when and for whom TCAs might be helpful.

When TCAs are used in the treatment of cocaine abuse, we recommend the same dosages as are used in the treatment of depression, that is, 150–300 mg/day. We start patients at 25–50 mg at bedtime and increase the dose 50–150 mg/week as clinically tolerated. We give the whole dose once a day at bedtime. Within one to three weeks, some patients report a reduction in the craving for cocaine and/or a blocking of the cocaine euphoria. Some patients report an unpleasant tremulousness after using cocaine while taking TCAs.

Lithium

There is substantial evidence from the animal literature to suggest that lithium antagonizes some actions of cocaine, perhaps via a serotonergic mechanism. This is reviewed in Chapter 3 by Nunes and Rosecan. Lithium carbonate was first advocated as a blocker of cocaine euphoria in several uncontrolled studies (Mandell & Knapp, 1977; Cronson & Flemenbaum, 1978). In these studies lithium also resulted in a decrease in cocaine abuse.

One controlled study (Resnick et al., 1977) showed, however, that lithium did not block the euphoria from intravenous cocaine in six methadone-maintained patients, although their cocaine use had reduced while they were on lithium.

The clinical rationale for using lithium in the treatment of cocaine abusers is as follows. Cocaine acutely produces a hypomanic state in many individuals, consisting of euphoria, talkativeness, loss of impulse control, grandiosity, and hypersexuality. This is often followed by a "crash" or "rebound depression" consisting of lethargy, overeating, oversleeping, and dysphoric mood. These cocaine-induced mood swings over time clinically resemble cyclothymia, which is responsive to lithium treatment. Some patients appear to have cyclothymia preceding their cocaine use.

In an uncontrolled study, Gawin and Kleber (1984) showed that lithium treatment helped nine cyclothymic cocaine abusers become abstinent. All patients reported a reduction in cocaine craving, but none reported a blocking of the cocaine euphoria. The five cocaine abusers who were not cyclothymic did not appear to benefit from lithium. The use of lithium in treatment of cocaine abusers requires further study before its effectiveness can be determined. At present, it appears that lithium may be effective only in the subpopulation of cocaine abusers with preexisting or coexisting cyclothymia or manic-depression. As with the TCAs, there have been no reports of adverse effects of the lithium-cocaine combination. We use therapeutic doses of lithium (600–1,800 mg/day) and monitor serum lithium levels carefully.

Stimulants

Khantzian (1985) has observed that some cocaine abusers may be self-medicating themselves for the adult residual syndrome of attention deficit disorder (ADD). ADD is a disorder of children and adolescents which consists of inattention, impulsivity, and hyperactivity. It often responds paradoxically to treatment with stimulants such as methylphenidate (Ritalin). Many children with this disorder appear to grow out of it in adolescence. However, some remain symptomatic into adulthood, and they may turn to abuse of stimulants, including cocaine, in an effort to self-medicate. Reestablishment of effective treatment such as methylphenidate may then eliminate the need for cocaine. Khantzian (1983) described an extreme case of cocaine dependence which responded to methylphenidate treatment. Three additional cocaine-abusing patients with histories of childhood ADD also responded to methylphenidate (Khantzian et al., 1984). Although methylphenidate is itself an abusable stimulant, none of these patients appeared to abuse it, and all were cocaine-free at six-month follow-up. There is one methylphenidate trial of non-ADD cocaine abusers (Gawin et al., 1985b), and none of the five patients in this study showed clinical improvement or decreased cocaine use. At present, we can recommend methylphenidate or other stimulants only for those cocaine abusers with clearly documented diagnoses of ADD. Since these stimulants are abusable, physicians should monitor the dose carefully and use them for the briefest period possible.

Bromocriptine

Bromocriptine (Parlodel) is a dopamine receptor agonist medication which has been used in the treatment of Parkinson's disease, of female infertility and galactorrhea (lactation), and of hyperprolactinemia (elevated levels of prolactin) found in some pituitary brain tumors. It has been advocated in the treatment of cocaine abuse by Dackis and Gold (1985), who have demonstrated that it reduced the cocaine craving in a small series of inpatients. The neurochemical rationale for this is as follows: Chronic cocaine abuse appears to cause a depletion of DA, the neurotransmitter that has been hypothesized to mediate cocaine euphoria and reward. This results in hyperprolactemia and supersensitivity of the DA receptor, which may underlie the craving for cocaine. Bromocriptine binds the supersensitive postsynaptic receptors, resulting in downregulation and normalization of prolactin levels. Bromocriptine side effects include nausea, headache, dizziness, sedation, abnormal involuntary movements, and psychosis, including hallucinations. These side effects may limit the use of bromocriptine, especially in outpatients. Further research is needed on this potential indication for bromocriptine, but it is probably justifiable in treatment-resistant cases, especially inpatients whose recovery is being hampered by severe craving. Bromocriptine is begun at low dosage (0.625 mg three times a day) and gradually increased to 7.5–12.5 mg/day as clinically tolerated.

Other Antidepressants

Trazodone (Desyrel), an antidepressant medication, was studied by Rowbotham et al. (1984) in eight subjects in a laboratory setting to test whether it antagonizes the physiological actions of cocaine. A single dose of 100 mg of trazodone appeared to attenuate the elevation in blood pressure, increase in pupil size, and decrease in skin temperature expected from the cocaine challenges their subjects received. Subjective effects of cocaine were not antagonized. Small and Purcell (1985) reported a case of cocaine abuse treated successfully with trazodone, with marked reduction in cocaine craving. Trazodone is primarily a seronter-gic antidepressant, and if these promising preliminary results are replicated in controlled treatment studies, current theories favoring dopaminergic and noradrenergic pathways in cocaine abuse neurochemistry and treatment may require revision.

We are aware anecdotally that monoamine oxidase inhibitors (MAOIs) have been used in the treatment of refractory cocaine abuse. However, there are no published reports. Such treatment would carry a high risk because the cocaine-MAOI combination may cause hypertensive crises and death. In one case series of 30 amphetamine abusers treated with MAOIs, a significant proportion suffered hypertensive crises (Maletzky, 1977).

There is a theoretical rationale for the use of MAOIs in the treatment of cocaine abuse. Klein, Quitkin, and colleagues have found that MAOIs appear to be more effective than other antidepressants (i.e., TCAs) in the treatment of a type of atypical depression characterized by overeating (especially carbohydrates), oversleeping, profound lethargy, and extreme sensitivity to rejection (see Klein et al., 1980). These patients frequently abuse stimulants, presumably as a self-medication attempt. In such patients, effective treatment of the underlying atypical depression with MAOIs may be necessary to eliminate the need for cocaine. Furthermore, the cocaine withdrawal syndrome of lethargy, depression, overeating, oversleeping, and cocaine craving clinically resembles atypical depression. MAOIs may effectively treat this unpleasant state and thus eliminate the need for cocaine. At present, however, we cannot recommend the use of MAOIs in the treatment of cocaine abuse because of the potentially lethal side effects of the cocaine-MAOI combination.

Antipsychotic (Neuroleptic) Medication

DA appears to mediate cocaine reward in animals, and antipsychotic medications, such as pimozide, which are DA receptor antagonists reduce or eliminate cocaine self-administration. These studies are reviewed by Geary in Chapter 2. In humans, there have been no studies of antipsychotic medication in the treatment of cocaine abusers, although several studies have shown that these medications are effective amphetamine blockers (Gunne et al., 1972; Angrist et al., 1974). This is confusing for the clinician since DA receptor agonists, such as bromocriptine, and DA receptor antagonists, such as haloperidol and pimozide, have opposite effects. Can both be used in the treatment of cocaine abuse? If one group of medications will reduce cocaine craving, will the other increase it? Until these questions can be answered through rigorous clinical trials, the authors reserve the use of antipsychotic medication to those cocaine abusers who are psychotic, although the typical cocaine-induced paranoid state in our experience resolves on its own within 24 hours of cessation of cocaine use.

Amino Acids

As noted in Chapter 2, chronic cocaine administration causes a depletion of NE, DA, and 5-HT from the brains of animals, with a resulting supersensitivity of their receptors. Rosecan (1983) and Gold et al. (1983) have advocated the use of amino acids, alone or in combination with TCAs, in the treatment of cocaine abusers. L-Tryptophan is the amino acid precursor of 5-HT, and L-tyrosine is the precursor of norepinephrine and dopamine (see Figures 10.1A and 10.1B).

The rationale is that they may promote the biosynthesis and restoration of depleted stores of neurotransmitters. The authors routinely recommended that cocaine abusers take L-tryptophan, 1–2 g at bedtime, and L-tyrosine, 1–2 g in the morning, although their efficacy has not been established. Amino acids are natural products which are purchased in health food stores and are taken enthusiastically by many of our patients who understand they might be reversing cocaine-induced chemical disruptions in their brains. Patients occasionally note mild sedation following L-tryptophan and mild stimulation following L-tyrosine. Gold and Vereby (1984) point out that cocaine abusers are often malnourished, with multiple vitamin and cofactor deficiencies. Tennant, who also recommends that his cocaine-abusing patients take L-tyrosine (personal communication), has found reduced tyrosine levels in cocaine abusers, although this was not statistically significant (Tennant, 1985). In summary, the treatment of cocaine abuse may be helped by active collaboration with nutritionists to identify and treat the vitamin, cofactor, and amino acid deficiencies found in these patients. Treatment of these deficiencies may help to stabilize patients medically and psychiatrically so that their substance abuse problems are more amenable to treatment.

SUMMARY

Cocaine abuse has recently been reconceptualized as both a physiological and psychological addiction, and several medications are showing promise as adjuncts to cocaine abuse treatment. This preliminary research is summarized in Table 10.1 (p. 259), and a decision-tree approach

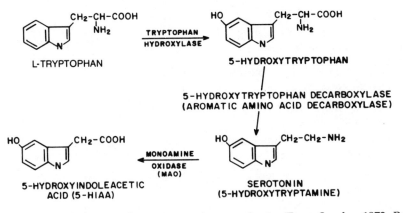

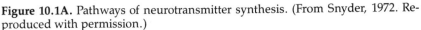

Figure 10.1A. Pathways of neurotransmitter synthesis. (From Snyder, 1972. Reproduced with permission.)

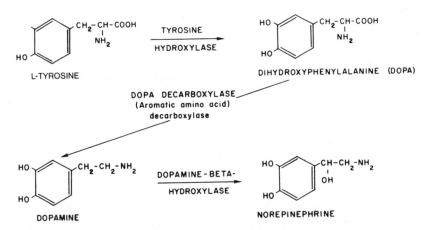

Figure 10.1B. Pathways of neurotransmitter synthesis. (From Snyder, 1967. Reproduced with permission.)

Table 10.3
Indications for Medication of Cocaine Abusers

Medication Indicated for:	
Preexisting or Coexisting Psychiatric Illness	Refractory Patient or Patient with Intense Cocaine Craving
1. Lithium indicated if cyclothymic or manic-depressive	1. TCAs (IMI or DMI)
2. TCAs (or trazedone) indicated for major depression	2. Possibly bromocriptine
3. Methylphenidate (or other stimulant) indicated for ADD	3. Possibly trazedone
4. Neuroleptic (antipsychotic) medication indicated for paranoid (or other) psychosis that doesn't resolve within 24 hours after cessation or cocaine use	4. Amino acids, vitamins, and cofactors

is presented in Table 10.3 to help the clinician decide if and when to use medication.

We conclude this chapter with a word of caution. The medication treatment of cocaine abuse is still in its infancy and is still to be considered experimental, even though the medications proposed have been safely used by physicians for decades in the treatment of various medical and psychiatric illnesses. Since cocaine abuse is now epidemic in the United States with no present sign of abating, the prevention and treatment of this problem should be given our highest national priority. The medication treatments reviewed in this chapter deserve further study based on these promising early results.

REFERENCES

Angrist B, Lee HK, Gershon S: The antagonism of amphetamine induced symptomatology by a neuroleptic. Am J Psychiatry 131:817, 1974.

Antelman SM, Kocan D, Rowland N, deGiiovanni L, Chiodo LA: Amitryptline provides long-lasting immunization against sudden cardiac death from cocaine. Eur J Pharmacol 69(1):119–120, 1981.

Byck R, ed: Cocaine Papers by Sigmund Freud, New York, Stonehill Publishing Company, 1974.

Charney DS, Menkes DB, Heninger GR: Receptor sensitivity and mechanism of action of antidepressant treatment. Arch Gen Psychiatry 38:1160–1180, 1981.

Charney DS, Riordan CE, Kleber HD, et al: Clonodine and naltrexone: a safe, effective and rapid treatment of abrupt withdrawal from methadone therapy. Arch Gen Psychiatry 39:1327–1333, 1982.

Cronson AJ, Flemenbaum A: Antagonism of cocaine highs by lithium. Am J Psychiatry 135(7):856–857, 1978.

Dackis CA, Gold MS: Bromocriptine as treatment of cocaine abuse (letter). Lancet 1151–1152, 1985.

Gawin FH, Kleber HD: Cocaine abuse treatment. Open pilot trial with desipramine and lithium carbonate. Arch Gen Psychiatry 41(9):903–909, 1984.

Gawin FH, Byck R, Kleber HD: Double-blind comparison of desipramine and placebo in cocaine abuse treatment. Presented at the 24th meeting of the American College of Neuropharmacology, Kaanapoli, Hawaii December 12, 1985a.

Gawin F, Riordan, Kleber H: Methylphenidate treatment of cocaine abusers without attention deficit disorder; a negative report. Am J Drug Alcohol Abuse 2:193–197, 1985b.

Gold MS, Verebey K: The psychopharmacology of cocaine. Psychiatr Ann 14:714–723, 1984.

Gold MS, Pottash ALC, Annitto WJ, Verebey K, Sweeney DR: Cocaine withdrawal: efficacy of tyrosine (abstract). Soc Neurosci 157, 1983.

Gunne LM, Anggard E, Johnson LE: Clinical trials with amphetamine blocking drugs. Psychiatr Neurol Neurochir 75:225–226, 1972.

Khantzian EJ: An extreme case of cocaine dependence and marked improvement with methylphenidate treatment. Am J Psychiatry 140:784–785, 1983.

Khantzian EJ: The self-medication hypothesis of addictive disorders: focus on heroin and cocaine dependence. Am J Psychiatry 142:11 1259–1264, 1985.

Khantzian EJ, Gawin F, Kleber HD, Riordan CE: Methylphenidate (Ritalin) treatment of cocaine dependence—a preliminary report. J Subst Abuse Treat 1(2):107–112, 1984.

Klein DF, Gittelman R, Quitkin F, Rifkin A: The Diagnosis and Drug Treatment of Psychiatric Disorders: Adults and Children, Baltimore/London, Williams & Williams, 1980, pp 440–441.

Maletzky BM: Phenelzine as a stimulant drug antagonist: A preliminary report. Int J Addictions 12:651–665, 1977.

Mandell AJ, Knapp S: Neurobiological antagonism of cocaine by lithium, in Ellinwood EH Jr, Kilby MM, eds: Cocaine and Other Stimulants, New York, Plenum Press, 1977.

Resnick RB, Washton AM, LaPlaca RW, Stone-Washton N: Lithium carbonate as potential treatment for compulsive cocaine use: a preliminary report. Presented at the 32nd annual meeting of the Society of Biological Psychiatry, Toronto, Canada, April 28–May 1, 1977.

Rosecan JS: The treatment of cocaine abuse with imipramine, L-tyrosine and L-tryptophan. Presented at VII World Congress of Psychiatry, Vienna, Austria July 13–19, 1983.

Rosecan JS, Klein DF: Imipramine blockade of cocaine euphoria with double-blind challenge. Presented at the 139th Annual Meeting of the American Psychiatric Association, Washington, DC, May 10–16, 1986.

Rowbotham MC, Jones RT, Benowitz NL, Jacob P III: Trazodone-oral cocaine interactions. Arch Gen Psychiatry 41(9)895–899, 1984.

Small GW, Purcell JJ: Trazodone and cocaine abuse (letter). Arch Gen Psychiatry 42:524, 1985.

Snyder SH: New developments in brain chemistry: Catecholamine metabolism and its relationship to the mechanism of action of psychotropic drugs. Am J Orthopsychiatry 37:864, 1967.

Snyder SH: Catecholamines and serotonin, in Albers RW, Siegal GI, Katzman R, Agranoff BW, eds: Basic Neurochemistry, Boston, Little, Brown & Co., 1972, p. 89.

Tennant FS Jr: Effect of cocaine dependence on plasma phenylalanine and tyrosine levels and on urinary MHPG excretion. Am J Psychiatry 142(10):1200–1201, 1985.

Tennant FS Jr, Rawson RA: Cocaine and amphetamine dependence treated with desipramine. Natl Inst Drug Abuse Res Monogr Ser; 43:351–355, 1983.

Tennant FS Jr, Tarver AL: Double-blind comparison of desipramine and placebo in withdrawal from cocaine dependence. NIDA Res Monogr Ser 55:159–163, 1984.

Wurmser L: Psychoanalytic considerations of the etiology of compulsive drug use. J Am Psychoanal Assoc 22:820–843, 1974.

IV
Future Directions

Chapter 11

Research Issues in Cocaine Abuse: Future Directions

Edward V. Nunes, M.D.,
and Donald F. Klein, M.D.

Cocaine abuse research is an exciting, important field. The epidemic of cocaine abuse, accompanied by tremendous personal and social costs, provides a strong research impetus. Further exploration of cocaine's effects promises to deepen our understanding of psychopathological processes at all levels.

In psychiatric research the underlying neurobiological and psychological systems are often vaguely understood. Therefore, most important advances stem from fortuitous astute clinical observations. Early in the development of psychopharmacology Abraham Wikler pointed out that clinical observations of drug effects can be a powerful tool for elucidating pharmacological mechanisms (Wikler, 1957). In cocaine abuse, even our knowledge of the clinical phenomena is rudimentary. Thus the clinician, armed with a knowledge of research issues, can play an especially important role in supplying clinical observations with possible relevance to underlying mechanisms. Conversely, the researcher can benefit from a knowledge of clinical phenomena.

This chapter will provide an overview of research in cocaine abuse. We will proceed through five levels of analysis—neurobiological, behavioral, clinical, psychological, and societal—formulating important research questions. The focus will be on how the findings from each level might explain clinical phenomena, and how clinical phenomena suggest underlying mechanisms.

NEUROBIOLOGY AND BASIC PHARMACOLOGY

Overview

The basic neurobiology and pharmacology of cocaine is reviewed in earlier chapters (Chapters 2 and 3) and elsewhere (Jones, 1984; Gilman et al., 1985; Kleber & Gawin, 1984; Gold et al., 1985). The following brief summary will provide a context for the discussion of research issues.

The pharmacological effects of cocaine on neural substrates are multiple, complicated, and incompletely understood. In cocaine's best-known action it blocks the presynaptic reuptake of catecholamines, norepinephrine (NE), and dopamine (DA). Like amphetamines, it may also facilitate release of these transmitters, although the evidence for this is mixed (Heikkila et al., 1975). It also increases the activity of tyrosine hydroxylase, the rate-limiting enzyme in the synthetic pathway of these transmitters, and increases their turnover rate. These actions, particularly within the mesolimbic and mesocortical DA pathways, are the likely basis for much of cocaine's euphoric and energizing effect.

Cocaine also has multiple effects on serotonin (5-HT) systems. It blocks the reuptake of serotonin and the uptake of its precursor tryptophan and decreases the activity of tryptophan hydroxlyase, resulting overall in serotonin depletion. Cocaine also may effect GABAergic (Gale, 1984) and cholinergic (Karpen et al., 1982) neurotransmission. Cocaine also has powerful local anesthetic activity, probably based on inhibition of sodium channels (Gilman et al., 1985; Matthews & Collins, 1983). The behavioral significance of these effects is poorly understood.

With repeated administration, cocaine causes depletion of presynaptic stores of NE, DA, and 5-HT. It also causes multiple neuroadaptations in receptor populations, such as upregulation of postsynaptic NE and DA receptors in a compensatory denervation supersensitivity effect. Phenomena such as acute tolerance, behavioral sensitization, psychosis, and postcocaine "craving" and dysphoria have been ascribed to these effects.

Cocaine may also cause "kindling"—a progressive increase in brain electrical activity and decrease in seizure threshold with repeated administration. Post and Contel (1983) have related this to its local anesthetic effects. This may underlie cocaine's alarming capacity to produce seizures and death with repeated high doses (Myers & Earnest, 1984; Mittleman & Wetli, 1984).

What Is the Basis of Cocaine's Stimulant Properties?

Clearly, much of cocaine's stimulant effect relates to its amphetamine-like influence on catecholamine systems, especially reuptake blockade. However, this is insufficient to explain its effects, since tricyclic antidepressants block reuptake but are not stimulating. Also, clinical experience suggests that cocaine is a unique stimulant, being more sought after by abusers than amphetamine or other stimulants despite its high price. The question is which among cocaine's other pharmacological effects are responsible for its stimulant properties.

Some local anesthetics are mildly reinforcing and are self-administered by animals (Johanson & Aigner, 1981; Ford & Balster, 1977). There is also conflicting evidence that humans experience mild euphoria from procaine and lidocaine and cannot distinguish them from low doses of cocaine (Fischman & Schuster, 1983a, 1983b; Van Dyck et al., 1979). The local anesthetic effect might potentiate the stimulant effects by lowering activity in inhibitory interneurons or by lowering the threshold to electrical activity via kindling.

Effects on other transmitter systems are also likely candidates. For instance, 5-HT is known to be an inhibitory transmitter centrally (Cooper et al., 1982). The 5-HT depletion and lowered 5-HT turnover following cocaine might then yield a functional shutdown of inhibitory 5-HT systems, thus enhancing activity in stimulatory catecholamine systems. GABA, the opioid system, other peptides such as vasopressin, and phenylethylamine might also play a role (see Chapter 3). Also, we are probably aware of only a fraction of the total number of neurotransmitters and effectors. Thus, there may be as yet unknown neurohumors that are important in cocaine neuropharmacology.

A related question is whether there are drugs that can attenuate cocaine's stimulant effect. Neuroleptics have cocaine-attenuating effects in some experimental paradigms (Wise, 1984). Lithium (Cronson, 1978), imipramine (Rosecan & Nunes, 1986), and trazodone (Rowbotham et al., 1984) may have some efficacy. However, to date there is no clear cocaine blocker. Further work on this is needed at both the basic and clinical levels.

What Is the Basis of Cocaine Withdrawal Phenomena?

Many cocaine abusers report that abstinence symptoms such as depression and "craving" drive their addictions. The question is which of the neuroadaptations thus far demonstrated in animals (or perhaps undemonstrated) might explain this. Preliminary work shows that bromocriptine, a direct-acting DA agonist, lessens craving in cocaine abusers (Dackis & Gold, 1985). This suggests that unoccupied supersensitive DA receptors underlie craving, which is reversed by occupation of those receptors by a DA agonist. Psychopharmacological interventions can be used as tools to help resolve this question.

Neurohormones may reflect transmitter depletion and receptor dysregulation thought to underlie abstinence phenomena. Early studies have shown abnormalities in prolactin, growth hormone, the TRH stimulation test, and the dexamethasone suppression test during early cocaine abstinence (Gawin & Kleber, 1985a; Dackis et al., 1984, 1985). The neuroendocrine window can be exploited in this area.

What Normal Hedonic Integrating Systems Might Be Affected by Cocaine?

Cocaine functions as a powerful source of pleasure or reward. This point has been manifest throughout the preceding chapters. Cocaine stimulus properties resemble those of stimulant drugs, such as amphetamine, but differ from those of other classes of rewarding drugs, such as opiates or sedatives. Cocaine is differentiated from the other classes by laboratory animals in discriminative stimulus experiments (see Chapter 2). Human drug users also discriminate drugs, and some clearly have preferences, many for cocaine as amply evidenced by the current cocaine abuse epidemic. The existence of several classes of drugs yielding different pleasure experiences suggests that each drug class may interact with a physiologically distinct pleasure system. Better understanding of such normal hedonic systems and their relationship to cocaine and other drugs of abuse would clearly be useful.

Klein (1986) has postulated the existence of two distinct pleasure systems based on his observations of depressed patients and addicts (see Figure 11.1). Addicts describe that heroin and cocaine both produce a strong "rush" of pleasure, but that the quality of the pleasure is quite distinct. Heroin addicts take a shot and become quiet, detached, and emotionally "cool" or imperturbable. They are satiated and for a period do not seek more drug. Klein likens this to certain natural pleasures such

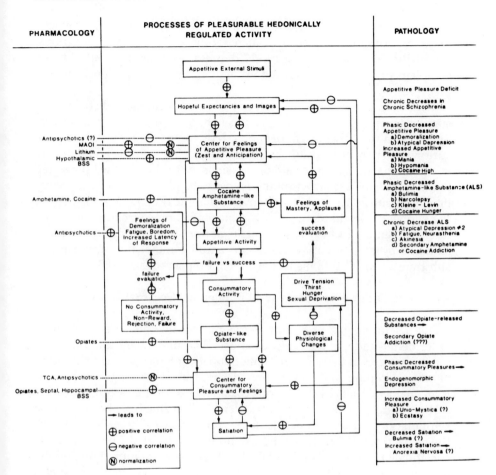

Figure 11.1

as eating and sexual orgasm, "pleasures of the feast," and terms it "consummatory pleasure."

Cocaine abusers, in contrast, become activated and constantly seek more and more drug. They do not satiate. Klein likens this to natural pursuit pleasures, such as foraging, socializing, and hunting, and terms it "appetitive pleasure."

Klein observed that endogenously depressed patients lose the capacity to experience satiating pleasures such as food and sex. Nonendogenous, especially "hysteroid" or "atypical," depressives retain this capacity, but complain of lethargy and boredom as if unable to experience pursuit pleasures.

Klein thus postulates the existence of two functionally distinct pleasure systems. The consummatory pleasure system may be activated by opiates and defective in endogenous depressions. The appetitive pleasure system may be activated by stimulants such as cocaine and defective in nonendogenous, "atypical" depressions. Klein has further suggested that the systems are structurally distinct with physiologically active endogenous substrates and that phenylethylamine (PEA) is a possibility for the endogenous stimulant. PEA is a biogenic amine structurally similar to amphetamine, which is present in normal brain, and which shares stimulus properties with cocaine and amphetamine. It is also a prime substrate for MAO-B (Sabelli et al., 1986; Colpaert et al., 1980).

Are There Cocaine Receptors and Endogenous Cocainelike Substances?

One useful source of hypotheses about cocaine abuse is analogy to other better-understood drugs of abuse. The understanding and treatment of opiate addiction were tremendously enhanced by the discovery of opiate receptors and endorphins. It is reasonable to ask whether there is an analogous set of endogenous cocainelike substances and receptors.

High-affinity binding sites for tritiated [3H]-cocaine have been found at serotonergic and dopaminergic nerve terminals closely associated with the respective 5-HT and DA reuptake pumps (Reith et al., 1983; Kennedy & Hanbauer, 1983). Other reuptake blockers, such as imipramine, inhibit cocaine binding at these sites. There is also tentative evidence that a peptide fraction interferes with binding at the 5-HT site. This implies an endogenous peptide ligand. Although the functional significance of these findings remains to be established, this clearly represents an important area for future research.

Is There Permanent Cocaine Neurotoxicity?

Chronic alcoholism can produce permanent organic brain damage, and it is reasonable to ask whether cocaine also does so. Cocaine abusers sometimes report that they have gradually lost the pleasure in the "high," cannot gain it back despite periods of abstinence, and thus do not understand why they continue to seek it. They may simply be experiencing tolerance or more sensitivity to cocaine's dysphoric effects or may be glorifying the past.

However, it is also possible that cocaine in high or sustained doses somehow poisons the very pleasure systems it stimulates. High-dose cocaine is known to cause ischemic heart damage, even to the point of heart attack and death, probably mediated by sympathetic overdrive (Schachne et al., 1984; Coleman et al., 1982; Nanji & Filipenko, 1984). Cocaine is also toxic to the liver, possibly by means of toxic cocaine metabolites (Kloss et al., 1984; Evans, 1983; Charkondian & Shuster, 1985). Is brain tissue damaged by similar mechanisms?

There is very little evidence on possible permanent toxic effects of chronic cocaine use in humans. One old case series suggests that dementia may result from chronic, high-dose cocaine use (Gordon, 1908). In another study among South American Indians, chronic coca chewers were compared to a control group of nonchewers on a battery of psychological tests. The chewers scored less well on several tests (Negrete & Murphy, 1976). However, the overall differences were subtle, and it is not clear that effects of acute cocaine intoxication were controlled for.

Long-term follow-up studies of cocaine abusers are needed to document enduring abnormalities in affective or cognitive functioning. Abnormalities in EEG, brain imaging, or neuroendocrine measures could also be identified and followed. Autopsy data would also be useful. Such studies might be most revealing among high dose free-base or intravenous abusers where toxicity would be most likely to develop. Animal studies of prolonged high dose exposure would also be useful in seeking evidence of permanent brain damage.

ANIMAL BEHAVIOR AND BEHAVIORAL PHARMACOLOGY

Overview

Studying the behavior of animals under controlled experimental conditions of cocaine availability is important because it provides models of the human process of cocaine abuse and addiction. This literature has been reviewed in Chapter 2 and elsewhere (Johanson, 1984). We will introduce the discussion of future research directions with an overview of those paradigms, with special relevance to clinical phenomena. The paradigms and their analogous clinical phenomena are summarized in Table 11.1.

In the self-administration model, an animal receives a dose of cocaine, usually intravenously, in return for some behavior such as bar-pressing.

Table 11.1

Human Analogs for Animal Models of Cocaine-Related Behavior

Animal Model	Analogous Behavior in Humans
1. Behavioral sensitization of hyper-activity and stereotypy	Hyperactivity, dysphoria, toxicity
2. Self-administration	Reward/euphoria, the cocaine binge, addiction and dependence
3. Self-administration with punish-ment	Continued cocaine use despite dire social or health consequences
4. Breaking point	Persistence of desire for cocaine and of drug-seeking behavior
5. Place conditioning	Craving, persistence of drug-seeking behavior, role of environmental setting
6. Discriminative stimulus properties	Subjective effects of cocaine, such as euphoria

The behavior can be linked to drug administration according to a wide variety of reinforcement schedules. The tendency of a drug to promote self-administration in animals strongly predicts its abuse potential in humans.

Interestingly, cocaine is self-administered by every species tested under a wide variety of reinforcement schedules. The ease with which it establishes self-administration has been known to behavioral scientists for several decades. This is to be contrasted with the common misconception that cocaine is "safe" and "only psychologically addictive."

More alarming are findings in monkeys and rats given unlimited supplies of cocaine for self-administration (Aigner & Balster, 1978; Deneau et al., 1969; Johanson & Balster, 1976; Bozarth & Wise, 1985). The animals typically shun food and even females in heat in preference for cocaine. Most go on to die if the cocaine supply is not cut off. This is unique among drugs of abuse. It suggests that alternative positive reinforcers are relatively ineffective at controlling cocaine-seeking behavior. The analogy to frenetic human freebasers incurring tremendous personal and financial costs, and even seizures, heart attacks, and death, is striking.

Another measure of the reinforcing power of a drug is the persistence of self-administration behavior despite progressively less frequent drug reward, known as the "breaking-point" paradigm. Animals continue to respond thousands of times between cocaine deliveries, which is more than for amphetamine. This again suggests that cocaine is a uniquely powerful reinforcer. It resembles the persistence of cocaine craving in many patients despite long intervals of abstinence.

The reinforcing power of a drug can also be gauged by delivering a punishment (usually electric shock) together with self-administered drug. Cocaine is relatively resistant to the effects of punishment. Punishment can suppress responding for cocaine, but the findings suggest that the punishment must be severe and that the suppressant effect can be easily overcome by raising the cocaine dose. This is reminiscent of patients who continue to take cocaine despite catastrophic personal, social, and financial consequences.

Cocaine administration to animals produces a range of psychomotor effects including hyperactivity, stereotypic movements, prolonged staring, dyskinesias, ataxia, and even convulsions. Most of these display behavioral sensitization in which repeated single doses over sequential days produce progressively greater psychomotor effects. These may serve as models for cocaine intoxication, toxicity, and craving and addiction.

Discriminative stimulus paradigms can be used to gauge the similarity between the subjective effects of cocaine and other drugs. This is especially helpful in attempts to delineate the neurobiological substrate for cocaine's effects.

Another behavioral paradigm of interest is so-called "place conditioning," in which an animal is permitted to choose between exploring two chambers in one of which it has received cocaine in the past. In the few studies that have been done, animals prefer a cocaine-associated chamber. This paradigm separates drug-seeking behavior from drug-taking behavior. It may serve as an analogy for drug-seeking behavior after a period of abstinence. It may thus reflect long-term memory for the drug.

The several paradigms provide models of different aspects of human cocaine abuse. These correspondences, as we see them, are compiled in Table 11.1. We suggest the following questions for clinically relevant future research.

Can Behavioral Paradigms Be Developed that Effectively Suppress Cocaine Self-Administration?

The bulk of the evidence suggests that behavioral paradigms are unlikely to suppress cocaine self-administration, since animals shun food and sex and withstand big shocks for cocaine. Severe punishments may have some efficacy (Johanson, 1984). However, elimination of the supply of cocaine may be the most effective strategy. Indeed, this has been a cornerstone of Alcoholics Anonymous, Narcotics Anonymous, and other traditional drug rehabilitation programs. Unfortunately, it will not always be practicable. Rather than behavioral interventions, pharmacological interventions capable of attenuating cocaine's rewarding properties may be crucial.

What Behavioral Strategies Are Clinically Effective?

Successful drug and alcohol rehabilitation programs employ a number of traditional strategies. Translation of their strategies into behavioral terms might help develop new innovations. For example, conventional wisdom holds that the abuser must "hit bottom" before becoming motivated to quit drugs. As with the animal data, it is as if drug taking must be linked with severe punishment in order to be suppressed. The technique of "contingency contracting" in effect links a severe punishment, such as loss of a professional license, to cocaine use, which is closely monitored with urine testing (Anker & Crowley, 1982). Research shows that many patients successfully treated with this method relapse after their contract ends (Crowley, 1982). Perhaps what is needed are extended negative contingencies. Also, clinical experience suggests that successfully rehabilitated patients rediscover sources of pleasure or reward in life that cocaine had usurped. Systematically incorporating reward contingencies into treatment programs might be useful.

What Is the Neurobiological Substrate for the Behavioral Paradigms?

It has been argued that because cocaine is such a powerful reinforcer, behavioral strategies alone are not likely to be effective in the treatment of cocaine abuse. Rather, interventions at the physiological level will need to be included in effective treatment strategies. To this end, it is important to better understand the neurobiological underpinnings of cocaine-related behavior. Cocaine self-administration has been subjected to brain lesioning and pharmacological manipulations in the laboratory (Wise, 1984). It may be mediated by the mesocortical DA pathways and can be blocked by high doses of neuroleptics in laboratory animals. Behavioral sensitization and cocaine stimulus properties also may be mediated by mesolimbic and mesocortical DA pathways (Chapter 2). Other aspects of cocaine-related behavior, such as place conditioning, may not be dopamine mediated (Gale, 1984; Spyraki et al., 1982). Also, other neurohumoral systems clearly must impact on the DA pathways.

Further elucidation of the neurobiological substrates for these effects is needed. This would be most helpful in suggesting pharmacotherapeutic interventions.

Are There Pharmacological Interventions That Help Suppress Cocaine-Seeking Behavior?

Animal experiments show that neuroleptics at low or intermediate doses may actually increase cocaine self-administration. Higher doses suppress it, but this may be a nonspecific sedation effect (Roberts & Vickers, 1984; De La Garza & Johanson, 1982; Woolverton & Balster, 1981). There is some evidence that lithium (Mandell & Knapp, 1977) and neuroleptics (Goeders & Smith, 1983) interfere with cocaine's reinforcing and stimulus properties in the laboratory. However, in general this is a neglected research area. The effects of various drugs in our current pharmacopoeia on the behavioral paradigms should be studied. Drugs that curb self-administration, place conditioning, or behavioral sensitization, or alter cocaine stimulus properties, or enhance the effects of punishment could then be considered for clinical applications.

Are There Strain Differences in Cocaine Self-Administration That Suggest a Genetic Vulnerability?

There is strong evidence that a vulnerability to alcoholism is genetically transmitted, explaining in part why most people can drink "socially" while some become alcoholic (Schuckit, 1986). Similarly, clinical experience and a small amount of prospective longitudinal data (Siegel, 1984) suggest that some people use cocaine in a "recreational" pattern, while others progress to abuse or addiction. Therefore, it is logical to ask whether some genetic vulnerability similarly underlies cocaine abuse.

Animals from highly inbred strains are virtual genetic clones of one another. Differences between such strains in response to a given drug can point the way to a genetic locus controlling the response or can help to elucidate the neurobiological substrate (Schuster, 1984). Several studies with rodents demonstrate strain and/or sex differences in cocaine-induced rotation behavior and liver toxicity (Glick & Hinds, 1984; Thompson et al., 1984; Glick et al., 1983). However, to our knowledge strain differences in cocaine self-administration have not been systematically explored. Identification of a self-administration resistant strain would be useful in terms of seeking neuropharmacological correlates of resistance to addiction.

CLINICAL PHENOMENA AND CLINICAL PHARMACOLOGY

In this section we will identify important avenues for future clinical research and explore how clinical phenomena may contribute to an understanding of the basic mechanisms of cocaine abuse.

Does Cocaine Abuse Depend on Preexisting Psychopathology?

Self-medication may be an important cause of drug abuse (Quitkin et al., 1972). Since cocaine is a powerful euphoriant, it has been postulated that cocaine abusers are self-medicating an underlying depression (Kleber & Gawin, 1984; Khantzian, 1985). The prevalance of psychiatric disorders among cocaine abusers has been reported in several small case series (Gawin & Kleber, 1986; Weiss et al., 1983; Nunes, 1985). They demonstrate high prevalences of both unipolar (about 30%) and bipolar (about 20%) affective illness. The unipolar disorders are largely dysthymic or atypical depressions, whereas the bipolar disorders are largely cyclothymic. A small percentage of attention deficit disorder, adult residual type, has also been found (Gawin & Kleber, 1986; Khantzian, 1983; Khantzian & Khantzian, 1984). Replications are needed in larger, diverse samples.

Such studies are problematic since cocaine causes depression during the withdrawal phase and a high that resembles hypomania. In practice, it can be difficult to sort out whether an affective disturbance is primary or secondary. In similar studies with alcoholics, disorders are called primary if their onset precedes that of the alcoholism. Refined historical methods are needed to separate transient, cocaine-induced affective disturbances from significant, autonomous affective illness (Nunes et al., 1986b).

Family history data have been used to clarify the relationship between alcoholism and affective illness (Schuckit, 1986), and the family history method should likewise be applied to cocaine addiction. Pedigrees with parents and children who are cocaine abusers are probably rare. However, sibling groups could be studied. Such studies would best take place in settings where cocaine is abundant and most individuals have been exposed to it. The familial assortment of cocaine abuse with other addictive disorders would also be of interest. Such studies might indicate whether persons inherit a broad vulnerability to addiction or specific predilection to cocaine.

Biological markers might also be useful in validating diagnosis in the setting of cocaine abuse. This approach will be limited by the many uncertainties in the field of biological markers at present. Early studies suggest that markers such as the dexamethasone suppression test and TRH stimulation test are confounded by chronic cocaine use (Gawin & Kleber, 1985b; Dackis & Gold, 1985; Dackis et al., 1985). Such studies must attempt to separate nonspecific cocaine effects from potential indicators of coexistent psychopathology.

Is There a Relationship Between Cocaine Abuse and Neurasthenia and Atypical Depression?

Our research group has had a long-standing interest in a type of atypical depression that is opposite in many respects to endogenous or melancholic depression (Liebowitz et al., 1984). These patients retain the capacity to enjoy food, sex, and other consummatory pleasures. They oversleep, overeat, gain weight, and feel extremely lethargic or "leaden." They also may become profoundly dysphoric in reaction to criticism or rejection such that they have difficulty handling relationships with superiors or loved ones. We have also observed that many of them abuse stimulants in the form of nose sprays, diet pills, caffeine, amphetamine, and lately cocaine. Klein postulates that these patients have a defect in a functionally and structurally distinct pleasure system which modulates pleasures of pursuit or "the hunt"—termed appetitive pleasures. He further postulates the existence of an endogenous agonist of this system, which cocaine and other stimulants may mimic (Klein, 1986). This theory has been outlined above in the discussion of normal hedonic systems that may be involved in cocaine effects.

We have observed that many cocaine abusers have profound rejection dysphoria, which they appear to self-medicate with cocaine. Many also complain of depression with lethargy and lack of motivation suggestive of an appetitive deficit (Nunes, 1985). We are currently attempting to confirm this observation by applying the structured interview for atypical depression, the ADDS-L, in our population of cocaine abusers (Nunes et al, 1986b). This distinction is important because evidence suggests that these depressives have chronic courses and often fail to respond to tricyclic antidepressants. Instead they respond to MAO-inhibitors (MAOIs) (Liebowitz et al., 1984). Giving MAOIs to amphetamine users was potentially dangerous in one case series where hypertensive reactions occurred during relapses of amphetamine use (Maletzky, 1977). We are aware anecdotally that MAOIs have been used to treat cocaine abusers. This deserves further study. Selective or reversible MAOIs or other relatively stimulating antidepressants might be tried if tricyclic antidepressants prove ineffective.

We suggest that other investigators and clinicians search systematically for this pattern of depression in their population of cocaine abusers. Positive, corroborating findings would be of theoretical interest and would spur the search for the neurobiological substrate of the appetitive system and for its putative endogenous neuromodulators.

Does Cocaine Cause Persistent Psychopathology?

Clinical experience suggests that most of the psychopathology induced by cocaine is short-lived. The acute euphoria, agitation, and paranoia reverse rapidly with abstinence. The withdrawal depression and lethargy usually disappear within a few days to a week. However, some patients describe feeling subtly different for up to months of abstinence. Many patients describe craving for weeks after quitting, and we have seen craving return after up to a year of abstinence. Gawin and Kleber, in their recent report on cocaine abstinence symptomatology, identify an "extinction" phase of indefinite length, consisting of episodes of craving for cocaine easily triggered by old conditioned cues (Gawin & Kleber, 1986). The possibility of cocaine neurotoxicity was discussed above in the neurobiology section. If there is relatively permanent pathology, this would have important implications for treatment and for preventive education. It would also have implications for our understanding of the disease process. For example, if cocaine were found to cause damage to pleasure centers, this would help explain compulsive use based on continuous self-medication of anhedonia.

What is needed are long-term follow-up data on cohorts of successfully treated cocaine abusers. The ideal would be to follow a large high-risk cohort prospectively, beginning before they become involved with cocaine.

What Proportion of Recreational Cocaine Users Convert to Abusers, and What Are the Risk Factors for Cocaine Abuse?

Not everyone who tries cocaine becomes an abuser. Furthermore, it is likely that some people can use cocaine sporadically and "recreationally" without compromising their health or functioning. Siegel conducted a longitudinal study of 99 "recreational" cocaine users (Siegel, 1984). He found that 50% remained recreational users over a 10-year follow-up. The other 50% went on to various degrees of habitual use—40% were mild abusers and 10% were severe freebase abusers. As cocaine supplies become more abundant, more individuals will be exposed to it. It would be very useful clinically to be able to identify persons at risk for progression from recreational use to abuse. Risk factors would also provide clues about the mechanism of the illness. Possible candidates would be persons with personal or family history of affective illness, personal or family history of other drug or alcohol abuse, family history of cocaine abuse, strength of subjective euphoria, relative resistance to the unpleasant aftereffects, ease of availability, peer acceptability, purity and average dose per episode, route (clinical experience suggests freebase or IV use always means serious abuse), financial status, and personality style. Large, prospective epidemiological studies are needed.

Are Pharmacological Treatments for Cocaine Abuse Effective?

This should be a high-priority area for research since clinical experience suggests that traditional drug rehabilitation methods for cocaine abuse frequently fail. Also, as already discussed, the animal behavior data suggest that interventions at the physiological level may be necessary to help curb cocaine related behavior. Potential pharmacological treatments are catalogued in Tables 11.2 and 11.3. Imipramine and desipramine (Gawin & Kleber, 1984; Rosecan, 1983; Tennant & Rawson, 1982), lithium (Gawin & Kleber, 1984), methylphenidate (Khantzian, 1983; Khantzian et al., 1984), and bromocriptine (Dackis et al., 1985) have shown efficacy in open trials. Two double-blind, placebo-controlled trials have been reported so far with desipramine. In one, drug was superior to placebo (Gawin & Kleber, 1985b), and in the other there was no difference (Tennant & Tarver, 1984). More double-blind, placebo-controlled trials are needed.

A complicating factor is that this population is likely to be heterogenous with respect to medication responsiveness. Methylphenidate may be effective only for those with a concurrent diagnosis of attention deficit disorder. Lithium may be effective only for those with a bipolar diathesis. Our experience with imipramine is that for some patients it dramatically blocks both the craving and the euphoria, but for others it does little. It is clearly important to identify homogeneous subgroups likely to respond to a given medication. However, this may be difficult in the setting of a placebo-controlled trial with a heterogeneous population, despite large numbers of subjects.

A potentially more efficient alternative is the double-blind placebo discontinuation design. Patients are treated openly, and responders only enter the double-blind trial, in which half remain on medication while half are switched to placebo. The hypothesis is that the relapse rate will be higher in the placebo group. This has the advantage of obtaining a

Table 11.2

Psychopharmacological Interventions in Cocaine Abuse

Medication	Rationales	Findings: Craving abstinence	Blocks euphoria	Comments
Desipramine	1. Treat underlying depression 2. Downregulate beta receptors 3. Interfere with cocaine binding	+	−	Supported by open clinical trials and 1 of 2 placebo-controlled trials
Imipramine	1. Treat underlying depression 2. Regulate 5-HT systems 3. Interfere with cocaine binding	+	+	Open clinical trials; blocking shown in one small placebo-controlled laboratory cocaine challenge
Trazodone	1. Treat underlying depression 2. Regulate 5-HT systems	+	?	Case reports; blocking of some cocaine effects in laboratory challenge
Lithium	1. Treat underlying bipolar disorder 2. Reverse cocaine effects on 5-HT systems	+	?	Cases, open clinical trials; blocking not confirmed by laboratory challenge; efficacy limited to bipolar patients?
Stimulants Methylphenidate Pemoline	1. Treat underlying ADD 2. Replace cocaine with more benign stimulant	+	−	Cases, open clinical trials; effect appears limited to ADD patients
Amino Acids Tryptophan	1. Promote 5-HT synthesis, combat depletion	?	−	Open clinical trials; data unclear
Tyrosine	1. Promote NE, DA synthesis, combat depletion	?	−	Open clinical trials; data unclear
Bromocriptine	1. Occupy supersensitive DA receptors	+	−	Small placebo-controlled trial

ADD = attention deficit disorder.

Table 11.3

Other Possible Psychopharmacological Interventions for Cocaine Abuse

Medication	Predicted Effects		Rationales
	Block Craving	Block Euphoria	
Imipramine plus bromocriptine	+	+	1. Regulate both DA and 5-HT systems
Monoamine oxidase inhibitors	+	−	1. Treat underlying AD 2. Counteract PEA deficit
Nomifensine (currently unavailable)	+	+	1. Treat underlying depression 2. Prevent cocaine binding to reuptake site on DA neurons
Phenylalanine	+	−	1. Counteract PEA deficit 2. Counteract catecholamine (DA or NE) deficit
Calcium channel blockers	−	+	1. Nonspecific antiadrenergic effects 2. Antagonize calcium-mediated cocaine effects
Physostigmine	?	+	1. Counteract cocaine antagonism of ACh
Lecithin	?	+	1. Counteract cocaine antagonism of ACh

DA = dopamine; 5-HT = serotonin; AD = atypical depression; PEA = phenylethylamine; NE = norepinephrine; ACh = acetylcholine.

more homogeneous sample of medication responders, so that the medication effect, if present, can be demonstrated with smaller numbers of subjects. The homogeneous group can also be studied for identifying criteria that would help clinicians target appropriate patients for treatment from the outset (Klein et al., 1980).

The neurobiology and animal behavior literature is an important source of hypotheses about medications that might be clinically useful. The rationale for trying lithium was based, in part, on evidence that it could suppress cocaine-related motor excitation in animals. The rationale for tricyclic antidepressants is, in part, that they may reverse receptor adaptations shown to occur in animals after chronic cocaine use (Kleber

& Gawin, 1984). Bromocriptine was hypothesized to work based in part on animal evidence that the mesolimbic dopamine pathways are involved in cocaine's effects (Dackis et al., 1985). Using the discontinuation trial model, it is easier to proceed from hypotheses to open trial to placebo-controlled test (Klein et al., 1980).

PSYCHOLOGICAL ISSUES AND PSYCHOTHERAPY

Does Personality Predispose to Cocaine Abuse?

Personality refers to stable, long-standing styles of coping with the world and other people. It is reasonable to ask whether persons with certain personality traits or disorders are more vulnerable to developing cocaine abuse. Attempts to document an "addictive personality" in alcoholics and heroin addicts have been disappointing. This may be due, in part, to limitations of the "pencil and paper" instruments such as the MMPI (Barnes, 1983). The few studies of personality measures in cocaine abusers are also inconclusive (Spotts & Shontz, 1984b; Helfrich et al., 1982). The advent of structured clinical interviews of personality disorders, such as the SCID-II (Spitzer & Williams, 1986), may be a significant advance. Such instruments should be applied to populations of cocaine abusers.

What Are the Psychodynamics of Cocaine Abuse?

Personality is inherently difficult to define and quantify, and personality scales and structured interviews have limitations. The personality constructs measured by such instruments may not adequately describe the psychological traits that predispose to cocaine abuse. Also, many traits might contribute in idiosyncratic ways from one individual to the next, making it difficult to arrive at generalizations about a population based on standardized criteria. In-depth psychodynamic study offers the distinct advantage of a rich, fine-grained level of apparent understanding about one individual. Conceptual similarities between cases can then be sought.

Current psychodynamic models hold that cocaine abusers have defects in ego structure (Spotts & Shontz, 1982, 1984a; Khantzian et al., 1984). Their drug use functions as a defense against external realities and internal feeling states that the faulty ego cannot handle. For example, cocaine, because it is a euphoriant, might substitute for ego deficit in handling feelings of rejection and loss. Through in-depth work with the patients at our clinic, we have observed that the theme of loss often figures prominently. Death of a loved one, or jilting by a spouse or lover, often accompanies the onset of cocaine overuse. Furthermore, these patients have usually been remarkably unable to acknowledge or express their feelings of loss. Difficulty negotiating developmental stages, such as leaving home, marriage, or having children, also frequently enters in (Nunes, 1985).

Clinicians can make an important contribution by seeking and documenting their patients' unique dynamics. This may contribute to more effective psychotherapy. Dynamic themes can also point the way to underlying biological mechanisms. For example, hypersensitivity to loss might indicate a biological diathesis toward depression or separation anxiety.

What Are the Family Dynamics of Cocaine Abuse?

The family systems approach asserts that substance abuse in an individual is linked to abnormalities in his family structure (Stanton & Todd, 1982; Kaufman, 1985). For example, an adolescent's drug abuse might function to divert attention from his parents' troubled marriage. The family tolerates and may even unwittingly promote or "enable" the drug abuse, because it stabilizes the family system. Conversely, in family therapy the family can be realigned in a way that pressures the abuser into sobriety. This method has found application in most successful drug and alcohol rehabilitation programs, including those that treat cocaine abusers. In our clinical experience, it is frequently a shift in the family, such as a threat of divorce or disownment, which first motivates a cocaine abuser for treatment. We have found family therapy a useful modality for treating cocaine abuse (Nunes, 1985).

An important question is whether the family dynamics with cocaine resemble those with other drugs, or whether there are unique patterns. The high cost of cocaine is one factor likely to have a unique impact on the family through their budget. The rapid development of symptoms such as paranoia and depression or failure at work or school might also have a unique impact. Clinicians should apply the family approach in this population and document their findings.

How Can the Efficacy of Psychotherapies for Cocaine Abuse Be Assessed?

A number of psychotherapies are available for cocaine abuse, including individual therapy, family therapy, group therapy, self-help groups like Narcotics Anonymous and Cocaine Anonymous and related groups for families, intensive inpatient rehabilitation programs, and therapeutic communities. The choice of one or a combination of modalities for an individual is at present a matter of clinical judgment. Studies are needed to determine what works best and for whom. This is particularly important in the current, cost-conscious economic climate.

Untreated or minimally treated control groups are probably not ethical. However, randomized trials using independent evaluators could be carried out to compare the efficacy of two or more treatments in a given population. Relevant comparisons would be inpatient versus outpatient, individual versus family versus group, directive/supportive versus interpretive styles, and psychotherapy versus pharmacotherapy. Patient variables could be regressed against outcome to develop models of which patient will respond to which treatment.

One problem is that individual studies will be able to address only a few of the many possible hypotheses. One solution to this is metaanalysis, which refers to a number of statistical techniques for combining similar studies into a single large study (Smith et al., 1980; Glass et al., 1981). However, this approach remains controversial.

SOCIAL AND CULTURAL FACTORS

How Do Peer Group and Culture Influence Cocaine Intake?

Peer group and social surroundings exert an obvious influence through the literal availability of cocaine. Social norms or peer pressure can also encourage cocaine abuse. Abusers often gravitate toward a subculture where the drug is condoned. An important therapeutic strategy is to get patients to avoid such environments. Conversely, group therapy and self-help groups use strong antidrug norms to influence members to reinforce abstinence (Yalom, 1985).

The nature of the link between group norms and drug-taking behavior is of interest and deserves further study. One theory is that the type of drug prevalent in a group or culture is related to its ideals for behavior and identity (see Table 11.4) (Wikler, 1953). For example, in Irish culture the ideal man is outspoken and aggressive. Alcohol promotes this kind of behavior, and alcoholism is indeed prevalent among the Irish. Oriental cultures, on the other hand, value a more controlled, contemplative comportment, such as that induced by opiates and hashish. Among middle-European Jews alcoholism is rare, whereas opiate addiction is more common, because for centuries they occupied a subservient niche in society where inflammatory aggressiveness would have been dangerous.

Table 11.4
Wikler's Theory of Cultural Determination of Drugs of Abuse

Culture	Cultural Ideal/Norm	Drug of Choice
Chinese	Contemplative, imperturbable	Opium
Irish	Gregarious, uninhibited	Alcohol
Middle-European Jewish	Unobtrusive, passive	Opiates
American	Aggressive, success oriented	Cocaine

It can be argued that today in America we value a hard-driving, high-energy, success-oriented ideal. This resembles the "type A" or "coronary-prone" behavior pattern (Jenkins, 1977). Cocaine temporarily promotes such a high-energy state and makes the user feel confident and powerful. It would be interesting to measure the type A behavior pattern or the extent of acceptance of type A norms in cocaine abusers.

It would also be important to identify other cultural or subcultural norms that contribute to cocaine abuse. For example, we have noted a high percentage of Italian Americans in our clinic population (Nunes, 1985). This may simply be an artifact of our referral pattern. However, it might be useful to study whether their group norms, the Italian "macho" concept perhaps, encourage cocaine abuse. Such knowledge could then be incorporated into treatment strategy.

What Interventions at the Societal Level Might Be Effective?

Given that many people are probably vulnerable to cocaine's powerful addictive properties, it would be ideal if cocaine was so disavowed by cultural norms that no one ever tried it. Law enforcement is one type of societal intervention (Caffrey, 1984). However, it is bound to be overwhelmed by the tremendous dollar value of cocaine and hence the economic incentives to the producers and dealers. Also, current efforts do not address the tremendous demand from our society for cocaine (Lieber, 1986). How could society intervene to curb the demand more effectively? One possibility would be more severe penalties (with enforcement) for simple cocaine use and possession. It will be recalled that punishment was an important method for curbing cocaine self-administration in laboratory animals. Widespread urine testing is now being proposed and might be an effective method of enforcement. This, however, raises sticky legal and ethical objections.

Another approach would be a massive public education campaign in an attempt to realign norms and attitudes about cocaine. Recent publicity about cocaine's dangers may already have brought this about to some degree. Both these approaches deserve further consideration and possible trial implementation.

A lot depends on the proportion of recreational cocaine users in society at large. A society with a high proportion of recreational users is not likely to be amenable to law enforcement or educational campaigns, much as alcohol prohibition was unsuccessful in the 1920s and 1930s.

CONCLUSIONS

This chapter points out the wide range of questions that remain to be answered about cocaine and cocaine abuse. The only way to dispel our current state of ignorance is through research. Researchers are needed to apply their skills to this field, and ample funding is needed to support them. A strong research effort will result in improved prevention and treatment of cocaine abuse. It will also advance our understanding of neurobiology. Aside from the humanitarian motive to relieve suffering, and the scientific motive to seek the truth, this also makes compelling economic sense. Cocaine abuse is very costly to society. It disables productive workers and drains resources spent on treating abusers, often ineffectively. A large investment in research is likely to yield a much larger savings on these debilitating costs.

REFERENCES

Aigner TG, Balster RL: Choice behavior in rhesus monkeys: cocaine versus food. Science 201:534–535, 1978.

Anker AL, Crowley TJ: Use of contingency in specialty clinics for cocaine abuse. NIDA Res Monogr Ser 41:452–459, 1982.

Barnes GE: Clinical and prealcoholic personality characteristics, in The Biology of Alcoholism; The Pathogenesis of Alcoholism, Psychosocial Factors, New York, Plenum Press, 1983, pp 113–195.

Bozarth MA, Wise RA: Toxicity associated with long term intravenous heroin and cocaine administration in the rat. JAMA 254:81–83, 1985.

Caffrey RJ: Counter-attack on cocaine trafficking: the strategy of drug law enforcement. Bull Narc 36:57–63, 1984.

Charkondian JC, Shuster L: Electrochemistry of norcocaine nitroxide and related compounds: implications for cocaine heptatotoxicity. Biochem Biophys Res Commun 130:1044–1051, 1985.

Coleman DL, Ross TF, Naughton JL: Myocardial ischemia and infarction related to recreational cocaine use. West J Med 136:444–446, 1982.

Colpaert FC, Niemegeers CJ, Janssen PA: Evidence that a preferred substrate for type B monoamine oxidase mediates stimulus properties of MAO inhibitors: a possible role for beta phenylethylamine in the cocaine cue. Pharmacol Biochem Behav 13:513–517, 1980.

Cooper JR, Bloom FE, Roth RH: The Biochemical Basis of Neuropharmacology, New York, Oxford, Oxford University Press, 1982.

Cronson AJ, Flemenbaum A: Antagonism of cocaine highs by lithium. Am J Psychiatry 135:856–857, 1978.

Crowley TJ: quoted in Reinforcing drug-free lifestyles. ADAMHA News, August 27, 1982, p. 3.

Dackis CA, Gold MS, Estroff TW, Sweeney DR: Hyperprolactinemia in cocaine abuse. Soci Neurosci Abstr 10:1099, 1984.

Dackis CA, Gold MS: Bromocriptine as a treatment for cocaine abuse. Lancet 2:1151–1152, 1985.

Dackis CA, Estroff TW, Sweeney DR, Pottash ALC, Gold MS: Specificity of the TRH stimulation test for major depression in patients with serious cocaine abuse. Am J Psychiatry 142:1097–1099, 1985.

De La Garza R, Johanson CE: Effects of haloperidol and physostigmine on self-administration of local anesthetics. Pharmacol Biochem Behav 17:1295–1299, 1982.

Deneau GA, Yanagita T, Seevers MH: Self-administration of psychoactive substances by the monkey. Psychopharmacologia 16:30–48, 1969.

Evans MA: Role of protein binding in cocaine-induced hepatic necrosis. J Pharmacol Exp Ther 224:73–79, 1983.

Fischman MW, Schuster CR: A comparison of the subjective and cardiovascular effects of cocaine and procaine in humans. Pharmacol Biochem Behav 18:711–716, 1983a.

Fischman MW, Schuster CR: A comparison of the subjective and cardiovascular effects of cocaine and lidocaine in humans. Pharmacol Biochem Behav 18:123–127, 1983b.

Ford RD, Balster RL: Reinforcing properties of intravenous procaine in rhesus monkeys. Pharmacol Biochem Behav 6(3):289–296, 1977.

Gale K: Catecholamine-independent behavioral and neurochemical effects of cocaine in rats. NIDA Res Monogr Ser 54:323–332, 1984.

Gawin FH, Kleber HD: Cocaine Abuse Treatment; open pilot trial with desipramine and lithium carbonate. Arch Gen Psychiatry 41:903–909, 1984.

Gawin FH, Kleber HD: Neuroendocrine findings in chronic cocaine abusers: a preliminary report. Br J Psychiatry 147:569–573, 1985a.

Gawin FH, Kleber HD: Desipramine in the treatment of cocaine abuse. Paper presented at the American College of Neuropsychopharmacology, Hawaii, December, 1985b.

Gawin FH, Kleber HD: Abstinence symptomalogy and psychiatric diagnosis in cocaine abusers. Arch Gen Psychiatry 43:107–113, 1986.

Gilman AG, Goodman LS, Rall TW, Murad F: The Pharmacologic Basis of Therapeutics, 7th ed, New York, Macmillan Publishing Company, 1985.

Glass GV, McGaw B, Smith ML: Meta-analysis in social research, Beverly Hills, CA, Sage Publications, 1981.

Glick SD, Hinds PA: Sex differences in sensitization to cocaine-induced rotation. Eur J Pharmacol 99:119–121, 1984.

Glick SD, Hinds PA, Shapiro RM: Cocaine-induced rotation: sex-dependent differences between left- and right-sided rats. Science 221:775–777, 1983.

Goeders NE, Smith JE: Cortical dopaminergic involvement in cocaine reinforcement. Science 22:773–775, 1983.

Gold MS, Washton AM, Dackis CA: Cocaine abuse: neurochemistry, phenomenology, and treatment. NIDA Res Monogr Ser 61:130–150, 1985.

Gordon A: Insanities caused by acute and chronic intoxication with opium and cocaine. A study of 171 cases. JAMA 51:97–101, 1908.

Heikkila RE, Orlansky H, Cohen G: Studies on the distinction between uptake inhibition and release of [3H]Dopamine in rat brain tissue slices. Biochem Pharmacol 24:847–852, 1975.

Helfrich AA, Crowley TJ, Atkinson CA, Post RD: A clinical profile of 136 cocaine abusers. NIDA Res Monogr Ser 43:343–350, 1982.

Jenkins CD: Recent evidence supporting psychologic and social risk factors for coronary disease (second of two parts). New Engl J Med 294:1033–1038, 1977.

Johanson CE: Assessment of the dependence potential of cocaine in animals. NIDA Res Monogr Ser 50:54–71, 1984.

Johanson CE, Aigner T: Comparison of the reinforcing properties of cocaine and procaine in rhesus monkeys. Pharmacol Biochem Behav 15(1):49–53, 1981.

Johanson CE, Balster RL, Bonese K: Self-administration of psychomotor stimulant drugs: the effects of unlimited access. Pharmacol Biochem Behav 4:45–51, 1976.

Jones RT: The pharmacology of cocaine. NIDA Res Monogr Ser 50:34–53, 1984.

Karpen JW, Aoshima H, Abood LG, Hess GP: Cocaine and phencyclidine inhibition of the acetylcholine receptor: analysis of the mechanisms of action based on measurements of ion flux in the millisecond-to-minute time region. Proc Natl Acad Sci USA 79(8):2509–2513, 1982.

Kaufman E: Substance Abuse and Family Therapy, New York, Grune & Stratton, 1985.

Kennedy LT, Hanbauer I: Sodium-sensitive cocaine binding to rat striatal membrane: possible relationship to dopamine uptake sites. J Neurochem 41(1):172–178, 1983.

Khantzian EJ: Cocaine dependence, an extreme case and marked improvement with methylphenidate treatment. Am J Psychiatry 140:784–785, 1983.

Khantzian EJ: The self-medication hypothesis of addictive disorders: focus on heroin and cocaine dependence. Am J Psychiatry 142:1259–1264, 1985.

Khantzian EJ, Khantzian BA: Cocaine Addiction: is there a psychological predisposition. Psychiatr Ann 14:753–759, 1984.

Khantzian EJ, Gawin RH, Riordan C, Kleber HD: Methylphenidate treatment in cocaine abuse—a preliminary report. J Substance Abuse Treatment 1:107–112, 1984.

Kleber HD, Gawin FH: Cocaine abuse: A review of current and experimental treatments. NIDA Res Monogr Ser 50:111–129, 1984.

Klein DF: Depression and anhedonia. Manscript in preparation, 1986.

Klein DF, Gittelman R, Quitkin F, Rifkin R: Diagnosis and Drug Treatment of Psychiatric Disorders: Adults and Children, 2nd ed, Baltimore, Williams & Wilkins, 1980, Chapter 20; Critique of Treatment Studies, pp 776–792.

Kloss MW, Rosen GM, Rauckman EJ: Cocaine-mediated hepatotoxicity. A critical review. Biochem Pharmacol 33:169–173, 1984.

Lieber J. Coping with cocaine. The Atlantic Monthly, January 1986, pp 39–48.

Liebowitz MR, Quitkin FM, Stewart JW, et al: Phenelzine versus imipramine in atypical depression: a preliminary report. Arch Gen Psychiatry 41:669–677, 1984.

Maletzky BM: Phenelzine as a stimulant drug antagonist: a preliminary report. Int J Addictions 12:651–665, 1977.

Mandell AJ, Knapp S: Neurobiological antagonism of cocaine by lithium in Ellinwood EH, Kilbey MM, eds: Cocaine and Other Stimulants, Plenum Press, pp 187–200.

Matthews JC, Collins A: Interactions of cocaine and cocaine congeners with sodium channels, Biochem Pharmacol 32(3):455–460, 1983.

Mittleman RE, Wetli CV: Death caused by recreational cocaine use. An update. JAMA 252(14):1889–1893, 1984.

Myers JA, Earnest MP: Generalized seizures and cocaine abuse, Neurology (NY) 34(5):675–676, 1984.

Nanji AA, Filipenko JD: Asystole and ventricular fibrillation associated with cocaine intoxication. Chest 85:132–133, 1984.

Negrete JC, Murphy HBM: Psychological deficits in chewers of coca leaf. Bull Narcotics, 19:11–17, 1967, in Cocaine—Summaries of Psychosocial Research, Rockville, MD, NIDA, 1976, pp 93–95.

Nunes EV: Treatment for cocaine abuse; a case series and review of the literature. Paper presented at the Taylor Manor Symposium. Ellicott City, MD, Sept. 28, 1985.

Nunes EV, Quitkin FQ, Klein DF: The self-medication model of substance abuse; predictions from the model and implications for treatment, unpublished manuscript, 1986a.

Nunes EV, Rosecan JS, Quitkin F: Psychiatric diagnosis in cocaine abuse; evidence for biological heterogeneity. Paper presented at the British Association of Psychopharmacology, Summer Meeting, Cambridge, England, July 14, 1986b.

Post RM, Contel NR: Human and animal studies of cocaine: implications for development and behavioral pathology, in Creese I, ed: Stimulants: Neurochemical, Behavioral, and Clinical Perspectives, New York, Raven Press, 1983, pp 169–203.

Quitkin FM, Rifkin A, Kaplan J, Klein DF: Phobic anxiety syndrome complicated by drug dependence and addiction; a treatable form of drug abuse. Arch Gen Psychiatry 27:159–162, 1972.

Reith ME, Sershen H, Allen DL, Lajtha A: A portion of [3H]cocaine binding is associated with serotonergic neurons. Mol Pharmacol 23(3):600–606, 1983.

Roberts DC, Vickers G: Atypical neuroleptics increase self-administration of cocaine: an evaluation of a behavioral screen for antipsychotic activity. Psychopharmacology 82:135–139, 1984.

Rosecan JS: The treatment of cocaine addiction with imipramine, L-tyrosine, and L-tryptophan. Paper presented at the VII World Congress of Psychiatry, Vienna, July 14, 1983.

Rosecan JS, Klein DF: Imipramine blockade of cocaine euphoria with double blind challenge. Presented at the 139th Annual Meeting of the American Psychiatric Association, Washington DC, May 10–16, 1986.

Rowbotham MC, Jones RT, Benowitz NL, Jacob P: Trazadone—oral cocaine interactions. Arch Gen Psychiatry 41:895–899, 1984.

Sabelli HC, Fawcett J, Gusovsky F, et al: Clinical studies on the phenylethylamine hypothesis of affective disorder: urine and blood phenylacetic acid and phenylaline dietary supplements. J Clin Psychiatry 47:66–70, 1986.

Schachne JS, Roberts BH, Thompson PD: Coronary artery spasm and myocardial infarction associated with cocaine use (letter). N Engl J Med 310:1665–1666, 1984.

Schuckit MA: Genetic and clinical implications of alcholism and affective disorder. Am J Psychiatry 143:140–147, 1986.

Shuster L: Genetic determinants of responses to drugs of abuse: an evaluation of research strategies. NIDA Res Monogr Ser 54:50–69, 1984.

Siegel RK: Changing patterns of cocaine use: longitudinal observations, consequences, and treatment. NIDA Res Monogr Ser 50:92–110, 1984.

Smith ML, Glass GV, Miller TI: The benefits of psychotherapy, Baltimore, Johns Hopkins University Press, 1980.

Spitzer RL, Williams JBW: Structured Clinical Interview for DSM-III-R Personality Disorders (SCID-II), 5/1/1986, Biometrics Research Department, New York State Psychiatric Institute, New York, 1986.

Spotts, JV, Shontz FC: Ego development, dragon fights, and chronic drug use. Int J Addictions 17:945–976, 1982.

Spotts JV, Shonz FC: Drugs-induced ego states. I. Cocaine: phenomenology and implications. Int J Addictions 19:119–151, 1984a.

Spotts JV, Shontz FC: Drugs and personality: extraversion-introversion. J Clin Psychol 40:624–628, 1984b.

Spyraki C, Fibiger HC, Phillips AG: Cocaine-induced place preference conditioning: lack of effects of neuroleptics and 6-hydroxydopamine lesions. Brain Res 253:195–203, 1982.

Stanton MD, Todd TC: The Family Therapy of Drug Abuse and Addiction, New York, Guilford Press, 1982.

Tennant FS, Rawson RA: Cocaine and amphetamine dependence treated with desipramine. NIDA Res Monogr Ser 43:351–355, 1982.

Thompson ML, Shuster L, Casey E, Kanel GC: Sex and strain differences in response to cocaine. Biochem Pharmacol 33:1299–1307, 1984.

Van Dyck C, Jatlow J, Ungerer P, Barash P, Byck R: Cocaine and lidocaine have similar psychological effects after intranasal application. Life Sci 24:271–274, 1979.

Weiss RD, Mirin SM, Michael JL: Psychopathology in chronic cocaine abusers. Paper presented at the 136th Annual Meeting of the American Psychiatric Association, New York, May 4, 1983.

Wikler A: Opiate Addiction: Psychological and Neurophysiological Aspects in Relation to Clinical Problems, Springfield, IL, Charles C Thomas, 1953, pp 56–57.

Wikler A: The Relationship of Psychiatry to Pharmacology, Baltimore, William & Wilkins, 1957.

Wise RA: Neural mechanisms of the reinforcing action of cocaine. NIDA Res Monogr Ser 50:15–33, 1984.

Woolverton WL, Balster RL: Effects of antipsychotic compounds in rhesus monkeys given a choice between cocaine and food. Drug Alcohol Depend 8:69–78, 1981.

Yalom ID: The theory and practice of group psychotherapy, 3rd ed, New York, Basic Books, 1985.

Chapter 12

Contemporary Issues in the Treatment of Cocaine Abuse

Jeffrey S. Rosecan, M.D.,
Henry I. Spitz, M.D.,
and Barbara Gross, M.A.

This final chapter concerns itself with several contemporary issues in the treatment of cocaine abuse where not enough scientific information or clinical experience is available to warrant a full chapter for each individual topic. This should not imply that these topics are any less important than those covered in previous chapters. In fact, they are often the topics that the general public reads about in the media daily. The issues to be covered are:

1. "Crack": the new cocaine epidemic
2. Women and cocaine
3. Cocaine, pregnancy, and the fetus
4. Cocaine and sports
5. Cocaine, the workplace, and urine testing
6. The cocaine-abusing health care professional

"CRACK": THE NEW COCAINE EPIDEMIC

The use of "crack," a highly purified form of cocaine that is smoked, appears to be reaching epidemic proportions in the United States, although no official figures are available. As described in Chapter 4, cocaine is commonly smoked in its "freebase" form by abusers. Crack is freebase cocaine that the user purchases in vials containing several pellets ("rocks") and smokes in a water pipe or cigarette. Cocaine powder cannot be smoked because of its lower vaporization point (Siegel, 1982). Crack is produced from cocaine hydrochloride powder, which is cooked in a mixture of sodium bicarbonate (baking soda) and water and then heat-dried. No flammable solvents such as ether are required in this simple chemical conversion:

Cocaine hydrochloride $(HCl) + HCO_3$ (sodium bicarbonate) $+ H_2O$

$$\Big\uparrow \Big\downarrow \quad heat$$

Cocaine CO_3 (crack or freebase) $+ HCl + H_2O$

Smoked cocaine (either crack or freebase) produces an immediate euphoria (the "rush"), which is soon followed by a dysphoric withdrawal (the "crash"). After smoking crack repeatedly, the user develops an intense craving for more. This craving is often uncontrollable, and the crack user will lie, steal, or even commit acts of violence in order to obtain more of the drug. Although it can take months or years for a nasal cocaine user to progress from recreational to compulsive use, this can happen within days to weeks with crack.

The rapidity with which compulsive use develops with crack is explained by the neurochemical changes produced by chronic cocaine use (see Chapter 3). Depletion of brain neurotransmitters and a supersensitivity of their receptors is presumably accelerated with crack because it is so potent. The personality changes and psychiatric disorders seen with chronic nasal cocaine use (i.e., depression, irritability, social withdrawal, paranoia) occur much sooner with crack, and the withdrawal syndrome seen with cessation of cocaine use (oversleeping, overeating, depression, and craving for more cocaine) is more pronounced and prolonged. These adverse psychiatric sequelae probably result from the cumulative neurochemical changes produced by cocaine. Since crack is much more potent than nasal cocaine, the chemical disruptions it produces in the brain are more deleterious. Based on our early clinical experience, crack is the most addicting form of our most addicting drug, cocaine.

Crack has many properties that make it appealing and accessible to the user. First, it is much less expensive than cocaine powder, costing $5–20 for several rocks. This puts it within reach of all age groups and socioeconomic classes. Because crack is precooked and prepackaged, it is convenient to buy, sell, and use. For some adolescents crack is the first drug of experimentation, before marijuana or even alcohol. For more experienced drug users, crack is often the first drug they are unable to control. Smoking crack can give users the false reassurance that because they are not using needles to inject the drug intravenously, it cannot be too dangerous and they cannot become addicted. Smoking a drug is also more socially acceptable than injecting it. All these factors are important in helping to explain the current popularity of crack, but what really makes it so appealing is the intense euphoria it produces, and the powerful need to repeat the experience.

Medical Complications

Crack is smoked and inhaled and is rapidly absorbed through the alveoli, the air sacs of the lungs, into the bloodstream. A single inhalation of freebase produces a marked rise in serum cocaine concentration, which corresponds to the subjective euphoria or "rush" reported by users (Perez-Reyes et al., 1982). The crack user commonly complains of respiratory difficulty and hoarseness, and there have been case reports of lung damage in chronic freebasers similar to emphysema (Itkonen et al., 1984). As with snorted or intravenous cocaine use, crack can produce seizures, cardiac arrhythmias, myocardial infarctions, and respiratory arrest, all of which can lead to death. Since crack is much more potent than snorted cocaine, these complications appear more frequently, and the incidence of crack-related emergencies is on the rise.

Treatment Considerations

Crack users are difficult to treat because their addictions are usually quite severe by the time they come to treatment, having suffered major disruptions at work and in their marriages and families. In spite of this, the treatment approaches outlined earlier in the text (Chapter 4) are generally effective. A period of inpatient or residential treatment may be necessary to initially remove the patient from the drug environment, making crack physically unavailable while the patient learns to make it psychologically unavailable.

Crack users usually also abuse central nervous system depressants (i.e., alcohol, marijuana, opiates, or tranquilizers) in order to relieve the agitation, insomnia, and dysphoria associated with crack use. If crack-abusing patients are physically dependent on any of these other drugs, a period of inpatient detoxification is indicated. Crack use per se is not an indication for inpatient treatment, since the cocaine withdrawal syndrome (lethargy, depression, overeating, cocaine craving) does not require the medical interventions needed with alcohol or heroin withdrawal.

The decision whether to treat the crack abuser as an inpatient or outpatient must be made on a case-by-case basis, where medical, psychological, and social factors are all taken into account. Outpatient treatment is possible if the patient's motivation is strong and family, friends, and/or co-workers can provide necessary supports. A structured outpatient substance abuse program with a specific cocaine component incorporating individual, group, and family psychotherapy is effective for many crack patients. An educational component should be part of the program, since patients and families are often misinformed about substance abuse in general, and cocaine specifically. Psychotropic medication adjuncts also appear to be helpful for selected crack abusers. Since crack probably produces a greater and more rapid neurochemical disruption than other forms of cocaine, medications and/or amino acids that reverse these chemical imbalances should be effective treatment adjuncts.

Preliminary data from our program using the antidepressant medication imipramine in combination with the amino acids L-tryptophan and L-tyrosine indicate that this might be the case. In an open clinical trial with 10 patients, these medications appeared to reduce the crack cravings and/or the euphoria in 80% (Rosecan & Nunes, 1986). Although further research needs to be done in large, carefully controlled clinical trials, at present the general guidelines (Chapter 10) for the use of medication in the treatment of cocaine abuse can be applied to crack patients as well.

Self-help groups such as Alcoholics Anonymous, Narcotics Anonymous, and especially Cocaine Anonymous are extremely helpful. These groups are widely available, without cost, on an ongoing basis. It is impressive to hear and see increasing numbers of recovering crack abusers who have been abstinent long-term and have successfully rebuilt their lives drug-free.

WOMEN AND COCAINE

The dramatic increase in the number of women abusing cocaine is forcing clinicians to examine the psychological issues that uniquely affect this group. The status and aura surrounding cocaine have made it particularly attractive to women from all backgrounds and socioeconomic groups. Women entering programs for cocaine abuse treatment present some problems that differ from those of men, and separate women's programs are evolving. Although we are aware of no studies in the scientific literature looking specifically at female cocaine abusers, it is widely accepted that their numbers are increasing.

As with men, underlying depression and low self-esteem are a common finding among women who abuse cocaine. A drug that can increase self-confidence and mood, even for a brief period of time, has a powerful draw for women in our culture. Just as cocaine helps some men feel more masculine, it helps some women feel more feminine and sexually less inhibited. A 1984 telephone survey of 165 women cocaine abusers showed that 87% had been introduced to cocaine by men, and 65% were continuing to receive it as gifts (Washton, 1985). Many of these women became dependent on men for cocaine. Paradoxically, women may be using cocaine to create a feeling of confidence and self-sufficiency, yet frequently become reliant on the men who provide the drug.

The relationship that develops around cocaine and the resulting problems that ensue include feelings of guilt, greater dependency, and a further loss of self-esteem.

Some women become trapped in a "superwoman" syndrome, struggling to be the primary caretaker of their children, maintain a career, as well as a successful marriage or relationship. As Blume (1985) has noted, "Women in American society are undervalued, underpaid and overstressed" (p. 625). If they begin to fail or perceive themselves as inadequate in any one area, this can lead to a global sense of diminished competence and eventual despair. Cocaine masks these problems while giving the woman the illusion of coping with them. Women are more likely to consider their problems or inability to cope as a weakness, and their success as an accident. When a woman does this, she sets the stage for being predisposed to feelings of depression.

Depression is more common in women than in men (Weissman et al., 1984); hence the self-medication hypothesis proposed by Khantzian (1985) would predict an increasing number of women cocaine abusers. Risk factors for depression include early parental loss, family history of depression, alcoholism, or drug abuse, physical or sexual abuse as a child, and history of suicide in a friend or family member. These general factors, combined with the status, availability, and euphoria-producing effects of cocaine, make women susceptible to addiction.

Cocaine initially acts as an antidepressant medication or "energizer" for many women, yet when it is abused chronically it can exacerbate depression. With continued use, the euphoric effects decrease and the dysphoria increases, causing the abuser to continue taking the drug in an attempt to recapture the "high." Each time a woman tries to withdraw from cocaine, the depression and cocaine withdrawal syndrome (irritability, oversleeping, overeating, cocaine craving) intensify. These dysphoric effects are often attributed to an emotional state rather than the drug per se; hence the drug use continues. Ongoing cocaine use serves to affirm the sense of inadequacy the woman is already feeling, and the depression worsens. She commonly becomes unable to function at work, her interest in sex decreases, and her marriage or relationship deteriorates. Parenting, usually the last function to fail in women substance abusers, may erode as well. She may begin to lie or deceive friends and family, and these vital support systems begin to break down. The woman patient will often deny that cocaine is the problem since it is still seen as a way to cope with the depression and emotional distress and not as their cause.

Another emerging area of interest concerning women centers around the possible relationship between eating disorders and cocaine use.

Anorexia nervosa and bulimia are eating disorders that mainly affect women, particularly adolescents and women in their early twenties. Although there have been no definitive links between eating disorders and cocaine abuse, there are certain overlapping characteristics. Cocaine is an appetite suppressant hence making it an appealing drug for a woman desirous of losing weight. Dissatisfaction with body size and distortions of body image, the hallmarks of anorexia nervosa, are often found in women who abuse cocaine. Binging that occurs in bulimia is similar to that of a cocaine binge. The preoccupation with food or cocaine can preclude dealing with emotional stresses and conflicts. There is a numbing or walling off of affect which leads to a substitute outlet provided by the food or drug. The compulsiveness seen in addictive disorders is similar to that in eating disorders, suggesting a similar internal mechanism that compels women to continue in what has become a self-destructive pattern.

Bruch (1985) discusses how the discipline in eating, as exhibited by anorectics, allows them a feeling of control in some area of their life. The use of cocaine parallels this in that the initial sense of confidence and euphoria will give the user a greater sense of competence and control. With the increasing numbers of adolescent and college age women abusing cocaine, there is likely to be an increase in the concurrent diagnoses of eating disorders and cocaine abuse. In a telephone survey by Jonas and Gold (1986) of 259 cocaine abusers, 22% met DSM-III criteria for bulimia, 7% for anorexia nervosa and bulimia, and 2% for anorexia nervosa alone. Clearly, more research needs to be done in this important area since cocaine abuse, eating disorders, and depression are affecting greater numbers of women today.

Treatment Considerations

The treatment approaches outlined in Chapter 4 are generally applicable to women. For all substance abusers, female or male, the first step is the acceptance that the drug use is out of control. Dealing with the addiction is the prerequisite to resolving the underlying psychological issues. For many women, these issues include low self-esteem, diminished social power, the need to use a stimulant to "push" oneself to function in anxiety-laden areas, internalization of problems, passivity and dependency issues, and conflicts with the demands that stem from the multiple roles of daughter, mother, wife, lover, and wage earner. The clinician must first deal with the addiction before psychotherapy, individual or group, can be effective.

The female patient's reaction to the realization that cocaine has become her major problem can be twofold. Initially, there is often a sense of relief that the depression, paranoia, irritability, sleeplessness, weight loss, and loss of libido are effects of the drug and are treatable. The second realization of being an addict is much more painful. The woman's level of self-confidence is already low and her vulnerability high. This must be dealt with in a supportive and safe environment. Family, individual, and group psychotherapy within a structured inpatient or outpatient treatment program can provide such an environment.

Some clinicians who treat women alcoholics feel that women's therapy groups are preferable to mixed-sex groups (Vannicelli, 1985). While these clinicians note that women are often inhibited about revealing their feelings and talking about sexual issues with men present, we have found that men in same-sex male groups report strikingly similar apprehensions. For some women (or men) whose anxiety level regarding the opposite sex is extreme, it makes good clinical sense to begin treatment in a group that is homogeneous for gender. It appears short-sighted, however, to restrict treatment exclusively to same-sex groups throughout the entire course of therapy. Particularly with cocaine abuse, where the tendency to avoid anxiety-filled situations is rampant, any successful psychotherapeutic approach cannot afford to exclude half the world's population. The authors favor mixed male/female groups as the ongoing group treatment. In this way, women are encouraged to deal with issues that historically have been coped with by resorting to excessive cocaine usage.

COCAINE, PREGNANCY, AND THE FETUS

The abuse of cocaine by women might have deleterious effects on a new group of victims, the fetus and newborn. There are remarkably few animal or human studies on the effects of cocaine in pregnancy and fetal development. The toxic fetal and newborn effects of alcohol (fetal alcohol syndrome), heroin and other opioids (neonatal withdrawal syndrome and respiratory depression), and cigarettes (low birth weight) have all been studied and documented.

There are conflicting studies on the effects of cocaine on both the animal and human fetus. Shah and co-workers (1980) found that radiolabeled cocaine passed through the placenta in pregnant mice since it was found in fetal liver and brain tissue. Mahalik and co-workers (1980) found teratogenic effects when pregnant mice were injected with cocaine; however, Fantel and Macphail (1982) found no teratogenic effects in rats or mice. In addition, no birth defects were noted, and the only consistent finding was a decrease in fetal weight. In a human study by Chasnoff et al. (1985), pregnant cocaine-abusing women had a higher rate of spontaneous abortion than controls. In addition, four women in this study had acute onset of labor with abruptio placentae immediately after intravenous cocaine use. Cocaine is a potent peripheral vasoconstrictor and causes an abrupt rise in blood pressure after administration. This can cause a reduction in blood flow to the fetus and an increase in maternal uterine contractions, which may explain both the higher rate of abortions and the abruptio placentae in these pregnant cocaine-abusing women.

Chasnoff et al. also found that the newborns of cocaine-abusing mothers were less reactive to environmental stimuli and that their interactive behavior was depressed. There did not appear to be any congenital abnormalities in these newborns. Madden et al. (1986) found no teratogenic effects or any abnormalities in eight infants born to women who had abused cocaine.

There is difficulty in interpreting the data available on the effects of cocaine on the fetus for the following reasons: small sample size, poly-drug abuse, and lack of long-term data. There were only eight women in the Madden study, and only 12 in the Chasnoff study were predominantly cocaine users. This factor alone makes it difficult to assess the dangers of cocaine use during pregnancy.

In the Cocaine Abuse Treatment Program at Columbia-Presbyterian Medical Center, New York City, almost 35% of the new patients in 1986 were women, up from 20% in 1983. No figures are available on the number of pregnant cocaine abusers, although almost all cocaine-abusing women are of childbearing age. Yoon (1986) claims that 75% of pregnant drug abusers at Bronx-Lebanon Hospital in New York City reported using cocaine, up from 25% in 1982.

This introduces the second problem with the human data, which is that many cocaine abusers are polydrug abusers, making it difficult to separate the teratogenic effects of cocaine from those of alcohol, cigarettes, and other drugs. Cocaine is a potent central nervous system stimulant which appears to cross the placenta and enter the fetal brain. The long-term neurobehavioral effects of cocaine have not been reported, although these studies are underway. One would predict that chronic cocaine abuse in pregnant women would produce neurobehavioral effects in their children, based on the known neurochemical actions of cocaine. What is not known is (1) what these effects might be, (2) how long-term they will be, and (3) whether they will be reversible.

As Huchings (1986) states, "The issue of drug safety and risk assessment goes far beyond structural defects and has come to encompass a whole range of adverse outcomes that include neurobehavioral as well as other functional effects." Drug-abusing parents can influence the development of a drug addiction in their children in many ways, including psychological development, genetic predisposition, as well as the direct action of maternal drug use on the fetus and newborn. Cocaine, which until recently was not classified as dangerous or addicting, must now be acknowledged as potentially dangerous to the fetus and newborn, especially when the cocaine abuse has been chronic. Further research is needed to determine what these risks are and what the long-term effects will be.

Guidelines for Clinicians

Clinicians who treat pregnant women or women trying to conceive should advise them not to use cocaine. If a woman is unable to stop using the drug, a referral to a specialized outpatient cocaine abuse treatment program should be made. If she is still unable to abstain, hospitalization or residential treatment at a drug rehabilitation facility is indicated.

Recently physicians have been faced with the dilemma of whether or not to recommend abortion for women who used cocaine before they realized they were pregnant. Washton (1986) has recommended that women who have used cocaine while pregnant have abortions. Clearly, more research is needed in this important clinical area before any definitive guidelines can be established.

COCAINE AND SPORTS

The use of cocaine by athletes, amateur and professional, has been widely publicized in the past few years. In this section, we will discuss the following issues:

1. What motivates athletes to use cocaine?
2. What are the medical, psychological, and societal dangers involved with cocaine abuse by athletes?
3. What solutions to this problem show promise?

Athletes use cocaine for the same reasons nonathletes use cocaine: for enjoyment, to help them perform, to cope with life stresses, because of peer pressure, and to reduce physical or emotional pain. The specific reasons in a given case depend on the individual. However, there are several factors that put athletes at special risk for abusing cocaine.

It is controversial whether cocaine improves athletic performance or merely gives the user the illusion of improved performance. As noted in Chapter 1, the only human experiment we are aware of that documents cocaine's effect on muscle strength and reaction time is Freud's 1885 study performed on himself (Freud, 1885). Freud found that cocaine decreased reaction time and increased muscle strength for four hours after cocaine administration (see Table 1.1 in Chapter 1, pp. 7–9).

Cocaine may improve performance initially, and many users gradually come to depend on it to perform, whether athletically, sexually, at a party, or at work. It also appears to reduce fatigue and increase mental alertness. These properties, however, are not unique to cocaine. Amphetamines have long been used to boost performance and reduce fatigue by athletes (e.g., bicyclists), students preparing for examinations, and long-distance truck drivers. They are banned from horse racing for this reason.

Cocaine is preferred over amphetamines by many athletes because its onset of action is much faster, producing a "burst" or energy and confidence. The problem with using cocaine to aid athletic performance is that once the athlete is convinced that this peak performance is related to cocaine (whether or not it is), it becomes difficult to perform without it. Cocaine becomes a crutch, and athletes who use cocaine to aid performance usually develop a psychological reliance on it which precedes the physiological dependence. When cocaine is used or abused chronically, performance invariably suffers. Some athletes may use more cocaine at this point in an effort to regain the initial improvement in performance. In this way they can become trapped in a cycle of increasing cocaine use and increasing depression, lethargy, paranoia, and cocaine craving.

Athletes require neurochemically intact central nervous systems to maintain peak musculoskeletal strength and fine-motor coordination. Baseball, basketball, football, hockey, and other sports require that that the athlete deal with milliseconds and millimeters with intense concentration. A misjudgment or mistake can lose a game or cause a serious injury. The chemical disruptions that repeated cocaine use produces in the brain will eventually impair the athlete's ability to perform, to withstand pain, and to endure extremes of physical and emotional stress.

The medical consequences of cocaine abuse are the same for athletes as they are for nonathletes, although they may be more apparent in athletes since their performance is measured. For example, a basketball player who smokes crack will soon notice a loss of endurance and a resulting drop in points scored or number of rebounds. There is no evidence that athletes are more prone to seizures or sudden cardiac death from cocaine abuse, although these cases are widely publicized when they occur.

Many top athletes are also predisposed to cocaine abuse because of their psychological makeup and their position in our society. In Western culture, athletes have been equated with the gods since the earliest days of recorded history. In contemporary America, athletes are often our heroes, yet the price of this adulation may be vulnerability to cocaine abuse. Athletes are usually young, and regardless of socioeconomic background are often sheltered psychologically.

Behind the wealth and celebrity there is often an adolescent naiveté. The athlete may believe that he is exempt from everyday obligations since he has become accustomed to special treatment. When the athlete is stopped for speeding, the officer may ask for an autograph rather than write a ticket. In college, it is difficult for a professor to flunk the star football quarterback and jeopardize his eligibility, so special "tutoring" is arranged. It is this sense of entitlement that leads some athletes to believe they are invulnerable to cocaine. Although there have been numerous widely publicized examples of athletes who have ruined their careers, been imprisoned, or even died because of cocaine abuse, the problem continues partly because of the individual athlete's refusal to believe this will happen to him.

Is there a solution to the problem of cocaine abuse in sports, amateur or professional? The answer depends on society's goal. If athletes are to be viewed as role models for youth and representatives of their schools or communities, society may decide to banish cocaine users from college or professional sports. This would require a comprehensive system of mandatory urine testing, with the many legal, practical, technical, and financial problems involved. This system would force drug-using athletes to abstain and could identify drug-abusing athletes unable to abstain.

Urine testing does not separate drug use from drug abuse; this can only be done with a comprehensive history and physical examination and the adjunctive use of urine and other laboratory testing.

Cocaine abuse programs geared to meet the unique circumstances and needs of the professional athlete are urgently required. Allied issues that require consideration in conjunction with the cocaine problem include the stance taken on the use of drugs other than cocaine. Should marijuana use exclude an athlete from sports? What about alcohol? These questions must be answered before policies and programs for the treatment of the athlete are adopted for implementation on a large scale.

Treatment Considerations

The cocaine-abusing athlete should receive the same treatment as the cocaine-abusing nonathlete. To offer special concessions would recreate the permissive environment and feelings of entitlement that may have contributed to the problem. Treatment should take into account, however, the athlete's needs; thus doctors, drug counselors, and self-help meetings in different cities must often be coordinated. Communication with coaches, agents, academic deans, managers, and owners is usually needed. Inpatient and outpatient treatment, adjunctive medication and amino acids, individual and group psychotherapy, and self-help groups such as Cocaine Anonymous have all been used successfully. Yet, as is the case with nonathletes, the athlete's motivation to change is the most important factor in successful treatment.

COCAINE, THE WORKPLACE, AND URINE TESTING

Drug and alcohol use in the workplace have long been problematic in the United States, and it is estimated that the annual direct cost exceeds 85 billion dollars a year (Cohen, 1984). The use of cocaine has increased dramatically in the past few years in all socioeconomic groups, age groups, and professions and is now considered the major drug problem in the workplace, second only to alcoholism. Accidents, poor job performance, absenteeism, pilferage, and embezzling are all directly related to the use of cocaine. Co-workers who do not use drugs, employers, and the general public all pay this price.

Why is cocaine use in the workplace so common? There are several reasons for this. Many cocaine-using employees came of age in the 1960s and have liberal attitudes toward the use of illicit drugs, particularly marijuana. As cocaine increased in popularity, it too became acceptable as a drug to be used recreationally without apparent ill effects. Cocaine's status as the "champagne of drugs" certainly helped to make it the drug of choice for many. Unlike alcohol or marijuana, cocaine can be used inconspicuously at the workplace, leaving no smell or hangover.

Cocaine initially may improve concentration and performance in some individuals, but with continued use performance invariably suffers. The Andean natives have chewed coca leaves for millennia in order to survive under adverse conditions. Otherwise, the high altitude and scarcity of food would make vigorous work impossible. The following case illustrates how cocaine can improve performance initially and mask problems in the workplace.

Case History

David is a 26-year-old attorney who was seen in consultation with a senior partner from his law firm and his mother.

David had a relatively normal suburban upper-middle-class childhood and adolescence. He had two younger sisters and was very protective of them. He excelled academically and had many friends and outside interests. Beginning in elementary school, David learned that good grades were rewarded. By the sixth grade he knew he wanted to be a lawyer like his father; by the time he was in high school he had a part-time job at his father's firm. He experimented with marijuana but, like his father, preferred to "wind down" with "several beers" after tennis or at a party. In David's last year of law school, his father died suddenly of a heart attack. Although David had applied for a prestigious clerkship in a federal agency, he withdrew his application and told his father's partners after the funeral that he would be joining the firm.

David's first year at the firm was a disappointment. He worked constantly, but never seemed to catch up, and the deadline on the case he was working on was approaching. He became anxious and lonely, lost contact with his college and law school friends, and his girlfriend left him for someone else. As the deadline approached, David began to panic and snorted a few lines of cocaine with a colleague. He felt relaxed and euphoric and was able to work all night. He was surprised how effortlessly he completed the project. David bought a gram of cocaine for himself and began to use it regularly. His mood was much better, he was talkative and outgoing, and he found his confidence and sense of humor returning.

After several months he began a romantic relationship with Susan, a 25-year-old lawyer from another firm, and began to socialize with her friends. Many of these new friends used cocaine socially, and Susan always seemed to have it around. David began using it several times a week, and after several months he needed it to wake up and get to work on time. He began having trouble sleeping and would smoke pot or have a few beers every night to get to sleep. Susan noticed that he became irritated easily, and they began to argue. When she suspected that David was more interested in using cocaine than having sex, she insisted that they both stop using cocaine "until things are better." While Susan was able to stop easily, David found the first week without cocaine terrible: he was lethargic, depressed, and irritable, and he called in sick twice because he couldn't get out of bed. Finally, he bought more cocaine and used it every morning, deceiving Susan. One evening Susan found a vial of cocaine in his pocket and confronted him. David broke down in tears and promised to seek professional help if he ever used cocaine again.

Over the next few days, David craved cocaine continuously. He felt tense and exhausted. He suspected that Susan was watching him constantly and believed she was talking behind his back at his firm. When he angrily confronted her, she denied everything, told him he was paranoid, and said she wanted to end their relationship. David was crushed. He felt numb but was unable to cry. He bought a quarter ounce of cocaine and snorted it continuously by himself; he called in sick three days in a row. He was despondent, he hadn't eaten or slept in days, and he had lost 15 pounds. He called a senior partner at work, one of his father's closest friends, and said he was quitting. He locked himself in his apartment, took the phone off the hook, and began to think that suicide would be better than facing his family or colleagues again. Several hours later the partner and David's mother arrived.

David entered a cocaine abuse treatment program and was started on antidepressant medication. He was seen in individual, group, and family therapy and began to improve after several weeks. His performance at work also improved, and after several months David decided to leave the firm and reapply to the federal agency in which he was originally interested.

In David's case, the problem was that he joined the firm for the wrong reasons. He was lucky that his relationship with his superiors was such that he wasn't fired when his cocaine dependence was discovered. His performance at work was certainly improved by cocaine initially, although he was nonfunctional eight months later. David's firm has since decided to set up an employee assistance program (EAP) to deal with the problems of alcohol and drug abuse.

EAPs have become a common way for corporations and unions to deal with alcohol- and drug-related problems among employees. EAPs provide job-based evaluation and referrals, and some also provide substance abuse treatment (Brill et al., 1985). EAPs are valuable for workers in that they provide a nonthreatening place to get drug and alcohol abuse information and counseling. They give employees the message that their companies would rather help them with their problems than fire them.

By definition, EAPs are in a difficult position: they are the advocate of the employee, yet at the same time they must protect the interests of the employer. They often serve as the intermediary between the two during the period of substance abuse treatment. As with all types of substance abuse treatment, patient confidentiality must be preserved. Yet, for the EAP to be effective, there has to be some degree of communication with the employee's supervisor, union, or personnel office. It is important that the guidelines for communications of this type be clear at the beginning of treatment. In most programs, the employer communicates with the EAP regarding job performance, and the EAP gives the employer periodic progress reports which do not divulge any confidential information.

Employers are generally in favor of the EAP system since they feel that in the long run it is more cost-effective to treat employees than to fire them and retrain new ones. It is also helpful for company morale to see recovering alcoholics and drugs abusers return to work, happier and more productive. Insurance companies are also generally in favor of EAPs since successful substance abuse treatment reduces overall medical costs.

It is our experience that many executives, upper-level managers and company presidents do not seek treatment for cocaine abuse through their EAPs. They often prefer to go to private off-site treatment programs or clinicians since (1) cocaine is illegal, (2) company morale would suffer if it became known that the president, for example, was a cocaine addict, and (3) it is difficult to be treated by someone you employ.

Urine Testing

Mandatory urine testing for illicit drugs, either as part of the preemployment physical examination or on a mandatory basis at the work site, has become an area of controversy over the past few years. In Table 12.1, the pros and cons of mandatory urine testing in the workplace are summarized. Many are in favor of mandatory urine testing since it will deter illicit drug use, whether at home or at work. Drug-using workers will be forced to stop, and drug-abusing workers unable to stop will be identified and referred to an EAP for evaluation and treatment. A safe, drug-free workplace has been viewed as a right, not a privilege, by both employees and management. Employees often feel that substance-abusing co-workers are jeopardizing everyone's safety (i.e., on an assembly line, in a power plant, etc.), and companies are aware of the magnitude of the financial loss due to absenteeism, pilferage, poor performance, and accidents. Many would like to see a drug-free workplace as the first step toward a drug-free society. Whether this is feasible or even desirable is a question that society as a whole must face.

Those who are opposed to mandatory urine testing say that it is in violation of constitutional rights protecting privacy. What an individual does in his or her private time, including taking drugs, is of no concern to the employer. Many feel that job performance, not presence or absence of drugs in the urine, is what is important.

An individual's right to privacy must be balanced with society's best interests. Should certain professions or occupations be drug-free, if the public safety is involved? For example, should airline pilots, air traffic controllers, or anesthesiologists be required to have mandatory urine testing? Society, through its legal and judicial system, will answer these questions.

Table 12.1
Mandatory Urine Testing for Drugs

Pros	Cons
1. Deterrent to drug use	1. May be unconstitutional
2. Permits early identification of abusers	2. Urine tests can be inaccurate
3. Drug-free workplace safer	3. Does not separate drug use from drug abuse
4. Drug-free occupations (i.e., airline pilot) promote public safety	4. Job performance, not drug use, should govern employment

An additional concern is the accuracy of the urine tests themselves. No matter how good the test is, it can be inaccurate, and a person's career, livelihood, and reputation can be jeopardized. It is possible to repeat all positive tests and then confirm them with serum tests, which are more accurate, but at present there is no guarantee that this will be done.

Urine tests do not distinguish drug use from drug abuse: this can only be done with a comprehensive history and physical examination. At best, laboratory tests are adjunctive and provide confirmation. It is accepted that urine testing is a useful adjunct in the treatment of cocaine abusers (see Chapter 4), but not all cocaine users are abusers.

Guidelines for Employers

How can you tell whether an employee has a cocaine problem? We commonly see personality changes in people who abuse cocaine. They become depressed and irritable, and sometimes quite paranoid. Mood swings and temper outbursts can occur for no apparent reason. Cocaine abusers often lose or gain weight and have insomnia while they are using cocaine and oversleep when they stop. People who were once industrious workers find that they have difficulty concentrating and staying alert. Marriages and relationships also suffer greatly, and financial problems invariably result because of the cocaine abuse.

Nosebleeds, sore throats, chronic sinusitis, skin excoriations, shortness of breath, and chronic cough (especially in cocaine smokers) are common. Cocaine dilates the pupils, raises the pulse and blood pressure, and can cause palpitations and profuse sweating.

Frequent unexplained absences, lateness, inability to sit still, and excessive trips to the restroom, combined with the above physical and psychological symptoms, should lead the employer to suspect cocaine abuse.

What should the employer do at this point? It is our experience that the employee must be confronted with the evidence. Denial of the problem is part of the cocaine abuse syndrome, and the denial must be confronted. If the employee is unwilling to be evaluated by a clinician experienced in the treatment of cocaine abuse, or refuses to go to the EAP, he may have to be threatened with the loss of his job if he doesn't seek help.

THE COCAINE-ABUSING HEALTH CARE PROFESSIONAL

The recent cocaine epidemic has affected all segments of society. Excessive cocaine use has infiltrated the ranks of those in the medical and mental health fields, forming the basis for serious public and professional concern.

The observation that chemical dependence is an occupational hazard among physicians, dentists, nurses, pharmacists, and others with ready access to drugs is well known. Alcoholism and addiction among members of the health care community has existed since the earliest days of the professions. Historical reports (Crothers, 1899) of substance abuse among health care professionals attest to the chronic and persistent nature of the problem. The search for effective identification of the substance-abusing professional and the creation of intervention programs that address the unique issues posed by this subculture form the basis for current efforts in the field.

Estimates concerning the scope of the substance abuse problem are described mainly for physicians and nurses and concentrate primarily on alcohol abuse and misuse of therapeutically prescribed drugs such as meperidine, benzodiazapines, anesthetic agents, amphetamines, and barbiturates. Studies regarding the incidence of cocaine use are rare. Maddux, Hoppe, and Costello (1986) note that in a survey of senior medical students, 20% acknowledged using cocaine at some point during their lives.

The data accumulated from studies of substance abuse among doctors and nurses suggest that the chance of developing a chemical dependency problem is extremely high. The incidence of alcoholism among doctors and nurses ranges from 7 to 10% of the total physician population (Bissell & Jones, 1976) and 8–12% of the total number of nurses (Buxton, Jessup, & Landry, 1985). Narcotic addiction for both physicians and nurses exceeds the rate of that for the general population.

Stress factors inherent in being a physician, nurse, or other health care practitioner strongly contribute to the development of excessive drug use as a coping mechanism. Chafetz (1976) reported that the ongoing pressure to perform at maximum efficiency, the demands on one's time, the stress related to keeping abreast of developments in one's field of practice, and the "susceptibility to depression that results from the gap between expectation and performance" (p. 122) predispose to the development of substance abuse in physicians.

Health care professionals may subscribe to the erroneous belief that their special training and knowledge about medication makes them immune to its misapplication and abuse. Physical illness, family pressures, working in a critical care setting (emergency room, intensive care unit, etc.), and the dual demands of parenting and career for professionals who have children, all become potential stressors related to the development of a drug problem. Buxton et al. (1985) describe the profile of "the nurse who experiences stress on the job, is pharmaceutically optimistic, has a positive family history of alcoholism or other drug dependency, and has access to psychoactive medication" (p. 135) as the amalgam of variables suggesting high risk for development of addiction.

An additional problem for substance-abusing physicians and nurses is the lack of belonging to a drug-using culture with which they can openly identify. Drug use is often private for fear of the repercussions on career if exposed publicly. The risk of isolation and the stress of secrecy are two other issues with which drug-abusing health care professionals often contend.

Compromised work performance typifies the way in which most impaired health professionals come to the attention of others. Irritability, interpersonal friction, moodiness, and isolation are some of the recognizable manifestations of the psychological consequences of excessive cocaine use. Inconsistency surrounding the performance of duties, along with lateness, absenteeism, and errors in judgment, suggests that cocaine use has reached proportions which dictate active intervention by colleagues, administration, and family.

Once identified as a cocaine user, a health care professional faces important decisions that influence his or her personal and professional fate. Local policy differs regarding whether the cocaine abuser will be treated legally and/or psychiatrically. Patients and consumers need to be protected from the inappropriate or potentially dangerous actions of the impaired care giver. At the same time, the addicted professional requires active and confidential management of his own "illness." As a result, many rehabilitative efforts strive to help cocaine users become abstinent and eventually return to a work setting. Structural treatment plans that ensure that no harm comes to those in the health professional's charge include initial removal from high-risk work circumstances and construction of a treatment contract dealing with the needs of the impaired professional and the patients and the hospital or facility in which the cocaine user is currently employed.

Common elements of an initial treatment contract include limit setting designed to place a ceiling on detrimental behavior resulting from cocaine abuse. Job retention is a function of successful participation in a lengthy rehabilitative process. Initial hospitalization followed by outpatient treatment which includes urine screening, NA/CA meetings, close follow-up by supervisory staff, peer support groups of addicted health professionals, and a comprehensive aftercare program are the bare essentials of many treatment and work reentry programs for cocaine abusers. Job reassignment rather than dismissal is a preferred means of initially dealing with the problem of cocaine dependence. Whenever possible, physicians and nurses who are cocaine dependent are encouraged to continue working in an effort to prevent serious demoralization and depression which may reach suicidal proportion. Reassignment of physicians and nurses to areas and duties which do not provide access to medications and which are less stressful and emotionally intense helps preserve self-esteem and facilitate compliance with treatment efforts.

The literature on the outcome of treatment efforts with impaired health professionals is encouraging. Herrington et al. (1982) and Morse et al. (1984) cite data from studies with alcoholic and drug-dependent physicians which suggest that physicians, including those with severe alcohol and narcotic addiction, who engage in comprehensive rehabilitative programs stand a high chance of full recovery and return to work. Successful treatment programs address the common reluctance on the part of health care professionals to assume the role of being a patient. Treatment models incorporate thoughtful mechanisms for providing face-saving entry into rehabilitation for the often isolated and frightened practitioner who desperately requires active and respectful intervention.

In the two cases that follow, some of the phenomenology of cocaine abuse in health care professionals illustrates the aforementioned principles.

Case 1. Florence N., R.N.

Florence N., a 32-year-old cardiac-intensive-care nurse, is currently divorced from her husband after 14 years of marriage. She is the second youngest of six children from a lower-middle-class Irish Catholic family. Her father, a skilled laborer, had a long-standing history of excessive drinking, during the course of which he was verbally abusive and physically violent with various family members. Following her father's death, Florence's mother and siblings disengaged and relocated to different parts of the country.

Florence began "snorting" cocaine during a period in her life that she described as "overwhelming." Traditionally an excellent worker, Florence began to call in sick and missed an uncharacteristically large number of days from work. Her usual stoic stance was altered by the impact of the simultaneous deaths of two patients with whom she had enjoyed a close relationship.

Her husband, a compulsive gambler, went into serious debt, blamed Florence and their two younger children for his difficulties, and left home to live with another woman. Despite the fact that her husband was only marginally involved with the children when at home, his departure intensified Florence's realization that the burden of parenting and probably the support of the family would now "officially" become hers.

Along with these pressures, Florence dreaded the prospect of having to reenter the "singles world" after such a protracted absence. The idea of having to meet new men mobilized her doubts and fears about her own desirability, social competence, attractiveness, and ability to sustain an intimate relationship. In order to offset the intensity of all these negative feelings, Florence began to experiment with a variety of mood-altering drugs.

At first, she began to take tranquilizers in the hopes that they would "take the edge off" her anxiety. This helped initially, but Florence soon found that the drugs were not sufficient to help with the persistent feelings of depression she was experiencing.

One evening at a party, a man offered her a "line" of cocaine. Florence's reaction was dramatic. She experienced an energizing effect and brief freedom from oppressive dysphoric emotions. Her desire to repeat this experience remained with her, and a period followed during which Florence planned how she could obtain cocaine on a consistent basis. Her drug use escalated to a point where she would have to use other medications to keep herself in psychological and physical balance. As part of this process, Florence resorted to stealing drugs from the medication cabinet at work and falsifying medication counts to cover her actions.

A nursing supervisor who had known Florence since her days as a nursing student, noted the personality changes and job performance gaps, which were increasing with continued cocaine use. These observations, coupled with objective evidence accumulated from colleagues, resulted in an undeniable picture of a capable person deep in the throes of a cocaine problem.

The supervisor, plus several friends and co-workers, planned an interventional meeting during which Florence was caringly confronted with the knowledge of a cocaine use. A treatment contract and initial abstinence plan were established wherein Florence was temporarily taken out of the intensive-care unit and reassigned to the student health service of the affiliated medical center. Along with this, Florence consented to a two-year rehabilitation plan which incorporated her attendance at Cocaine Anonymous meetings daily plus a twice-weekly support group composed exclusively of nurses with substance abuse problems. Routine urine screening for drugs formed a nonnegotiable element of the recovery program, as were mandatory weekly meetings with hospital supervisory staff to monitor her work performance.

Florence did well with this basic plan and required additional individual psychotherapy to deal with personality issues and stress factors that emerged once drug-taking behavior had ceased. Two years later, Florence returned to her original position, met a man with whom she was having a serious relationship, and described herself as a "cocaine addict in recovery."

Case 2. Dr. D. K.

Dr. D. K. is a 46-year-old oral surgeon who had been divorced twice and is currently separated from his third wife. The oldest child of four and only son in an enmeshed upper-middle-class Jewish family, Dr. D. K. described his first depressive episode occurring during adolescence shortly after his father committed suicide. He felt compelled to be "the man" in the family and took a paternal role with his sisters and mother to fill in the gap left by his father's death.

After successfully completing dental training, Dr. D. K opened a practice employing two of his sisters as office staff and his mother as bookkeeper. His extroverted nature and professional competence brought him quick career rewards and financial success. He began to enjoy life in the "fast lane," which exposed him to a variety of temptations, most notably recreational drugs and extramarital sexual possibilities.

Although outwardly poised and self-assured, Dr. D. K. struggled with lifelong feelings of inadequacy concerning his sexual capabilities. Up to this point in his life, his only drug use was marijuana and Quaaludes, both of which he employed for their sexual side effects in reducing his anxiety about approaching women and being able to function with them in a sexual context. Cocaine held the same initial appeal for Dr. D. K. He employed it as "bait" to help seduce women who he felt would not otherwise consider him as a sexual partner. Ironically, but not uncommonly, Dr. D. K.'s continued use of cocaine resulted in his being more involved with the drug than with the women he desired.

His habit of doing things to excess took him rapidly from intranasal use to freebasing. He spent thousands of dollars arranging for "parties" in which he supplied cocaine for his guests. Once involved with regular freebasing, Dr. D. K. began a progressively deteriorating course. His drug use brought with it the accumulation of debts and threats from drug dealers and the cocaine underworld. His current wife decided that she had to separate from him since his unpredictability, infidelity, massive denial, and refusal to seek treatment were more than she could bear.

Dr. D. K.'s office staff and family were able to "cover" for him with his patients and colleagues up until the point where he collapsed in the rear of his office after being up for three nights "binging" on cocaine. He was hospitalized in a rehabilitation program for addicted physicians and dentists. Dr. D. K. left this program prematurely and against the advice of the staff, citing his opinion that he had things "under control" and was eager to return to work. Following this aborted treatment experience, he attempted to remain drug free but very shortly resumed his contacts with his cocaine-using network. His freebase use resumed, and the cycle of decompensation ensued again. Dr. D. K. was rehospitalized in a 28-day detoxification-rehabilitation program and, this time, remained in the hospital for the full stay.

Upon discharge, Dr. D. K. agreed to attend Cocaine Anonymous meetings and to be in a psychotherapy/support group not restricted solely to health care professionals. He was seen in psychiatric consultation and started on imipramine in the hopes of helping him resist his tendency to return to heavy cocaine use. Family sessions with key members of Dr. D. K.'s network were employed to discuss "enabling" behaviors in family members and to utilize family resources to help maintain a drug-free system.

Dr. D. K. progressed in "fits and starts" until one solid period of six months of abstinence passed. With sufficient distance from cocaine, Dr. D. K. was able to reflect and take a personal inventory of the type not possible during active cocaine use. He came to enjoy the feelings of physical and emotional well-being he had long forgotten and observed how his desire to "rescue" and please everyone contributed to the stress that made cocaine an appealing alternative.

At present, Dr. D. K. is back at his practice, out of debt, and on better terms with his wife, children, and original family members. He continues to attend weekly group sessions in conjunction with Cocaine Anonymous meetings.

SUMMARY AND CONCLUSIONS

The issues raised in this chapter represent a small sample of the growing concerns posed by the cocaine problem. The attempt in this chapter, and throughout the book, has been to help define and illuminate cocaine-related diagnostic, theraputic, and research issues.

While society awaits the results of further study from the scientific community, clinicians are faced with the immediate task of treating those people who have a major involvement with cocaine. The thrust of this volume has been to try to expand the knowledge base available to these practitioners.

At the start of their training, medical students are taught that the physician who does not familiarize him/herself with the existence and characteristics of a specific disease entity will be unlikely to help patients suffering from that condition. The psychologically minded clinician who has had minimal exposure to cocaine abuse becomes a prime candidate to fall into this trap.

The information and ideas contained in this text have been collected and presented in the spirit of trying to advance the state of awareness about cocaine, improve the quality of theraputic interventions, and point the way to the frontiers of promising research of the future.

REFERENCES

Bissell L, Jones RW: The alcoholic physician: a survey. Am J Psychiatry 133:1142–1146, 1976.

Blume SB: Women and alcohol, in Bratter TE, Forrest GG, eds: Alcoholism and Substance Abuse: Strategies for Clinical Intervention, New York, The Free Press, 1985.

Brill P, Herzberg J, Speller JL: Employee assistance programs: an overview and suggested roles for psychiatrists. Hosp Community Psychiatry 36:727–732, 1985.

Bruch H: Four decades of eating disorders, in Garner, DM, Garfinkel PE, eds: Handbook of Psychotherapy for Anorexia Nervosa and Bulimia, New York, Guilford Press, 1985, pp 7–18.

Buxton M, Jessup M, Landry MJ: Treatment of the chemically dependent health professional, in Milkman HB, Shaffer HJ, ed: The Addictions: Multidisciplinary Perspectives and Treatments, Lexington, MA, Lexington Books, D.C. Heath and Co., 1985.

Chafetz MS: Alcoholism and health professionals. Psychiatr Ann 6:120–124, 1976.

Chasnoff IJ, Burns WJ, Schnoll SH, Burns KA: Cocaine use in pregnancy, N Engl J Med 313:666–669, 1985.

Cohen S: Drugs in the workplace. J Clin Psychiatry 45:4–8, 1984.

Crothers TD: Morphinism among physicians. Med Rec 55:784–786, 1899.

Fantel AG, Macphail BJ: Teratogenicity of cocaine. Teratology 26:17–19, 1982.

Freud S: Contribution to the knowledge of the effect of cocaine. Wien Mec Wochenschr 35:129–1133, 1885.

Herrington RE, Benzer DG, Jacobson GR, Hawkins MR: Treating substance-use disorders among physicians. JAMA 243:2253–2257, 1982.

Hutchings DE: Drug abuse during pregnancy: embryopathic and neurobehavioral effects, in Braudl H. and Zimmerman P. eds: Genetic and Perinatal Effects of Abused Substances, Orlando, FL, Academic Press, in press, 1986.

Itkonen J, Schnoll S, Glassroth J: Pulmonary dysfunction in freebase cocaine users. Arch Intern Med 144:2195, 1984.

Jonas JM, Gold MS: Cocaine abuse and eating disorders (letter). Lancet 2:390, 1986.

Khantzian EJ: The self-medication hypothesis of addictive disorders: focus on heroin and cocaine dependence. Am J Psychiatry 142:1259–1264, 1985.

Madden JD, Payne TF, Miller S: Maternal cocaine abuse and effect on the newborn. Pediatrics 77:209–211, 1986.

Maddux JF, Hoppe SIC, Costello RM: Psychoactive substance use among medical students. Am J Psychiatry 143:187–191, 1986.

Mahalik MP, Gautier RF, Mann DE: Teratogenic potential of cocaine hydrochloride in CF-1 mice. J Pharm Sci 69:703–706, 1980.

Morse RM, Martin MA, Swenson WM, Niven RE: Prognosis of physicians treated for alcoholism and drug dependence. JAMA 251:743–746, 1984.

Perez-Reyes M, DiGuiseppi BS, Ondrusek G, Jeffcoat AR: Freebase cocaine smoking. Clin Pharmacol Ther 32:459, 1982.

Rosecan J, Nunes E: The treatment of crack (cocaine smoking) abuse: a preliminary report. submitted for publication, 1986.

Shah NS, May DA, Yates J: Disposition of levo-CH-1 cocaine in pregnant and nonpregnant mice. Toxicol Appl Pharmacol 53:279–284, 1980.

Siegel RK: Cocaine smoking. J Psychoactive Drugs 14:271, 1982.

Vannicelli M: Treatment outcome of alcoholic women: the state of the art in relation to sex bias and expectancy effects, in Wilson KSC, Beckman LJ, eds: Alcohol Problems in Women, New York, Guilford Press, 1985, pp 369–412.

Washton A, in Brozan N: Women and cocaine: a growing problem. New York Times, p C18, Feb. 18, 1985.

Washton A, quoted in Gross J: Rise in cocaine abuse poses threat to infants. New York Times, p B1, Feb. 4, 1986.

Weissman MM, Leaf PJ, Holzer CE, Myers JK, Tischler GL: The epidemiology of depression: an update on sex differences and rates. J Affective Disorders 7:179–188, 1984.

Yoon J: Cocaine infants: a new arrival at hospital's step? Hospitals, p 96, April 5, 1986.

Name Index

Subject Index

331